Y0-BYV-028

Diagnosis and Treatment of Polyostotic Spinal Tumors

Diagnosis and Treatment of Polyostotic Spinal Tumors

By

KENT K. WU, M.D.

Senior Orthopaedic Surgeon
Department of Orthopaedic Surgeon
Henry Ford Hospital
Detroit, Michigan

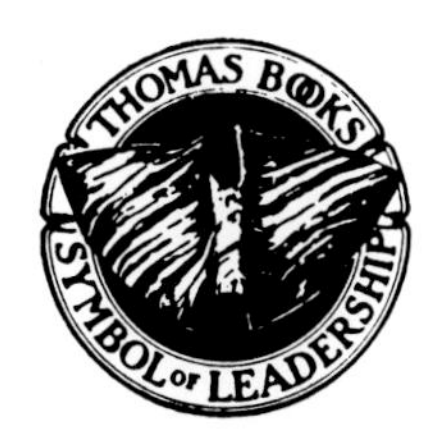

Charles C Thomas • Publisher
Springfield • Illinois • U.S.A.

Published and Distributed Throughout the World by

CHARLES C THOMAS • PUBLISHER
2600 South First Street
Springfield, Illinois 62717 U.S.A.

ISBN 0-398-04671-9

Library of Congress Catalog Card Number: 81-23425

With THOMAS BOOKS careful attention is given to all details of manufacturing and design. It is the Publisher's desire to present books that are satisfactory as to their physical qualities and artistic possibilities and appropriate for their particular use. THOMAS BOOKS will be true to those laws of quality that assure a good name and good will.

Library of Congress Cataloging in Publication Data

Wu, Kent K.
Diagnosis and treatment of polyostotic spinal tumors.

Bibliography: p.
Includes index.
1. Spine — Tumors. I. Title. [DNLM:
1. Spinal neoplasms — Diagnosis. 2. Spinal neoplasms — Therapy. WE 725 W959d]
RC280.S72W8 616.99'2711 81-23425
ISBN 0-398-04671-9 AACR2

Printed in the United States of America
C-1

to my wife, Judith
and my children, Jonathan, Richard, and Kimberly
whose love and understanding make life an unforgettable experience

Preface

WITH THE EXCEPTION of metastases and multiple myeloma, benign and malignant tumors of the spine are rarely encountered in clinical practice. The cases presented in this book represent a very unusual collection of spinal tumors, which my predecessors and my contemporary medical colleagues at Henry Ford Hospital had the foresight of preserving in our institutional teaching files during the past thirty-five years.

It is planned to have two separate books to cover this subject. This first book deals with the classification and general consideration of spinal tumors; the different modalities of spinal tumor therapy; and the incidence, clinical symptoms and signs, laboratory findings, roentgenographic manifestations, pathology, treatment, and prognosis of metastasis, malignant lymphomas, leukemia, myeloma, and chordoma of the spine that tend to show polyostotic involvement and systemic symptoms and frequently require nonsurgical treatments.

In contrast, the second book will cover the remainder of the spinal tumors, which usually exist in the monostotic form with rare systemic symptoms prior to their metastases. Eradicative surgical procedures coupled with reconstructive spinal stabilization procedures are commonly the treatment of choice for these tumors, and medical treatments tend to play a secondary role. Consequently, two special chapters, one dealing with surgical exposure of the spine, and the other with different spinal stabilization procedures, are included in the second book.

I am indebted to Doctors C. Leslie Mitchell, Harold M. Frost, Edwin R. Guise, and Robert Knighton for allowing me to use their cases, which form a substantial portion of the cases presented in this book. I am grateful to Doctor Ghaus M. Malik, James Ausman, and J. Speed Rogers of our Department of Neurosurgery for cooperating with me in our attempts to eradicate different spinal tumors; Doctors Joseph W. Lewis and Donald J. Magilligan of our Department of Thoracic Surgery for helping us in transthoracic and transthoraco-abdominal exposure of the spinal column; Doctors William R. Eyler, William A. Reynolds, and Roushdy S. Boulos of our Department of Radiology for assisting me in interpreting many roentgenograms; and Doctors John W. Rebuck, Gerald Fine, and Julius M. Ohorodnik of our Department of Pathology for aiding me in verifying the diagnosis of spinal tumor slides. I also wish to give my sincere thanks to Jay Knipstein for his superb illustrations on surgical exposure and different stabilization procedures of the spine; and Arthur Bowden, Walter Harlan, and John Worsham for making the numerous photomicrographs for me. Finally, I am obliged to my outstanding secretary, Mrs. Justine Frankfurth, who tirelessly and meticulously typed the whole manuscript and skillfully handled the office of my very busy orthopaedic practice at the same time.

KENT K. WU, M.D.

Introduction

EXCLUDING metastatic tumors and myeloma of the spine, spinal tumors are uncommon lesions. A great variety of spinal tumors reported in the medical literature consists of single case reports.[1-18] The fact that the author was able to publish a chordoma of the atlas,[19] an osteochondroma of the atlas,[20] and an unicameral bone cyst of the lumbar spine[21] in two leading orthopaedic journals clearly illustrates the point. Dahlin's book, *Bone Tumors: General Aspects and Data on 6,221 Cases,*[22] provides us with a rough estimate of the relative frequency of occurrence of various types of spinal tumors. This is presented in Table I.

Although Table I shows that only myeloma, malignant lymphoma, and chordoma exceed 1 percent of the total number of tumors, the whole spinal tumor group comprises 12.65 percent (or roughly one-eighth) of the entire tumor group. This is a sizable and unique tumor group, deserving special medical attention. The same table also indicates that chordoma, osteoblastoma, myeloma, fibrous histiocytoma, and hemangioma, in descending order, show significant predilection for the spinal column.

Anatomically, the spinal column lies in the deepest portion of the body and is surrounded by various bony, visceral, myofascial, and cutaneous structures, which, when coupled with the relatively small size of spinal tumors, make these tumors hard to detect by either physical or roentgenographic examination. In addition, owing to the fact that most spinal tumors are osteolytic in nature and frequently produce compression fractures that immediately obliterate all the traces of any distinctive intraosseous architecture, very different tumors can look surprisingly alike in the

Table I

THE RELATIVE FREQUENCY OF OCCURRENCE OF BENIGN AND MALIGNANT SPINAL TUMORS IN 4,277 CASES OF BONE TUMORS.

	Type of Tumor	*Frequency of Occurrence Within the Individual Tumor Group (in percent)*	*Frequency of Occurrence Within the Entire Tumor Group (in percent)*
BENIGN TUMORS	Osteochondroma	3.28	0.40
	Chondroma	4.41	0.14
	Chondroblastoma	2.27	0.02
	Chondromyxoid Fibroma	3.33	0.02
	Osteoid Osteoma	5.69	0.21
	Benign Osteoblastoma	44.19	0.44
	Giant Cell Tumor	12.03	0.75
	Fibrous Histiocytoma	28.57	0.05
	Fibroma	0	0
	Desmoplastic Fibroma	0	0
	Hemangioma	24.64	0.39
	Lipoma	0	0
	Neurilemmoma	10	0.02
MALIGNANT TUMORS	Myeloma	38.71	3.53
	Malignant Lymphoma	14.07	1.08
	Primary Chondrosarcoma	8.94	0.87
	Secondary Chondrosarcoma	9.62	0.12
	Mesenchymal Chondrosarcoma	6.67	0.02
	Osteosarcoma	2.91	0.65
	Parosteal Osteosarcoma	0	0
	Ewing's Sarcoma	7.36	0.51
	Malignant Giant Cell Tumor	10	0.05
	Adamantinoma	0	0
	Fibrous Histiocytoma	0	0
	Fibrosarcoma	9.49	0.35
	Chordoma	63.59	2.89
	Hemangioendothelioma	20	0.12
	Hemangiopericytoma	20	0.02
Total			12.65

absence of adequate histological examination. Consequently, every effort should be made to make use of all the available clinical information in order to maximize the chances of arriving at a correct diagnosis and formulating a logical course of treatment. For example, past history of cancer surgery; exposure to excessive ionizing radiation, cytotoxic substances, and carcinogenic drugs; or the presence of diseases with tendency to exhibit malignant transformation (such as neurofibromatosis, Ollier's disease, heredity multiple exostosis, and Maffuci's syndrome) in patients with unexplained spinal symptoms should alert the clinicians of the possible existence of benign or malignant spinal tumors. Particular attention should be paid to patients' complaints of neck and back pain; paresthesia, weakness and paralysis of upper or lower extremities; and disturbances of the normal bowel or bladder functions, which all suggest impairment of spinal cord and nerve functions and mandate prompt medical attention in order to prevent permanent disability or a potentially fatal outcome. Furthermore, the presence of constitutional symptoms, such as weight loss, anorexia, malaise, ease of fatigue, fever, night sweats, etc., favors the diagnosis of metastases, especially in patients with known history of cancer.

In examining patients suspected of having spinal tumors, one should try to find the point of maximal tenderness; the presence or absence of muscle spasm, list, sensory or motor deficit, pathological reflexes, clonus, muscular atrophy and fasciculation, and palpable mass; asymmetrical, decreased, or absent deep tendon reflexes; decreased range of motion of the spine, etc., which will enable the examiner to localize the exact level of spinal involvement and the extent of neurological dysfunction.

Roentgenographically, ill-defined and inconspicuous spinal tumors are usually not well demonstrated by routine x-rays; consequently special studies, such as laminography, myelography, angiography, bone scan, and CAT scan, are often indispensable in clearly delineating the size, shape, and the extent of the spinal involvement by the tumor under consideration. This will not only improve the accuracy of a preoperative diagnosis, but can also greatly enhance the chances of a safe and complete removal of the spinal tumor by competent surgeons. In addition, preoperative laboratory studies can also provide valuable information on the nature of the spinal tumor in question. Some specific examples are elevated serum acid phosphatase in association with metastatic prostatic carcinoma; elevated catecholamine with metastatic neuroblastoma; the presence of Bence-Jones protein and typical electrophoretic curve with multiple myeloma; increased histologically distinct but abnormal cells in blood or bone marrow with leukemias; and abnormal proliferation of malignant lymphomatous cells in lymph nodes with lymphomas. Other less specific abnormal laboratory studies, including anemia, thrombocytopenia, hypercalcemia, hyperuricemia, leukocytosis, elevated erythrocyte sedimentation rate, and alkaline phosphatase caused by destruction of tumor cells and the invaded normal tissues, are the common features shared by several malignant diseases, such as metastatic carcinomas, malignant lymphomas, multiple myeloma, leukemias, etc.

Needless to say, definitive diagnosis of any spinal tumor requires adequate tissue biopsy, which will enable pathologists to identify the types of cells in the spinal tumor and the intercellular substance associated with these cells whose shape, number, variations, and staining characteristics help to differentiate malignant lesions from benign ones. Generally speaking, all spinal tumors fall under two categories: intrinsic and extrinsic tumors. The intrinsic are tumors originating in the spinal column; extrinsic tumors are metastatic tumors from distant primary sites or invading tumors from various adjacent soft tissues and bones. A complete list of tumors of the spine can be easily obtained if one will only remember that they are no more than the benign and malignant counterparts of various tissues present in bone, which include bone, cartilage, fibrous tissue, nerve, blood vessel, bone marrow elements, fat, etc. A comprehensive classification of benign and malignant tumors of the spine is presented in Table II.

TABLE II
CLASSIFICATION OF SPINAL TUMORS

	Tissue Type	*Malignant Tumor*	*Benign Tumor*
Intrinsic spinal tumors	Osteogenic tissue	Osteogenic sarcoma Parosteal osteogenic sarcoma	Osteoid osteoma Osteoblastoma
	Chondrogenic tissue	Chondrosarcoma	Osteochondroma Chondroblastoma Chondroma Chondromyxoid Fibroma
	Fibrogenic tissue	Fibrosarcoma	Fibrous cortical defect, non-ossifying fibroma, unicameral bone cyst, fibrous dysplasia
	Vasogenic tissue	Malignant hemangio-endothelioma Malignant hemangio-pericytoma	Hemangioma Benign hemangiopericytoma
	Neurogenic tissue	Neurogenic sarcoma (malignant Schwannoma, neurofibrosarcoma)	Neurilemmoma Neurofibroma
	Myelogenic tissue	Myeloma, Hodgkin's disease, Non-Hodgkin's lymphomas, Leukemias	None
	Lipogenic tissue	Liposarcoma	Lipoma
	Reticuloendothelial tissue	Malignant giant cell tumor Malignant fibrous histiocytoma	Benign giant cell tumor Benign histiocytoma
	Notochordal tissue	Chordoma	None
	Uncertain tissue	Ewing's sarcoma, Adamantioma	None
Extrinsic spinal tumors		Metastatic tumors	
		Invading malignant tumors from adjacent soft tissues and bones	

Once the diagnosis of a particular spinal tumor has been firmly established, the treatment naturally depends on the nature, site, and the extent of involvement of the spinal tumor. As a rule of thumb, tumors with polyostotic involvement of the spine, such as myeloma, lymphomas, leukemias, and metastases, usually do not readily lend themselves to radical surgical eradication except for limited decompression procedure to relieve pressure on the spinal cord or nerves and stabilization procedure to prevent disastrous collapse of the vertebral column. In contrast, well-localized benign and malignant spinal tumors should be removed as completely as possible in order to prevent recurrence and metastasis, and the resulting defect should be stabilized if spinal instability has been created by the surgery. In dealing with large spinal tumors with significant soft tissue and bone involvement, complete eradication may not be practical because of the danger of damaging vital organs. Under this circumstance, every attempt should be made to remove as much tumor tissue as possible in order to restore the normal functions of the impaired organs. This palliative surgical procedure may have to be repeated when the spinal tumor recurs. Adjuvant radiotherapy and chemotherapy should be employed to treat spinal tumors which are not amendable to radical surgical ablation or highly malignant spinal tumors with high potential of producing local recurrence and distal metastases. It should again be emphasized that owing to the fact that malignant spinal tumors do invade the surrounding neurovascular and visceral structures and produce distant metastases, specialists of different medical fields, such as orthopaedists, neurosurgeons, thoracic surgeons, vascular surgeons, general surgeons, radiologists, pathologists, oncologists, etc., should closely cooperate with each other in a multidisciplinary approach to strive for the highest probability of a complete tumor eradication and the minimal degrees of functional impairment at the same time.

REFERENCES

1. Blaylock, R. L., and Kempe, L. G.: Chondrosarcoma of the cervical spine. Case report. *J Neurosurg, 44:*500-503, 1976.
2. Buraczewski, J., Lysakowska, J., and Rudowski, W.: Chondroblastoma (Codman's tumour) of the thoracic spine. *J Bone and Joint Surg, 39-B:*705, 1957.
3. Dowdle, J. A., Jr., Winter, R. B., and Dehner, L. P.: Postradiation osteosarcoma of the cervical spine in childhood. A case report. *J Bone & Joint Surg, 59-A:*969-971, 1977.
4. Fink, L. H., and Meriwether, M. W.: Primary epidural Ewing's sarcoma presenting as a lumbar disc protrusion. Case report. *J Neurosurgery, 51:*120-123, 1979.
5. Gertzbein, S. D., Cruickshank, B., Hoffman, H., Taylor, G. A., and Cooper, P. W.: Recurrent benign osteoblastoma of the second thoracic vertebra. A case report. *J Bone and Joint Surg, 55-B:*841-847, 1973.
6. Gonem, M. N.: Osteoclastoma of the thoracic spine. Case report. *J Neurosurg, 44:*748-752, 1976.
7. Guarnaschelli, J. J., Wehry, S. M., Serratoni, F. T., and Dzenitis, A. J.: A typical fibrous histiocytoma of the thoracic spine. *J Neurosurg, 51:*415-416, 1979.

8. Hemmy, D. C., McGee, D. M., Armbrust, F. H., and Larson, S. J.: Resection of a vertebral hemangioma after preoperative embolization. *J Neurosurg, 47:*282-285, 1977.
9. Hvorslev, V., and Reiter, S.: A case of neurofibromatosis with severe osseous disease of the thoracic spine. *Pediatr Radiol, 8:*251-253, 1979.
10. Inglis, A. E., Rubin, R. M., Lewis, R. J., and Villacin, A.: Osteochondroma of the cervical spine. Case report. *Clin Orthop, 126:*127-129, 1977.
11. Mandell, G. A.: Resolution of Hodgkin's induced ivory vertebrae. *Pediat Radiol, 7:*178-179, 1978.
12. Merli, G. A., Angiari, P., Botticelli, A., Galli, V., and Peserico, L.: Chondromyxoid fibroma with spinal cord compression. *Surg Neurol, 10:*123-125, 1978.
13. Nag, T. K., and Falconer, M. A.: Enchondroma of the vertebral body. *Brit J Surg, 53:*1067-1071, 1966.
14. Polkey, C. E.: Intraosseous neurilemmoma of the cervical spine causing paraparesis and treated by resection and grafting. *J Neurol Neurosurg & Psychiat, 38:*776-781, 1975.
15. Regen, E. M., and Haber, A.: Giant-cell tumor of cervical vertebra with unusual symptoms. *J Bone & Joint Surg, 39-A:*196-200, 1957.
16. Rinsky, L. A., Goris, M., Bleck, E. E., Halpern, A., and Hirshman, P.: Intraoperative skeletal scintigraphy for localization of osteoid-osteoma in the spine. Case report. *J Bone & Joint Surg, 62-A:*143-144, 1980.
17. Shannon, F. T., and Hopkins, J. S.: Paget's sarcoma of the vertebral column with neurological complications. *Acta Orthop Scand, 48:*385-390, 1977.
18. Stern, M. B., Grode, M. L., and Goodman, D.: Hemangiopericytoma of the cervical spine: Report of an unusual case. *Clin Orthop, 151:*201-204, 1980.
19. Wu, K. K., Mitchell, D. C., and Guise, E. R.: Chordoma of the atlas. *J Bone & Joint Surg, 61-A:*140-141, 1979.
20. Wu, K. K., and Guise, E. R.: Osteochondroma of the atlas: A case report. *Clin Orthop, 136:*160-162, 1978.
21. Wu, K. K., and Guise, E. R.: Unicameral bone cyst of the spine. *J Bone & Joint Surg, 63-A:*176-178, 1981.
22. Dahlin, D. C.: *Bone Tumors: General Aspects and Data on 6,221 Cases,* 3rd Ed. Springfield, Illinois, Charles C Thomas, 1978.

Contents

Diagnosis and Treatment of Polyostotic Spinal Tumors

Chapter 1

The Armamentarium of the Different Treatments of Primary and Metastatic Tumors of the Spine

MANY DIFFERENT KINDS of malignant and benign primary bone tumors originate in the spine, which is also one of the favorite sites for metastatic carcinomas and sarcomas. A comprehensive understanding of the basic principles of various modalities of cancer therapy appears to be quite desirable prior to the detailed discussion of each individual kind of spinal tumors. From a practical point of view, there are seven basic methods of treating cancers, which include surgery, chemotherapy, hormonal therapy, radiotherapy, immunotherapy, hyperthermic therapy, and cryotherapy. As a rule of thumb, surgery, radiotherapy, hyperthermia, and cryotherapy are usually used in treating localized tumors, whereas chemotherapy, hormonal therapy, and immunotherapy are more applicable to metastatic tumors. However, there are exceptions to the rules, such as intrathecal spinal or pleural injection of immunotherapeutic and chemotherapeutic agents, systemic hyperthermic therapy, whole body irradiation, etc.

Surgery

Before any definitive surgical procedure is taken to eradicate a certain spinal tumor, the exact nature of the tumor, the extent of the spinal tumor's bony and soft tissue involvements, which can be demonstrated preoperatively by CAT scan, myelography and angiography, the presence or absence of metastasis, the patient's general health, etc., should be thoroughly investigated. It should be strongly emphasized that eradicative spinal tumor surgery is often very technically demanding. It should never be attempted by inexperienced surgeons. Not only complicated and time consuming, spinal tumor surgery requires the close cooperation of orthopaedist, neurosurgeon, thoracic surgeon, and anesthesiologist and requires many units of blood transfusions. In addition, the patient often needs to spend the first two to three postoperative days in the surgical intensive care unit where he or she can be closely watched in order to minimize any preventable postoperative complications. The indications for spinal tumor surgery, the surgical approaches to the spine, and the various techniques in stabilizing the defects created by the removal of the diseased vertebrae will be discussed in details in subsequent chapters.

Chemotherapy[1-7]

An intelligent choice of particular chemotherapeutic agents requires a thorough understanding of the mechanisms of action of these agents on the different stages of the cell cycle. The life cycle of the cell consists of two phases: a short period of actual cell division, the so-called D (division) or M (mitosis) phase, and a relatively longer period, the so-called resting phase, during which the replication of the DNA is accomplished. The resting phase can be subdivided into the G1, S, and G2 phases. The G1 phase follows the D (or M) phase and is responsible for synthesis of RNA, histone proteins, and enzymes needed for subsequent DNA synthesis. The G1 phase is followed by the S phase, during which DNA synthesis is achieved by replication and polymerization of DNA components. The S phase is followed by the G2 phase, during which RNA synthesis and production of specialized proteins for mitotic spindle apparatus and specialized DNA needed during mitosis take place. The antitumor activity of different chemotherapeutic agents depends on their ability to impair the vital biochemical reactions that occur during one or more phases of the cell cycle. Generally speaking, the great majority of the antineoplastic drugs can be segregated into two big families: the cell cycle (phase) specific drugs and the cell cycle (phase) nonspecific drugs. Cell cycle specific drugs usually act on a particular phase of the cell cycle and are effective in treating small tumors with high rate of tumor cell proliferation and should be given in multiple repeated doses (schedule dependent). In contrast, cell cycle nonspecific drugs can attack tumor cells in both resting and proliferating state and are effective against large tumors with relatively low proliferative activity as well as small tumors with high mitotic activity. In addition, these cell cycle nonspecific agents' ability to kill tumor cells is directly proportional to the absolute dose given, and multiple, repeated small doses, totalling to one large single, dose have no significant advantage over the same large dose given in a single administration.

Cell Cycle (Phase) Specific, Dose-independent, Drugs

M-PHASE (OR D-PHASE) SPECIFIC DRUGS. They are the vinca alkaloids derived from the periwinkle plant *(Vinca rosea).* Vincristine (Oncovin®) and vinblastine (Velban®) are the two plant alkaloids in clinical use.[8-26] Their mechanism of action appears to depend on their ability to bind and cause crystallization of the microtubular protein of the mitotic spindle, producing mitotic arrest in metaphase. However, at high concentrations they can also inhibit G1 and S phases.

G1 — PHASE SPECIFIC DRUGS. L-asparaginase (Elspar®),[27-40] an enzyme derived from several different microorganisms, can hydrolyze the amino acid, asparagine, to asparatic acid and ammonia and thus deprive the tumor cells of an indispensable amino acid for asparagine-dependent protein synthesis, in the absence of which, subsequent DNA and RNA synthesis and tumor cell proliferation are severely impaired.

S-PHASE SPECIFIC DRUGS. These agents are called antimetabolites whose chemical structures are so similar to those of normal DNA precursors (metabolites) that they can substitute for a normal metabolite in a key molecule, occupy the catalytic site of a key enzyme, and act at an enzyme regulatory site to change the catalytic activity of the enzyme. There are four main types of antimetabolites: folate analogues — methotrexate,[41-59] dichloromethotrexate, etc.; purine analogues — azathioprine,[60-66] 6-mercaptopurine,[67-75] 6-thioguanine, etc.;[76-87] pyrimidine analogues — 5-fluorouracil,[88-104] 5-azacytidine,[105-115] cytosine arabinoside (Cytarabine®), etc.;[116-126] hydroxyurea (Hydrea®).[127-137] It should be mentioned that leucovorin (citrovorum factor),[138-147] a folic acid derivative, is commonly used to "rescue" cells with high proliferative activity, e.g. bone marrow and gastrointestinal epithelium, from the severe cytotoxic effects of Methotrexate.

A G2-PHASE SPECIFIC DRUGS. Bleomycin (Blenoxane®)[148-167] and razoxane (ICRF-159)[168-181] appear to interfere with the biochemical reactions of the G2-phase of the cell cycle and thus inhibit cell progression out of G2 phase. However, bleomycin also binds DNA and causes a break of the DNA molecule, resulting in impaired DNA, RNA and protein syntheses which make Bleomycin a cell cycle nonspecific agent. On the other hand, when Razoxane is given during the premitotic and early mitotic phases of the cell cycle, it can cause mitotic arrest, making it cell-phase specific for the M phase as well.

Cell Cycle (Phase) Nonspecific, Dose-dependent, Drugs

ALKYLATING AGENTS. These antitumor agents have the ability of substituting an alkyl group ($R - CH_2 - CH_2^+$) for hydrogen atoms of many organic compounds. Aklylation of DNA causes breakage of DNA molecule and cross linkage of its double strands, resulting in severe impairments of DNA replication and transcriptions. Alkylating agents can be classified into the following types: nitrogen mustard derivatives — cyclophosphamide (Cytoxan®),[182-199] chlorambucil (Leukeran®,[200-212] melphalan (Alkaran®), etc.;[213-222] ethylenimine derivatives — triethylenethiophosphoramide (Thiotepa);[223-233] alkyl sulfonates — busulfan (Myleran®),[234-243] Yoshi-864, etc.;[244-248] triazene derivatives — dacarbazine (DTIC-Dome®);[249-257] nitrosoureas — carmustine (BCNU),[258-274] lomustine (CCNU)[275-290] semustine (methyl-CCNU), etc.[291-299]

ANTITUMOR ANTIBIOTICS. They include doxorubicin (Adriamycin®),[300-318] daunorubicin (Cerubidine®),[319-326] actinomycin-D (dactinomycin),[327-333] mithramycin (Mithracin®),[334-342] mitomycin-C (Mutamycin®), etc.,[343-358] whose mechanism of tumoricidal action is to bind DNA and, therefore, interferes with DNA-directed DNA, RNA, and protein synthesis.

MISCELLANEOUS CELL CYCLE (PHASE). Nonspecific drugs — cisplatin,[359-379] streptozotocin,[380-395] galactitol (dianhydro-galactitol), etc.[396-403] — are antineoplastic agents, which attack multiple phases of the cell cycle and are thus dose-dependent drugs.

Although many anticancer drugs are employed as single agents in treating cancers, multi-drug combination chemotherapy[404-412] is becoming more and more popular. The basic principles of combination chemotherapy should include drugs with active cytotoxic effects against the particular tumor under consideration and agents with different, but synergistic, mechanisms of antitumor action and noncumulative toxicities to the hosts; maximal effective doses can thus be employed to achieve high tumoricidal effects and minimize the emergence of drug resistance[413-419] without causing severe impairment of the recipients' normal body functions. In addition, adjuvant chemotherapy is commonly employed to eradicate disseminated micrometastases after surgery or irradiation of the primary malignant lesions. Intrathecal administration of chemotherapeutic agents in treating central nervous system leukemias and malignant pleural effusions can provide significantly symptomatic relief. However, since all cytotoxic chemotherapeutic agents attack one or more phases of the cell cycle, normal cells with high proliferative activities, such as cells of bone marrow, gastrointestinal epithelium, hair follicles, and gonads, are markedly affected by these agents. Consequently, bone marrow depression, nausea, vomiting, GI hemorrhage, alopecia, sterility, and possible chromosomal abnormalities of the germinal cells are some of the more common complications of chemotherapy.[420-425] In addition, neurologic, pulmonary, renal, hepatic, cardiac, dermatologic, ocular and endocrinologic toxicities, growth disturbances, and teratogenic and oncogenic effects are the other sequelae associated with antineoplastic chemotherapy.[426-434]

Hormonal Therapy

Hormonal therapy is a special kind of chemotherapy that takes advantage of the fact that several human cancers, e.g. carcinomas of the breast, prostate, endometrium, etc., originate in tissues that are ordinarily under hormonal control. Surgical or medical ablation of these hormone-secreting sites,[435-438] e.g. hypophysectomy, adrenalectomy, orchiectomy, and oophorectomy, and administration of compounds antagonistic to the actions of these hormones tend to inhibit the growth of hormonally sensitive tumors. The pharmacologic mechanism of action of anticancer hormones and antihormonal agents seems to act at nuclear and cytoplasmic levels through specific cell hormone receptor proteins. A few agents can also directly block the biochemical pathways of hormone synthesis, thus depriving the tumor cells of the hormonal growth stimulus. However, in spite of the powerfully palliative effects of these hormones or hormonelike agents against hormonally dependent tumors, their antitumor power is usually not curative due to the lack of direct cytotoxicity. It explains why these antitumor hormones are frequently combined with powerful cytotoxic chemotherapeutic agents in treating many different kinds of cancer. A list of drugs clinically useful in treating hormonally-sensitive cancers is presented in Table 1-I.

TABLE 1-I
HORMONES USED IN TREATING CANCERS

Hormone or Agent	*Clinical Use*
Estrogens[439-458]	Breast, prostate and sometimes ovarian carcinomas
Androgens[459-467]	Breast and occasionally renal carcinomas
Progestins[468-480]	Endometrial, breast and renal carcinomas
Adrenal Corticosteroids[481-487]	Leukemias, lymphomas and breast cancer
Antiestrogens (1) Nafoxidine[488-491] (2) Tamoxifen[492-508]	Breast and endometrial carcinomas
Antiadrenal Agents (1) Mitotane (O,P′-DDD)[509-515] (2) Aminoglutethimide[516-527]	Adrenal and breast carcinomas

Radiotherapy[528-534]

To take full advantage of what radiotherapy has to offer, a comprehensive understanding of the basic principles of radiation biology and physics is indispensable.

Types of Ionizing Radiations

ELECTROMAGNETIC. X-rays from x-ray machines and gamma-rays from Cobalt 60, Cesium 137, etc.

PARTICULATE. Beams composed of alpha particles, beta-particles (electrons), and neutrons.

Sources of Radiation

X-RAY MACHINES.

Grenz rays — 10 kv. (kilovolts)
Superficial x-rays — 40-100 kv
Orthovoltage x-rays (conventional x-rays or deep x-rays) — 250 kv

RADIOISOTOPE TELETHERAPY MACHINES. Radioisotopes are placed in these machines at a fixed distance from the patients.

Cesium 137 (^{137}Cs) — 600 kv and up
Cobalt 60 (^{60}Co) — up to 2 MEV (million electron volts)

LINEAR ACCELERATORS. 4-8 MEV.

BETATRONS. Greater than 20 MEV.

NEUTRON GENERATORS (D-T GENERATORS AND CYCLOTRONS). Up to 30 MEV.

OTHER RADIOISOTOPES AND THEIR CLINICAL APPLICATIONS.

Radium 226(^{226}Ra), Tantalum 182 (^{182}Ta), and Iridium 192 (^{192}Ir)— Brachytherapy (small sources of radiation used in close contact with tumors) of cancers

Strontium 90 (^{90}Sr) — Contact therapy for superficial lesions

Sodium 24 (^{24}Na) — Treatment of bladder cancer by means of intravesicular balloon

Phosphorus 32 (^{32}P) — Treatment of polycythemia rubra vera and metastatic breast and prostate carcinomas plus diagnosis of intraocular tumors

Iodine 131 (^{131}I) — Localization and treatment of primary and metastatic thyroid carcinoma and hyperthyroidism plus diagnosis of different thyroid disorders for which both ^{131}I and ^{123}I are useful

Chromium 51 (^{51}Cr) — Determination of erythrocyte volume and survival time

Cobalt 57 (^{57}Co) — Cobalt 57 tagged vitamin B12 is used in the diagnosis of pernicious anemia

Gold 198 (^{198}Au) — Liver scanning

Iron 59 (^{59}Fe) — Study of iron absorption and utilization and anemia
Mercury 197 (^{197}Hg) — Brain and kidney scanning
Selenium 75 (^{75}Se) — Pancreas and parathyroid scanning
Technetium 99m (^{99m}Tc) — Brain, thyroid, liver, lung, bone, and placenta scanning

Methods of Radiotherapy

EXTERNAL BEAM THERAPY. Electromagnetic radiations or particle beams from an external source of radiation such as x-ray tubes, linear accelerator, betatron, neutron generator, etc., or from a radioisotope teletherapy machine, using cobalt 60 and cesium 137, which are powerful sources of radiation.

INTERSTITIAL RADIOTHERAPY. Direct implantation of radioactive substances into the tumor proper, e.g. radium needles, gold grains, tantalum wires, etc.

INTRACAVITARY AND MOULD THERAPY AND SURFACE APPLICATORS. Radium, cobalt, strontium, etc., are the radioactive sources used in close contact with the small, superficial, and accessible tumors.

SYSTEMIC ADMINISTRATION OF RADIOISOTOPES. Radioactive iodine (^{131}I) can be taken up by both the primary and metastatic thyroid carcinoma cells. Radioactive phosphorus (^{32}P) atoms can substitute for the normal phosphorus atoms in the DNA and RNA molecules and are thus useful in treating metastatic breast and prostate carcinomas and leukemias.

Biophysical Parameters of Radiotherapy

UNITS OF RADIATION

Roentgen — A measure of the amount of radiation delivered to a particular area.

Rad — A measure of the amount of radiation absorbed by a particular area. In biophysical terms, one rad is equal to the radiation energy absorption of 100 ergs per one gram of irradiated tissue.

Gray — Equivalent to 100 rads or 1 joule per kilogram of irradiated matter.

TUMOR DOSE. It is the absorbed dose of radiation in rads at a particular location of a tumor. Needless to say, a portion of the given radiation is scattered and does not contribute to the tumoricidal effect.

QUALITY OF RADIATION. It refers to the penetrating power and the composition of the electromagnetic waves of the x-rays. The quality of x-rays can be improved by means of filters, which are made of tin and copper and tin, and have the ability of removing low energy radiation with relatively long wave lengths from the incident radiation, thus creating a x-ray beam of higher quality with better penetrating power.

ARTIFICIAL RADIOISOTOPES (RADIONUCLIDES). They are produced by bombarding the stable nuclides with subatomic particles such as deuterons or neutrons in a cyclotron or nuclear reactor. When the nucleus of a bombarded atom captures a neutron or a deuteron, it becomes unstable and spontaneously undergoes degradation by emitting alpha particles (helium ions), beta particles (electrons), or gamma-rays (electromagnetic waves).

Biological Effects of Radiation[535-554]

Ionizing radiations such as x-rays, gamma-rays, electron beam, neutron beam, etc., have the ability to displace electrons from atoms of matter in their path. These atoms become positively charged ions and the displaced electrons can ionize other atoms, combine with neutral atoms to produce negatively charged ions, or recombine with positively charged ions to form neutral atoms. In addition, since water is a major component of all living things, ionizing radiations can produce hydroxy radical from water, which, like many free radicals, is a highly reactive molecule and can attach and damage many vital components of the living cells.

Therefore, ionization of cellular components; changes in permeability of cellular membrane; ionization of circulating minerals and their effects on the electrolyte, water, acid-base balance; disturbances of blood supply; damages to DNA, RNA, enzymes, proteins, other organic and inorganic compounds, etc., can all in one way or another contribute to subsequent cellular deaths. These cell deaths can take the form of immediate death, or delayed death from disintegration of protoplasm, inhibition of cell division due to destruction of centrioles, suppression of cell mobility caused by damage to the motor center of the cells, abortive anomalies of mitosis brought about by destruction of nuclear chromatin, and hereditary malformations due to gene damage of gonadal germinal cells.

Generally speaking, radiosensitivity of a tumor refers to its responsiveness to radiation and is not synonymous with radiocurability, which implies that the tumor can be completely and permanently eradicated by radiation alone. The following is a list of different cell types arranged in order of decreasing radiosensitivity.

IN DECREASING RADIOSENSITIVITY ↓

- Lymphocytes
- Bone marrow cells
- Germinal cells of the gonads
- Lens
- Lung tissue cells
- Squamous mucous epithelial cells
- Cornea
- Squamous epithelial cells of the skin
- Bone and cartilage cells
- Muscle cells
- Thyroid cells
- Pituitary cells
- Nerve cells
- Hepatic cells
- Mature erythrocytes

By the same token, radiosensitivity of tumors seems to bear some resemblance to the radiosensitivity of the tissues which give rise to these tumors.

IN DECREASING RADIOSENSITIVITY ↓

- Malignant lymphomas and multiple myeloma
- Lymphoepitheliomas of the upper respiratory system
- Seminomas and dysgerminomas of the gonads
- Ewing's sarcoma
- Cutaneous basal cell carcinomas
- Squamous carcinomas of skin, mucous membrane or metaplasia from columnar epithelium
- Endometrial, mammary, gastrointestinal and endocrine adenocarcinomas
- Soft tissue sarcomas
- Chondrosarcomas
- Neurogenic sarcomas
- Osteogenic sarcoma
- Malignant melanoma

The radiosensitivity of a tumor depends on many factors, which include the following:

1. Histological type.
2. Degrees of maturation and differentiation. (The poorly differentiated and less mature cells are more radiosensitive.)
3. Number of mitosis per unit of tumor tissue. (Tumors with high mitotic activity seem to be more radiosensitive.)

4. The relative length of mitotic phase. (The tumor cells with longer mitotic phase are more vulnerable to radiotherapy.)
5. The degree of oxygenation. (Anoxic tumor cells are more radioresistant.)
6. Size of the tumor. (Larger tumors are more radioresistant due to poor blood supply and necrosis at their central portions.)

Clinical Applications of Radiotherapy[555-565]

Radiotherapy has been extensively employed in treating primary and metastatic tumors throughout the body. The following is a brief description of the various clinical uses of radiotherapy.

CURATIVE RADIOTHERAPY. Tumors curable by radiotherapy must be radiosensitive. For instance, basal cell and squamous cell carcinomas of the skin are radiocurable tumors. However, before radiotherapy is chosen, the attending physician has to consider all the alternative treatments such as surgery, in order to be certain that radiotherapy is indeed the treatment of choice, which implies that the treatment is the most effective and the simplest and has the least possibility of immediate and long-term morbidity and mortality.

PALLIATIVE RADIOTHERAPY. This mode of radiotherapy is intended to relieve patients of distressful symptoms and impending life threatening situations caused by incurable tumors. For examples, properly administered radiotherapy can provide significant relief of bone pain and spinal cord and nerve compression from primary or metastatic carcinomas and sarcomas; control of frequency, dysuria and hematuria of bladder carcinoma; and amelioration of distressing coughs, dyspnea and hemoptysis from bronchogenic carcinoma.

PREOPERATIVE RADIOTHERAPY. Owing to the fact that radiation does reduce the vascularity, size and inflammation of a tumor, preoperative radiotherapy can materially facilitate the subsequent surgical removal of the tumor in question. In addition, the destruction of the tumor by the radiation may produce certain antigens from the tumor that may stimulate the host's immune system to produce specific antitumor antibodies against the tumor.

POSTOPERATIVE RADIOTHERAPY. This modality of radiotherapy is used when a complete eradication of a particular tumor is not feasible or when there are reasonable chances of having residual tumor cells left in the tumor bed after attempted surgical eradication. If these remaining tumor cells can be killed by the postoperative radiotherapy, future local recurrence and distant metastasis can be prevented.

THE ROLE OF RADIOTHERAPY IN COMBINATION CANCER THERAPY. In addition to combining surgery and radiotherapy, radiotherapy is frequently combined with chemotherapy in treating a wide variety of malignant tumors, especially the ones with metastatic involvements. By the same token, it is perfectly conceivable to combine radiotherapy with immunotherapy, cryotherapy and hyperthermia when the proper indications are present.

Complications of Radiotherapy.[566-600]

Although radiotherapy is a very useful anticancer tool, improper or excessive administration of radiotherapy can cause death or permanent damages to every conceivable organ in the body. The so-called irradiation sickness consisting of anorexia, nausea, vomiting, lassitude, pallor, and profuse perspiration can sometimes be observed during the course of radiotherapy. The long-term complications of radiotherapy such as permanent damage to radiosensitive organs, sterility, growth disturbances, congenital anomalies associated with radiation-induced chromosomal aberrations, oncogenic effects (radiation-induced carcinomas and sarcomas), shortening of life expectancy, etc., should always be borne in mind whenever radiotherapy is utilized as the anticancer agent.

Immunotherapy

Immunotherapy[601-605] of cancer is based on the premise that it can stimulate the host's natural defenses, e.g. body's immune and phagocytic systems, to eradicate residual cancer cells concurrently with or after other modalities of cancer treatments such as surgery, chemotherapy, and radiotherapy. The human immune system is a cell-mediated response in which lymphocytes (both T and B lymphocytes), monocytes, and macrophages play the vital roles. There are three types of immunotherapy: passive immunotherapy, adoptive immunotherapy, and active immunotherapy.

Passive immunotherapy[606-607] involves administration of antibodies produced by other human beings or animals to the cancer victims who, in a strict sense, do not actively participate in the immunotherapeutic process.

Adoptive immunotherapy[608-613] calls for the administration of immunocompetent cells (leukocytes, lymphocytes and macrophages) from closely related or unrelated individuals. These cells may be sensitized *in vivo* or *in vitro,* e.g. cultured lymphoid cells, to patient's tumor, other tumors, or oncogenic viruses to potentiate their immunotherapeutic power. In addition, adoptive immunotherapy also employs subcellular components, such as transfer factor and "immune" RNA in the fight against cancers.

Active immunotherapy is the most promising area of immunotherapy. The cancer patients play an active role in the initiation and modulation of their body immune responses. There are two main methods of activating the active immunotherapeutic mechanisms: specific active immunotherapy and nonspecific active immunotherapy.

SPECIFIC ACTIVE IMMUNOTHERAPY.[614-629] The cancer patients are immunized with modified or unmodified tumor cells from their own bodies or donors with histologically similar tumors. The antigenicity of these tumor cells can be augmented by first treating them with enzymes, such as neuraminidase in order to increase their immunogenicity.

NONSPECIFIC ACTIVE IMMUNOTHERAPY. It employs a variety of biological and biochemical agents to induce an overall augmentation of the host immune responses that are not specifically directed at any particular neoplastic cells. The following is a partial list of nonspecific active immunotherapeutic agents.

- Bacillus calmette-Guerin (BCG)[630-645] — a vaccine made of whole, attenuated bovine mycobacterium tuberculosis, which can be administered locally proximal to the local tumor site or given systemically via the regional lymphatic system by means of dermal scarification.
- Methanol extraction residue of BCG (MER).[646-658]
- BCG cell walls.[659-660]
- Coryne bacterium parvum[661-679] — a vaccine made of whole, killed gram-negative bacteria, which is usually administered intravenously.
- Levamisole[680-700] — anthelmintic agent with immunorestorative activity.
- Thymosin[701-710] — extract of thymic tissue, which promotes maturation of thymus-derived cells, e.g. T-lymphocytes.
- Interferon-inducers[711-718] — interferonogens such as naturally occurring and synthetic polynucleotides, phytohemagglutinin and some co-polymers.
- Neuraminidase[719-722] — enzyme produced by microorganisms.

Cryotherapy[723-727]

Medical cryogenics is a special scientific field in which the physical, chemical, and functional properties of living tissues are subjected to subfreezing temperature and studied. The clinical application of the cryogenic principles obtained from experiments in subhuman species enables us to treat a wide spectrum of benign and malignant human diseases with encouraging results.

Cryogenic Sources[728-739]

LIQUID CRYOGENS. Liquid nitrogen, air, oxygen, carbon dioxide, freon-12 (Dichlorodifluoromethane, C Cl_2 F_2), Freon-22 (Chlorodifluoromethane, $CHClF_2$), and nitrous oxide (N_2O).

SOLID CRYOGEN. Solid carbon dioxide.

MECHANICALLY GENERATED LOW TEMPERATURE. This method of cooling is achieved by evaporation of a liquid, melting or sublimation of a solid, or expansion of a liquid or a gas through an expansion valve or a miniature turbine, all of which increases the molecular kinetic energy of the employed agent and thus removes heat from the median and eventually produces the desired cooling effect.

THERMOELECTRIC COOLING. By passing a direct electric current through a whole series of two dissimilar conductors or semiconductors (thermocouples), a wide temperature difference can be maintained across the entire thermocoupling junction.

Methods of Applying Cryotherapy

Cryogens such as liquid nitrogen and air can be directly applied to the tumors by means of applicators or by pouring into the tumor cavity that has been carefully isolated from the surrounding normal tissues. A better method of applying the cryogenic agent to the tumors is by the use of different cryosurgery probes, which can be connected to different cryogenic sources to produce the desired hypothermia. Needless to say, an ideal cryogen should have reproducible tumoricidal effect, sharp delineation, hemostatic ability, flexibility, safety, simplicity, and rapidity of application.

The Cellular Response to Subzero Hypothermia

Although tissue destruction caused by exposure to cold such as frost bite and immersion foot is well known to us. The real mechanisms of cold injury to living tissues are rather complex. The several possible factors that may directly and indirectly contribute to tissue injury by cold are the rapidity of cooling and thawing, changes in cellular membrane permeability, the thermal shock, the presence or absence of protective agents, and vascular stasis with resulting tissue necrosis.

RAPIDITY OF COOLING AND THAWING.[740-761] When living tissue is slowly cooled to below 0 degrees C., large ice crystals begin to form in the extracellular space. The resulting increased extracellular solute concentration draws water from the cell interior across the cell membrane, contributing to further extracellular ice crystal formation, which may cause mechanical injury to the already shrunken cells. However, with rapid cooling, minute intracytoplasmic and intranuclear ice crystals are formed. With the presence of intracellular ice crystals, Stowell et al. (1965)[761] noted marked degree of intracellular vacuolation. Sherman and Kim (1967)[755] observed chromosomal clumping, most likely caused by ice crystal formation in chromosomes. During the thawing process, slow thawing of the rapidly frozen tissues is always more detrimental than rapid thawing because slow thawing causes the small intracellular ice crystals to undergo a recrystallization process to form larger ice crystals. These are particularly harmful to the surviving cells by virtue of the fact that their total volume may exceed the elasticity limit of the cell and nuclear membranes, resulting in cell rupture and death. In addition, slow thawing also exposes the surviving cells to the toxic concentrated solute for a longer period of time which can be very harmful to these cells. The combination of rapid freezing and slow thawing appears to be most lethal to living cells and should be employed in cryosurgery for cancers. In animal experiments, Cahan (1965)[741] implanted cryogenically treated and untreated walker carcinoma cells into littermates of rats. Within a few weeks, the rats who received unfrozen tumor implants all died from extensive carcinomatosis while the control littermates who were implanted with frozen carcinoma cells had no evidence of malignancy even after careful examination at autopsy. In a similar experiment, Asahina and Emura (1966)[740] injected slowly frozen and rapidly frozen ascites sarcoma cells into rats and sacrificed these animals after several weeks. A specially designed, refrigerated microscope was used to observe the intracellular ice formations found in the rats injected with the rapidly frozen acites sarcoma cells. They were all completely free of the tumor. Only extracellular ice formation was present in the rats injected with slowly frozen ascites sarcoma cells, and they all died from the implanted tumor. These two experiments strongly suggest that rapid cooling in association with intracellular ice formation is indispensable for tumor eradication.

CHANGES IN CELLULAR MEMBRANE PERMEABILITY.[762-770] Cell, nucleus, mitochondria, microsomes and lysosomes are enclosed by membranes in which lipid-protein complexes of various compositions are the indispensable components. The lipid-protein complexes are held together by relatively weak bonds that can be broken by drastic temperature change such as subzero freezing. During rapid freezing, intracellular ice crystal formation locks up the water and produces high concentration of electrolytes within the cell, which makes the cell membrane and the lesser membranes, e.g. membranes of nucleus, mitochondria, microsomes, lysosomes, etc., more permeable. Lovelock (1957)[766] feels that the solvent action of the concentrated electrolytes is responsible for dispersion and dissociation of lipids and lipid-proteins from the cell membrane. In addition, as freezing rapidly proceeds, the cell buffering salts crystallize out, pH of the medium changes, and substances like urea and dissolved gases may increase to cytotoxic levels to hasten cell death.

THERMAL SHOCK.[771-772] Although cryotherapy usually implies subzero freezing of living tissues, sudden and precipitous drop of temperature to subnormal level above 0 degrees C. can also be detrimental to many different living cells due to gelation of protoplasmic components and expulsion of fluid from the cell.

CRYOPROTECTIVE AGENTS.[773-780] Compounds like glycerol, dimethyl sulphoxide, ethylene glycol, acetamide, polyvinyl pyrrolidone, dextran, albumen, etc., reduce the electrolyte concentration levels at any particular temperature during equilibrium freezing. This decreases the tendency for cells to take in electrolytes and may also influence the start of the leak in the cell membrane. If the protective agent can enter the cells prior to the freezing process, it will reduce the cellular shrinkage during freezing. On the other hand, if the protective agent has high molecular weight and cannot penetrate the cells, e.g. polyvinyl pyrrolidone, dextran, albumen, etc., it will cause cell shrinkage and thus reduce the chances of intracellular ice formation during rapid freezing. These protective agents are used to protect spermatozoa, red cells and tissue culture cells at low temperature.

VASCULAR STASIS LEADING TO TISSUE NECROSIS.[781-784] Although arteries and veins are quite resistant to the destructive effects of freezing and thawing, arterioles, venules, and capillaries are remarkably vulnerable to the freezing process that first causes vasoconstriction and then produces vasodilation, capillary permeability, formation of intraluminal clot and rupture of the walls of arterioles, capillaries, and venules, resulting in tissue ischemia and necrosis.

Immunological Aspect of Cryotherapy[785-796]

Cryogenically induced rupture or change in permeability of the tumor cell membrane and lesser membranes and denaturation of the molecules of various cellular components make many antigenic substances available to the body's immune mechanisms that can be stimulated to produce specific antibodies against the tumor cells. In clinical practice, it is of interest to note that Gonder et al. (1969)[791] and Ablin et al. (1969)[786] observed remission of metastatic growths from prostatic carcinoma in several patients who had previously undergone cryosurgical prostatectomy, suggesting that cryoimmunization may play a therapeutic role in these patients.

Clinical Applications of Cryotherapy

The tumoricidal and hemostatic effects of cryosurgery coupled with its relatively low morbidity and mortality make it a useful tool in treating a wide variety of benign and malignant diseases. The following is an incomplete list of the clinical applications of cryosurgery in different medical specialities.

- Neurosurgery[797-803] — Brain tumors and dysfunction of basal ganglia.

- Otolaryngology[804-816] — Tonsillectomy; labyrinth surgery; and head, neck, mouth, nose, and throat tumors.
- Urology[817-821] — Prostate and bladder cancers.
- Dermatology[822-827] — Various cutaneous malignancies and growths.
- Ophthalmology[828-837] — Malignancies of eyelid, retinal detachment, cataract extraction and viral keratitis.
- Thoracic surgery[838] — Pulmonary neoplasms.
- Gynecology[839-847] — Inflammatory and neoplastic diseases of the uterus and vulva.
- Oral surgery[848-852] — Intraoral and mandibular tumors.
- Orthopaedic surgery[853-860] — Primary and metastatic tumors.
- General surgery[861-867] — Various tumors of the gastrointestinal tract and hemorrhoidectomy.

Hyperthermia

Modern hyperthermic cancer therapy is a relatively new, but potentially promising, method of combating various forms of primary and metastatic cancers. The advantages of hyperthermia include relatively low therapy-related morbidity and mortality, virtual absence of oncogenic effects, preservation of the normal tissues adjacent to the tumors, wide spectrum of clinical applications in treating different primary and metastatic carcinomas and sarcomas, flexibility in its local or whole-body treatment, and its synergistic or complimentary anticancer action when combined with surgery, chemotherapy, radiotherapy, etc. Generally speaking, clinically useful hyperthermia is restricted to a narrow spread of temperature elevation — 41 degrees C. to 45 degrees C. Prolonged hyperthermia above 45 degrees C. causes indiscriminating protein denaturation of both tumor and normal cells. Hyperthermia below 41 degrees C. merely increases blood flow and oxygen concentration to the heated region, which may not contribute much to the tumoricidal effects of hyperthermia, but it can significantly enhance the efficacy of radiotherapy and chemotherapy. The clinical value of hyperthermia can be better appreciated only when the clinicians have acquired the fundamental working knowledge of hyperthermia.

Historical Background of Hyperthermia

The first documented therapeutic value of hyperthermia dated back to 1866 when Busch described the disappearance of a sarcoma in a patient caused by hyperthermia during erysipelas.[868] Similar observations were subsequently made by Bruns (1887)[869] and Coley (1893)[870] Westermark (1899)[871] inserted hot water circulating cisterns into uteri with advanced carcinomas and reported palliative destruction of some of these incurable uterine tumors. Warren (1935)[872] applied heat from infrared and high frequency currents to "hopeless" tumors and was able to produce remissions in some of his tumor cases. Recently, Suer et al. (1980)[873] also reported lysis of Burkitt's lymphoma following malignant hyperthermia.

Sources of Hyperthermia and Their Administration

MICROWAVE HYPERTHERMIA.[874-880] Clinical microwave generators can generate electromagnetic waves up to 2450 megahertz (MHZ or million cycles per second). They can be delivered to tumors by means of specially designed applicators or thermocouples that can be placed over the skin surface or inserted into the depth of the tumor.

RADIOFREQUENCY HYPERTHERMIA.[881-885] Clinical radiofrequency generators can produce electromagnetic waves with lower frequency and longer wave length than microwave (usually under 30 megahertz). Both microwave and radiofrequency transfer their electromagnetic energy to the molecules of the irradiated tumor or normal tissue cells to increase their kinetic energy, which, in turn, produces heat energy.

ULTRASOUND HYPERTHERMIA.[886-891] Ultrasound generators produce inaudible mechanical sound waves that impart their mechanical energy to the molecules of irradiated tissues, resulting in increased molecular kinetic energy, which produces heat.

INTRAVASCULAR PERFUSION AND EXTRAVASCULAR IMMERSION AND IRRIGATION WITH HYPERTHERMIC FLUIDS.[892-895] Upper and lower extremities with malignant tumors can be isolated and perfused with heated blood through cannulated axillary and iliac (or femoral) arteries and veins. In addition, regional hyperthermia can be obtained by extravascular fluid immersion and irrigation with heated fluids.

TOTAL BODY HYPERTHERMIA.[896-902] Cavaliere et al. (1981)[892] successfully perfused heated blood to achieve total body hyperthermia by using aortal-caval shunts in a limited number of patients. Total body hyperthermia can also be accomplished by immersing the body in a carefully controlled hyperthermic liquid or gas medium.

Biological Effects of Hyperthermia on Normal and Tumor Tissues[903-921]

Although heating of normal and tumor tissues from body temperature to 41 degrees C. results in significant increase in blood flow and oxygen tension in both tissues, a further rise in temperature produces different behavior in normal and tumor tissue that provides the clinical basis for the application of hyperthermia. Several studies have shown that the pH of fluid in human and animal tumors is lower than that of normal tissue pH of 7.4.[922-923]

Hyperthermia beyond 41 degrees causes a decrease in blood flow and oxygen concentration to a much greater degree in the tumor tissue than in the surrounding normal tissue, which is intrinsically more capable of dissipating the applied heat. This decline of blood flow can be brought about by a reduction of red cell deformability, multiple microthrombi, and occlusion of microvessels. In addition, elevated temperature affects the cellular buffering processes and increases cellular metabolic rate and the production of acidic metabolites such as lactic and pyruvic acids. The acidic metabolites tend to accumulate in the hyperthermic tumor cells with impaired blood circulation, driving the pH of tumor cells to an even lower level.[924-929]

In short, the relative vulnerability of tumor cells to collapse in blood flow, lower oxygen tension, and a shift of the tissue pH toward acidosis from the already low pH values present in tumors makes hyperthermia a potentially promising anticancer agent. It should also be mentioned that hyperthermia alters both DNA and RNA synthesis and inhibits cellular enzymatic systems needed for cell metabolism and division, all of which can contribute to the final lethality of the heat-treated cancer cells.

Clinical Application of Hyperthermia in Combined Cancer Therapy

HYPERTHERMIA AND RADIOTHERAPY.[930-944] Hyperthermia is very frequently combined with radiotherapy because of their proven synergistic effects. From normal body temperature to 41 degrees C., hyperthermia can improve vascularity of the tumor tissue, which makes it more radiosensitive. However, hyperthermia exerts its maximal tumoricidal effects when temperatures are beyond 41 degrees C., because, although the hypoxic tumor cells are less radiosensitive, the microcirculation, oxygenation, and pH of the tumor cells are depressed. Furthermore, hyperthermia seems to be effective in inhibiting the biochemical processes of the S(synthesis) phase of the cell cycle which happens to be the most radioresistant phase. Consequently, hyperthermia can not only increase the tumor cell killing power of radiotherapy, but can also reduce the total amount of radiation needed to achieve a reliable tumor eradication effect and thus decrease the short and long term radiation-related morbidity and mortality.

HYPERTHERMIA AND CHEMOTHERAPY.[945-951] Owing to the fact that hyperthermia initially increases the tumor blood flow, which naturally brings more biological substrates and chemotherapeutic agents to the tumor tissue, the higher concentration of these anticancer agents coupled with the increase in substrate supply which tends to enhance the recruitment of cancer cells belonging to the dormant Go-fraction will undoubtedly bring about a higher degree of cancer cell killing action.

HYPERTHERMIA AND SURGERY. The ability of hyperthermia in eradicating microscopic amounts of tumor cells left after en-bloc resection of highly malignant tumor enables cancer victims to preserve the tumor bearing limb, especially in young and vigorous patients. Of the nine patients with osteogenic sarcoma of the extremities treated with en-bloc resection of the tumor plus hyperthermic perfusion of the involved extremities, Cavalier et al. (1981)[892] found complete absence of the initial tumor in five patients for a period ranging between nineteen and fifty-one months. On the other hand, surgery can expose inaccessible areas, e.g. intracranial and intraspinal structures, for hyperthermia to exert its maximal effects.

HYPERTHERMIA AND IMMUNOTHERAPY. It has been demonstrated that hyperthermia increases cell and lysosome membrane permeability, which will expose many intracellular antigens to the host's immune system. In addition, any thermally damaged tumor cellular components may act like new specific antigens to induce the production of specific antibodies against these tumor cells. Goldenberg and Langner (1971)[952] implanted human colonic tumors to bilateral hamster cheek pouches and applied shortwave diathermy to only one pouch per animal. They found that the growth of these colonic tumors was inhibited in both the thermally treated and normothermic pouches, suggesting that the generalized tumor regression was most likely mediated by the hosts' immune system. In a different animal experiment, Hahn et al. (1975)[948] found that the delayed killing of sarcoma cells implanted in mice was very likely caused by the stimulation of a tumor-directed immune response secondary to the direct effect of hyperthermia.

REFERENCES

1. Cline, M. J., and Haskell, C. M.: *Cancer Chemotherapy,* ed. 2. Philadelphia, W. B. Saunders, 1980.
2. Door, R. T., and Fritz, W. L.: *Cancer Chemotherapy Handbook.* New York, Elsevier, 1980.
3. Garattini, S., and Franchi, G. (Eds.): *Chemotherapy of Cancer Dissemination and Metastasis.* New York, Raven Press, 1973.
4. Greenspan, E. (Ed.): *The Pharmacological Basis of Therapeutics,* ed 5. New York, MacMillan, 1975.
5. Greenspan, E. (Ed.): *Clinical Cancer Chemotherapy.* New York, Raven Press, 1975.
6. Holland, J. F., and Frei, E., III (Eds.): *Cancer Medicine.* Philadelphia, Lea & Febiger, 1973.
7. Rubin, P. (Ed.): *Current Concepts in Cancer.* Chicago, American Medical Association, 1974.
8. Bender, R., Castle, M., Margileth, D., and Oliverio, V.: The pharmacokinetics of (^{3}H)-Vincristine in man. *Clin Pharmacol Ther, 22:*430-438, 1977.
9. Bohannon, R. A., Miller, D. G., and Diamond, H. D.: Vincristine in the treatment of lymphomas and leukemias. *Cancer Res, 23:*613-621, 1963.
10. Brook, J., and Schreiber, W.: Vocal cord paralysis: A toxic reaction to Vinblastine (NSC-49842) therapy *Cancer Chemother Rep, 55:*591-593, 1971.
11. Byrd, R. L., Rohrbaugh, T. M., Raney, R. B., Jr., and Norris, D. G.: Transient cortical blindness secondary to Vincristine therapy in childhood malignancies. *Cancer, 47:*37-40, 1981.

12. Camplejohn, R. S.: A critical review of the use of Vincristine (VCR) as a tumour cell synchronizing agent in cancer therapy. *Cell Tissue Kinet, 13:*327-335, 1980.
13. Carpentieri, U., and Lockhart, L. H.: Ataxia and athetosis as side effects of chemotherapy with Vincristine in non-Hodgkin's lymphoma. *Cancer Treat Rep, 62:*561-562, 1978.
14. Creasey, W. A.: Modifications in biochemical pathways produced by the vinca alkaloids. *Cancer Chemother Rep, 52:*501, 1968.
15. Donigan, D. W., and Owellen, R. J.: Interaction of Vinblastic, Vincristine and Colchicine with serum proteins. *Biochem Pharmacol, 22:*2113-2119, 1973.
16. Einhorn, L. H., and Donahue, J.: Cis-diammine Dichloroplatinum, Vinblastine and Bleomycin combination chemotherapy in disseminated testicular cancer. *Ann Intern Med, 87:*293-298, 1977.
17. Gomez, G. A., and Sokal, J. E.: Use of Vinblastine in the terminal phase of chronic myelocytic leukemia. *Cancer Treat Rep, 63:*1385-1387, 1979.
18. Hansen, M. M., Bloomfield, C. D., Jorgensen, J., Ersboll, J., Pedersen-Bjergaard, J., Blom, J., and Nissen, N. I.: VP-16-213 in combination with Cyclophosphamide, Doxorubicin, Vincristine, and Prednisone in the treatment of non-Hodgkin's lymphoma. *Cancer Treat Rep, 64:*1135-1137, 1980.
19. Johnson, I. S.: Plant Alkaloids. In Holland, J. F., and Frei, E., III (Eds.): Cancer Medicine. Philadelphia, Lea and Febiger, 1973, pp. 840-850.
20. Lu, K., Yap, H. Y., Watts, S., and Loo, T. L.: Comparative clinical pharmacology of Vinblastine (VLB) in patients with advanced breast cancer: Single versus continuous infusion. *Proc Am Assoc Cancer Res, 20:*371, 1979.
21. Noble, R. L., Beer, C. T.: Experimental observations concerning the mode of action of vinca alkaloids. In Skedded, W. I. H. (Ed.): *Vinca Alkaloids in the Chemotherapy of Malignant Disease.* Alburcham, England, John Sherratt and Sons, 1968, pp. 4-11.
22. Owellen, R. J., Hartke, C. A., and Hains, F. O.: Pharmacokinetics of Vindesine and Vincristine in humans. *Cancer Res, 37:*2597, 1977.
23. Owellen, R. J., Root, M. A., and Hains, F. O.: Pharmacokinetics of Vindesine and Vincristine in humans. *Cancer Res, 37:*2603, 1977.
24. Rosenthal, S., and Kaufman, S.: Vincristin neurotoxicity. *Ann Intern Med, 80:*733, 1974.
25. Solan, A. J., Greenwald, E. S., and Silvay, O.: Long-term complete remissions of Kaposi's sarcoma with Vinglastine therapy. *Cancer, 47:*637-639, 1981.
26. Yap, H., Blumenschein, G. R., Hortobagyi, G. N., Tashima, C. K., and Loo, T. L.: Continuous 5-day infusion Vinblastine (VLB) in treatment of refractory advanced breast cancer. *Proc Am Assoc Cancer Res, 20:*334, 1979.
27. Adamson, R. H.: Antitumor activity and other biological properties of L-Asparaginase: A review. *Cancer Chemother Rep, 52:*617, 1968.
28. Capizzi, R. L.: Improvement in the therapeutic index of methotrexate (NSC-740) by L-Asparaginase NSC-10922. *Cancer Chemother Rep, 6:*37-41, 1975.
29. Capizzi, R. L., Bertino, J. R., and Handschumacher, R. E.: L-Asparaginase. *Ann Rev Med, 21:*2433-2444, 1970.
30. Ertel, I. J., Nesbit, M. E., Hammond, D., Weiner, J., and Sather, H.: Effective dose of L-Asparaginase for induction of remission in previously treated children with acute lymphocytic leukemia: A report from childrens cancer study group. *Cancer Res, 39:*3893-3891, 1979.
31. Lobel, J. S., O'Brien, R. T., McIntosh, S., Aspnes, G. T., and Capizzi, R. L.: Methotrexate and Asparaginase combination chemotherapy in refractory acute lymphoblastic leukemia in childhood. *Cancer, 43:*1089-1094, 1979.

32. Mathe, G., Amiel, J. L., Clarysse, A., Hayat, M., and Schwarzenburg, L.: The place of L-Asparaginase in the treatment of acute leukemias. *Recent Results in Cancer Res, 33:*279-287, 1970.
33. Miller, H. K., Slaser, J. S., and Balis, M. E.: Amino acid levels following L-Asparagincaminohydrolase therapy. *Cancer Res, 29:*183-187, 1969.
34. Ramsay, N. K. C., Coccia, P. F., Krivit, W., Nesbit, M. E., and Edson, J. R.: The effect of L-Asparaginase on plasma coagulation factors in acute lymphoblastic leukemia. *Cancer, 40:*1398-1401, 1977.
35. Schwartz, M. K., Lash, E. D., Oettgen, H. F., and Tomao, F. A.: L-Asparaginase activity in plasma and other biological fluids. *Cancer, 25:*244-252, 1970.
36. Spiegel, R. J., Echelberger, C. K., and Poplack, D. G.: Delayed allergic reactions following intramuscular L-Asparaginase. *Med Pediatr Oncol, 8:*123-125, 1980.
37. Tallal, L., Tan, C., Dettgen, H., Wollner, N., McCarthy, M., Helson, L., Burchenal, J., Karnofsky, D., and Murphy, L.: E. Coli Asparaginase in the treatment of leukemia and solid tumors in 131 children. *Cancer, 25:*306-320, 1970.
38. Tan, C., and Oettgen, H.: Clinical experience with L-Asparaginase administered intrathecally. *Proc Am Assoc Cancer Res, 10:*92, 1969.
39. Yap, H. Y., Benjamin, R. S., Blumenschein, G. R., Hortobagyi, G. N., Tashima, C. K., Buzdar, A. U., and Bodey, G. P.: Phase II study with sequential L-Asparaginase and Methotrexate in advanced refractory breast cancer. *Cancer Treat Rep, 63:*77-83, 1979.
40. Zubrod, C. G.: The clinical toxicities of L-Asparaginase: In treatment of leukemia and lymphoma. *Pediatrics, 45:*555-559, 1970.
41. Abelson, H. T., Ensminger, W. D., and Rosowsky, A.: Serum and cerebrospinal fluid (CSF) pharmacokinetic studies of high dose methotrexate (MTX) — Carboxypeptidase G (CPDG). *Proc Am Assoc Cancer Res, 20:*213, 1979.
42. Aherne, G. W., Piall, E., Marks, V., Mould, G., and White, W. F.: Prolongation and enhancement of serum Methotrexate concentrations by Probenecid. *Br Med J, 1:*1097-1099, 1978.
43. Bender, J. F., Grove, W. R., and Fortner, C. L.: High-dose Methotrexate with Folinic acid rescue. *Am J Hosp Pharm, 34:*961-965, 1977.
44. Bode, U., Magrath, I., Bleyer, N., Poplack, D., and Glaubiger, D.: Mechanism for Methotrexate (MTX) efflux from cerebrospinal fluid (CSF) in man. *Proc Am Assoc Cancer Res, 20:*375, 1979.
45. Chabner, B. A., and Young, R. C.: Threshold Methotrexate concentration for *in vivo* inhibition of DNA synthesis in normal and tumorous target tissues. *J Clin Invest, 52:*1804-1811, 1973.
46. Chello, P. L., Sirotnak, F. M., and Dorick, D. M.: Kinetics and growth phase dependence of Methotrexate and folic acid transport by L-1210 leukemia cells. *Proc Am Assoc Cancer Res, 20:*219, 1979.
47. Djerassi, I., Ohanissian, H., Kim, J. S., Mills, K., Cerdan, A., Cerdan, C., and Joshua, H.: A new approach to massive Methotrexate-citrovorum rescue — A nontoxic dose schedule for Methotrexate assistant tumors in poor risk patients. *Proc Am Assoc Cancer Res, 20:*398, 1979.
48. Ettinger, D. S., Stanley, K. E., and Nystrom, J. S.: Phase II study of high-dose Methotrexate in the treatment of patients with non-small cell carcinoma of the lung: An eastern cooperative group study. *Cancer Treat Rep, 64:*1017-1021, 1980.
49. Frei, E., Jaffe, N., Tattersal, M., Pitman, S., and Parker, L.: New approaches to cancer chemotherapy with Methotrexate. *N Engl J Med, 292:*846-851, 1975.
50. Goldman, I. D.: The membrane transport of Methotrexate (NSC-740) and other

folate compounds: Relevance to rescue protocols. *Cancer Chemother Rep, 6:*63-72, 1975.

51. Goldman, I. D.: Effects of Methotrexate on cellular metabolism: Some critical elements in the drug-cell interactions. *Cancer Treat Rep, 71:*549-558, 1977.
52. Jaffe, N., Frei, E., III, Watts, H., and Straggis, D.: High dose Methotrexate in osteogenic sarcoma: A 5-year experience. *Cancer Treat Rep, 62:*259-264, 1978.
53. Natale, R. B., Yagoda, A., Watson, R. C., Whitmore, W. F., Blumenreich, M., and Braun, D. W., Jr.: Methotrexate: An active drug in bladder cancer. *Cancer, 47:*1246-1250, 1981.
54. Nirenberg, A., Mosende, C., Mehta, B. M., Gisolfi, A. L., and Rosen, G.: High-dose Methotrexate with citrovorum factor rescue: Predictive value of serum Methotrexate concentrations and corrective measures to avert toxicity. *Cancer Treat Rep, 61:*779-783, 1977.
55. Shapiro, W. R., Young, D. F., and Mehta, B. M.: Methotrexate: Distribution in cerebrospinal fluid after intravenous ventricular and lumbar injections. *N Engl J Med, 293:*161-166, 1975.
56. Stroller, R. G., Kaplan, H. G., Cummings, F. J. and Calabresi, P.: A clinical and pharmacological study of high-dose Methotrexate with minimal leucovorin rescue. *Cancer Res, 39:*908-912, 1979.
57. White, J. C., and Goldman, I. D.: Inhibition and reversal of ^{3}H-Methotrexate (MTX) binding to dihydrofolate reductase (DHFR) by dihydrofolate (H_3F): Relationship of intracellular (IC) events. *Proc Am Assoc Cancer Res, 20:*263, 1979.
58. Yap, B., McCredie, K. B., Benjamin, R. S., Bodey, G. P., and Freireich, E. J.: Refractory acute leukaemia in adults treated with sequential colaspase and high-dose Methotrexate. *Br Med J, 2:*791-793, 1978.
59. Zaharko, D. S., and Dedrick, R. L.: Antifolate: *In vivo* kinetic considerations. *Cancer Treat Rep, 61:*513-518, 1977.
60. Erkman, J., and Blythe, J. G.: Azathioprine therapy complicated by pregnancy. *Obstet Gynecol, 40:*708-710, 1972.
61. Jensen, M. K.: Effect of Azathioprine on the chromosome compliment of human bone marrow cells. *Int J Cancer, 5:*147-151, 1970.
62. Lewis, P., Hazelman, B. L., Hanka, R., and Roberts, S.: Cause of death in patients with rheumatoid arthritis with particular reference to Azathioprine. *Ann Rheum Dis, 39:*457-461, 1980.
63. McGrath, B. P., Ibels, I. S., Raik, E., Hargrave, M., Mahony, J. F., and Stewart, J. H.: Erythroid toxicity of Azathioprine. *Q J Med, 44:*57-63, 1975.
64. Paloyan, D., Levin, B., and Simonowitz, D.: Azathioprine-associated acute pancreatitis. *Am J Dig Dis, 22:*839-840, 1977.
65. Rosman, M., and Bertino, J. R.: Azathioprine. *Ann Intern Med, 79:*694-700, 1973.
66. Rubin, G., Baume, P., and Vandenberg, R.: Azathioprine and acute restrictive lung disease. *Aust N Z J Med, 2:*272-274, 1972.
67. Butler, H. E., Jr., Morgan, J. M., and Smythe, C. M.: Mercaptopurine and acquired tubular dysfunction in adult nephrosis. *Ann Intern Med, 116:*856, 1965.
68. Clark, P. A., Hsia, Y. E., and Huntsman, R. G.: Toxic complications of treatment with 6-Mercaptopurine: Two cases with hepatic necrosis and intestinal ulceration. *Br Med J, 1:*393-395, 1960.
69. Coffey, J. J., White, C. A., and Lesk, A. B.: Effects of allopurinol on the pharmacokinetics of 6-Mercaptopurine: Two cases with hepatic necrosis and intestinal ulceration. *Br Med J, 1:*393-395, 1960.
70. Einhorn, M., and Davidson, I.: Hepatoxicity of Mercaptopurine. *JAMA, 188:*802-806, 1964.

71. Esterhay, R., Aisner, J., Levi, J. A., and Wiernik, P. H.: High-dose 6-Mercaptopurine in advanced refractory cancer. *Cancer Treat Rep, 62:*1229-1231, 1978.
72. Loo, T. L., Luce, J. K., Sullivan, M. P., and Frei, E., III: Clinical pharmacologic observations on 6-Mercaptopurine and 6-Methyl Thiopurine Ribonucleoside. *Clin Pharmacol Ther, 9:*180-194, 1968.
73. Tidd, D. M., and Paterson, A. R. P.: A biochemical mechanism for the delayed cytotoxic reaction of 6-Mercaptopurine. *Cancer Res, 34:*738, 1974.
74. Tterlikkis, L., Ortega, E., Solomon, R., and Day, J.: Pharmacokinetics of Mercaptopurine. *J Pharm Sci, 66:*1454-1457, 1977.
75. Wiernik, P. H., and Serpick, A. A.: A randomized clinical trial of Daunorubicin and a combination of Prednisone, Vincristine, 6-Mercaptopurine and Methotrexate in adult acute nonlymphocytic leukemia. *Cancer Res, 32:*2023-2026, 1972.
76. Denes, A., and Presant, C.: 6-Thioguanine (TG): A phase 1 study of intermittant oral (P.O.) and Intravenous (I.V.) therapy in solid tumor (ST). *Proc Am Assoc Cancer Res, 20:*107, 1979.
77. Finkel, J. M.: Fluorometric assay of Thioguanine. *J Pharm Sci, 64:*121-122, 1975.
78. Krakoff, I. H., Ellison, R. R., and Tan, C. T. C.: Clinical evaluation of Thioguanosine. *Cancer Res, 21:*1015-1018, 1961.
79. LePage, G. A., and Whitecar, J. P., Jr.: Pharmacology of 6-Thioguanine in man. *Cancer Res, 31:*1627, 1971.
80. Lewis, J. P., Unman, J. W., Marshall, G. J., Pajar, T. F., and Bateman, J. R.: Randomized clinical trial of Cytosine Arabinoside and 6-Thioguanine in remission induction and consolidation of adult non-lymphocytic acute leukemia. *Cancer, 39:*1387-1396, 1977.
81. Moore, E. C., and Lepage, G. A.: The metabolism of 6-Thioguanine and neoplastic tissue. *Cancer Res, 18:*1075-1083, 1958.
82. Nelson, J. A., Carpenter, J. W., and Rose, L. M.: Mechanisms of action of 6-Thioguanine, 6-Mercaptopurine, and 8-Azaguanine. *Cancer Res, 35:*2872-2878, 1975.
83. Pandya, K. J., Tormey, D. C., Davis, T. E., Falkson, G., Banerjee, T. K., and Crowley, J.: Phase II trial of 6-Thioguanine in metastatic breast cancer. *Cancer Treat Rep, 64:*191-192, 1980.
84. Philips, F. S., Sternberg, S. S., Hamilton, L., and Clark, D. A.: Effects of Thioguanine in mammals. *Cancer, 9:*1092-1102, 1956.
85. Presant, G. A., Denes, A. E., Klein, L., Garrett, S., and Metter, G. E.: Phase I and preliminary phase II observations of high-dose intermittent 6-Thioguanine. *Cancer Treat Rep, 64:*1109-1113, 1980.
86. Spiers, A. S., Kaur, J., Galton, D. A. G., and Goldman, J. M.: Thioguanine as primary treatment for chronic granulocytic leukemia. *Lancet, 1:*829-833, 1975.
87. Valeriote, F., Vietti, T., and Edelstein, M.: Combined effect of Cytosine Arabinoside and Thiopurines. *Cancer Treat Rep, 60:*1925-1934, 1976.
88. Baker, L. H., Talley, R. W., and Matter, R.: Phase III comparison of the treatment of advanced gastrointestinal cancer with Bolus weekly 5-Fu vs. Methyl-CCNU plus Bolus weekly 5-FU. *Cancer, 138:*1-7, 1976.
89. Bateman, J. R., and Moertel, C. G.: Oral vs. intravenous administration of Fluorouracil. *JAMA, 229:*1109, 1974.
90. Cohen, J. L., Irwin, L. E., Darvey, H., and Bateman, J. R.: Clinical pharmacology of oral and intravenous 5-Fluorouracil (NSC 19893). *Cancer Chemother Rep, 58:*723-731, 1974.
91. Frey, C., Twomey, P., Keehn, R., Elliott, D., and Higgins, G.: Randomized study of 5-FU and CCNU in pancreatic cancer: Report of the Veterans Administration Surgical Adjuvant Cancer Chemotherapy Study Group. *Cancer, 47:*27-31, 1981.

92. Heidelberger, C., and Ansfield, F. J.: Experimental and clinical uses of fluorinated pyrimidines in cancer chemotherapy. *Cancer Res, 23:*1226, 1963.
93. Jacobs, E. M., Luce, J. K., and Woods, D. A.: Treatment of cancer with weekly intravenous 5-Fluorouracil. *Cancer, 22:*1233, 1968.
94. Kaufman, S.: 5-Fluorouracil in the treatment of gastrointestinal neoplasia. *N Engl J Med, 288:*199-201, 1973.
95. Klein, E., Stoll, H. L., Miller, E., Milgrom, H., Helm, F., and Burgess, G.: The effects of 5-Fluorouracil (5-FU) ointment in the treatment of neoplastic dermatoses. *Dermatologica, 144:*21-33, 1970.
96. LaHiri, S. R., Boileau, G., and Hall, T. C.: Treatment of metastatic colorectal carcinoma with 5-Fluorouracil by mouth. *Cancer, 28:*902-906, 1971.
97. MacMillan, W. E., Wolberg, W. H., and Welling, P. G.: Pharmacokinetics of Fluorouracil in humans. *Cancer Res, 38:*3479-3482, 1978.
98. Martin, D. S., Stolfi, R. L., Spiegelman, S.: Striking augmentation of the *in vivo* anticancer activity of 5-Fluorouracil (FU) by combination with pyrimidine nucleosides: A RNA effect. *Proc Am Assoc Cancer Res, 19:*221, 1978.
99. Miller, E.: The metabolism and pharmacology of 5-Fluorouracil. *J Surg Oncol, 8:*309-315, 1971.
100. Moayeri, H., DiBenedetto, J., Jr., and Mittelman, A.: Metastatic colorectal cancer. Combination chemotherapy in patients previously treated with 5-Fluorouracil. *N Y State J Med, 80:*1220-1224, 1980.
101. Seifert, P., Baker, L. H., Reed, M. L., and Vaitke Vicius, V. K.: Comparison of continuously infused 5-Fluorouracil with Bolus injection in treatment of patients with colorectal adenocarcinoma. *Cancer, 36:*123-128, 1975.
102. Stolinsky, D. C., Pugh, R. P., and Bateman, J. R.: 5-Fluorouracil (NSC-19893) therapy for pancreatic carcinoma: Comparison of oral and intravenous routes. *Cancer Treat Rep, 59:*1031-1033, 1975.
103. Tandon, R. N., Bunnel, I. L., and Cooper, R. G.: The treatment of metastatic carcinoma of the liver by percutaneous selective hepatic artery infusion of 5-Fluorouracil. *Surg, 73:*118-121, 1973.
104. Tattersall, M. H. N., Jackson, R. C., Connors, T. A., and Harrap, K. R.: Combination chemotherapy: The interaction of Methotrexate and 5-Fluorouracil. *Eur J Cancer, 9:*733-739, 1973.
105. Bergy, M. E., and Herr, R. R.: Microbiological production of 5-Azacytidine. II. Isolation and chemical structure. *Antimicrob Agents Chemother, 6:*625-630, 1966.
106. Israili, Z. H., Vogler, W. R., Mingioli, E. S., Pirkle, J. L., Smithwick, R. W., and Goldstein, J. H.: The disposition and pharmacokinetics in humans of 5-Azacytidine administered intravenously as a bolus or by continuous infusion. *Cancer Res, 36:*1453-1461, 1976.
107. Koeffler, H. P., and Haskell, C. M.: Rhabdomyolysis is a complication of 5-Azacytidine. *Cancer Treat Rep, 62:*573-574, 1978.
108. Levi, J. A., and Wiernik, P. H.: A comparative study of 5-Azacytidine and Guanazole in previously treated adult acute non-lymphocytic leukemia. *Cancer Chemother Rep, 59:*1043-1045, 1975.
109. Lomen, P. L., Khilanani, P., and Kessel, D.: Phase I study using combination of Hydroxyurea and 5-Azacytidine (NSC-102816). *Neoplasma, 27:*101-106, 1980.
110. McCredie, K. B., Bodey, G. P., Burgess, M. A., Gutterman, J. U., Rodriguez, V., Jordan, U., Sullivan, M. P., and Freireich, E. J.: Treatment of acute leukemia with 5-Azacytidine (NSC-102816). *Cancer Chemother Rep, 57:*319-323, 1973.
111. Moertel, C. G., Schott, A. J., Reitemeier, R. J., and Hahn, R. G.: Phase II study of

5-Azacytidine (NSC-102816) in the treatment of advanced gastrointestinal cancer. *Cancer Chemother Rep, 56:*649-652, 1972.

112. Omura, G. A., Vogler, W. R., Bartolucci, A., Neely, C. L., and Silberman, H.: Treatment of refractory adult acute leukemia with 5-Azacytidine plus Beta-2-Deoxythioguanosine. *Cancer Treat Rep, 63:*209-210, 1979.
113. Troetel, W. M., Weiss, A. J., and Stambaugh, J. E.: Absorption, distribution and excretion of 5-Azacytidine (NSC-102816) in man. *Cancer Chemother Rep, 56:*405-411, 1972.
114. Vogler, W. R., Miller, D., and Keller, J. W.: Remission induction in refractory myeloblastic leukemia with continuous infusion of 5-Azacytidine. *Proc Am Assoc Cancer Res, 16:*155, 1975.
115. Von Hoff, D., Slavik, M., and Muggia, F.: 5-Azacytidine — a new anticancer drug with effectiveness in acute myelogenous leukemia. *Ann Intern Med, 85:*237-245, 1976.
116. Body, G. P., Freireich, E. J., Hewlett, J. S., and Monto, R. W.: Cytosine Arabinoside (NSC-63878) therapy for acute leukemia in adults. *Cancer Chemother Rep, 53:*59-66, 1969.
117. Coleman, C. N., Johns, D. G., and Chabner, B. A.: Studies on mechanisms of resistance to Cytosine Arabinoside: Problems in the determination of related enzyme activities in leukemic cells. *Ann N Y Acad Sci, 255:*247-251, 1975.
118. Edelstein, M., Vietti, J., and Valeriote, F.: The enhanced cytotoxicity of combinations of 1-B-D-Arabinofuranosylcytosine and Methotrexate. *Cancer Res, 35:*1555-1558, 1975.
119. Eden, O. B., Goldie, W., Wood, T., and Etucubanas, E.: Seizures following intrathecal Cytosine Arabinoside in young children with acute lymphoblastic leukemia. *Cancer, 42:*53-58, 1978.
120. Furth, J. J., and Cohen, S. S.: Inhibition of mammalian DNA polymerase by the 5′-Triphosphate of 1-B-D-Arabinofuranosylcytosine and the 5′-Triphosphate of 9-B-D-Arabinofuranosyladene. *Cancer Res, 28:*2061, 1968.
121. Ho, D. H. W., and Frei, E., III: Clinical pharmacology of 1-B-D-Arabinofuranosylcytosine. *Clin Pharmacol Ther, 12:*944-954, 1971.
122. Skipper, H. E., Schabel, F. M., and Wilcox, W. S.: Experimental evaluation of potential anticancer agents. XXI. Scheduling of Arabinosylcytosine to take advantage of its S-phase specificity against leukemic cells. *Cancer Chemother Rep, 51:*125-141, 1967.
123. Tattersall, M. H. N., and Harrap, K. R.: Combination chemotherapy: The antagonism of Methotrexate and Cytosine Arabinoside. *Eur J Cancer, 9:*229-232, 1973.
124. Van Prooijen, R., Kleijn, E. V. D., and Haanen, C.: Pharmacokinetics of Cytosine Arabinoside in acute myeloid leukemia. *Clin Pharmacol Ther, 21:*744-750, 1977.
125. Wang, J. J., and Pratt, C. B.: Intrathecal Arabinosylcytosine in meningeal leukemia. *Cancer, 25:*531-534, 1970.
126. Wolff, L., Zighelboim, J., and Gale, R. P.: Paraplegia following intrathecal Cytosine Arabinoside. *Cancer, 43:*83-85, 1979.
127. Ariel, J. M.: Treatment of disseminated cancer by intravenous Hydroxyurea and autogenous bone-marrow transplants: Experience with 35 patients. *J Surg Oncol, 7:*331-335, 1975.
128. Belt, R. J., Haas, C. D., Kennedy, J., and Taylor, S.: Studies of Hydroxyurea administered by continuous infusion: Toxicity, pharmacokinetics, and cell synchronization. *Cancer, 46:*455-462, 1980.
129. Bloedow, C. E.: Phase II studies of Hydroxyurea in adults: Miscellaneous tumor. *Cancer Chemother Rep, 40:*39, 1964.

130. Kennedy, B. J.: Hydroxyurea therapy in chronic myelogenic leukemia. *Cancer, 29:*1052-1056, 1972.

131. Krakoff, I. H., Brown, N. C., and Reichard, P.: Inhibition of ribonucleoside diphosphate reductase by Hydroxyurea. *Cancer Res, 28:*1559-1569, 1968.

132. Lerner, H. F., and Malloy, T. O.: Hydroxyurea in stage D carcinoma of the prostate. *Urology, 10:*35-38, 1977.

133. Lokich, J. J., Pitman, S. W., and Skarin, A. T.: Combined 5-Fluorouracil and Hydroxyurea therapy for gastrointestinal cancer. *Oncology, 32:*34-37, 1975.

134. Rominger, D. J.: Hydroxyurea and radiation therapy in advanced neoplasms of head and neck. *Am J Roentgenol Rad Ther Nucl Med, 111:*103, 1971.

135. Schwartz, J. H., and Canellos, G. P.: Hydroxyurea in the management of the hematologic complications of chronic granulocytic leukemia. *Blood, 46:*11, 1975.

136. Stefani, S., Eels, R. W., and Abbate, J.: Hydroxyurea and radiotherapy in head and neck cancer — Results of a prospective controlled study in 126 patients. *Radiology, 101:*391, 1971.

137. Young, C. W., Schochetman, G., Hadas, S., and Balis, M. E.: Inhibition of DNA synthesis by hydroxyurea: Structure — activity relationships. *Cancer Res, 27:*535-540, 1967.

138. Bertino, J. R.: "Rescue" techniques in cancer chemotherapy: Use of Leucovorin and other rescue agents after Methotrexate treatment. *Semin Oncol, 4:*203, 1977.

139. Djerassi, L., Abir, E., and Roger, G. L., Jr.: Long term remission in childhood acute leukemia; use of infrequent infusions of Methotrexate: Supportive role of platelet transfusions and Citrovorum factor. *Clin Pediatr, 5:*502-509, 1966.

140. Jaffe, N.: Progress report on high dose Methotrexate (NSC-740) with Citrovorum rescue in the treatment of metastatic bone tumors. *Cancer Chemother Rep, 58:*275-280, 1974.

141. Kirschner, E. A., Nixon, P. F., and Bertino, J. R.: Metabolism of methyltetrahydrofolate in man. *Clin Res, 16:*537, 1968.

142. Lauper, R. D.: Leucovorin calcium administration and preparation. *Am J Hosp Pharm, 35:*377-378, 1978.

143. Lefkowitz, E., Papac, R. J., and Bertino, J. R.: Head and neck cancer. III. Toxicity of 24 hour infusions of Methotrexate and protection by Leucovorin in patients with epidermoid carcinomas. *Cancer Chemother Rep, 51:*305-311, 1967.

144. Mattsson, W., Arwidi, A., Von Eyben, F., and Lindholm, C. E.: Phase II study of combined Vincristine, Adriamycin, Cyclophosphamide, and Methotrexate with Citrovorum factor rescue in metastatic breast cancer. *Cancer Treat Rep, 61:*1527-1531, 1977.

145. Mehta, B. M., Gisolfi, A. L., Hutchison, D. J., Nerenberg, A., Kellick, M. G., Rosen, G.: Serum distribution of Citrovorum factor and 5-Methyltetrahydrofolate following oral and IM administration of calcium Leucovorin in normals. *Cancer Treat Rep, 12:*345-350, 1978.

146. Nixon, P. F., and Bertino, T. R.: Effective absorption and utilization of oral Formyltetrahydrofolate in man. *N Engl J Med, 286:*175-179, 1972.

147. Vogler, W. R., Israili, Z. H., Soliman, A. G. M., Moffitt, S., and Barlogie, B.: Marrow cell kinetics in patients treated with Methotrexate and Citrovorum factor. *Cancer, 47:*215-223, 1981.

148. Alberts, D. S., and Peng, Y. M.: Effective simulation of the minimum cytotoxic concentration of continuous Bleomycin with multiple subcutaneous injections in cancer patients. *Proc Am Assoc Cancer Res, 20:*432, 1979.

149. Barranco, S. C., Kue, J. K., Romsdahl, M. M., and Humphrey, R. M.: Bleomycin as a possible synchronizing agent for human tumor cells in vivo. *Cancer Res, 33:*882-887, 1973.

150. Bearden, J., Jr., and Haidle, C. W.: Stimulation of Bleomycin-induced fragmentation of DNA by intercalating agents. *Biochem Biophys Res Commun, 65:*371, 1975.
151. Bishun, N. P., Smith, N. S., and Williams, D. C.: Bleomycin (review). *Oncology, 35:*228-234, 1978.
152. Blum, R. H., Carter, S. K., and Agre, K.: A clinical review of Bleomycin — a new, antineoplastic agent. *Cancer, 31:*903-914, 1973.
153. Catane, R., Schwade, J. G., Turrisi, A. T., III, Webber, B. L., and Muggia, F. M.: Pulmonary toxicity after radiation and Bleomycin: A review. *Int J Radiat Oncol Biol Phys, 5:*1513-1518, 1979.
154. Freedman, M. A.: A review of the Bleomycin experience in the United States. *Recent Results Cancer Res, 63:*152-168, 1978.
155. Ginsberg, S. J., Gottlieb, A. J., Bloomfield, C. D., Blom, J., and Crooke, S. T.: Combination chemotherapy with continuous infusion, low dose Bleomycin in lymphoma. *Proc Am Assoc Cancer Res, 20:*322, 1979.
156. Haidle, C. W., Weiss, K. K., and Klo, M. T.: Release of free bases from deoxyribonucleic acid after reaction with Bleomycin. *Molec Pharmacol, 8:*531-537, 1972.
157. Hall, S. W., Boughton, A., Strong, J. E., and Benjamin, R. S.: Clinical pharmacology of Bleomycin by radioimmunoassay. *Clin Res, 25:*407, 1977.
158. Kondi, E. S., Allitano, A. L., Eviy, J. J., and Barnard, D. E.: Prolonged survival in a patient with hepatic malignant melanoma treated by intra-arterial Bleomycin and oral hydroxyurea. *Am J Surg, 128:*85-87, 1974.
159. Nachman, J. B., Baum, E. S., White, H., and Crussii, F. G.: Bleumycin-induced pulmonary fibrosis mimicking recurrent metastatic disease in a patient with testicular carcinoma: Case report of the CT scan appearance. *Cancer, 47:*236-239, 1981.
160. Leichman, L. P., Baker, L. H., Stanhope, C. R., Samson, M. K., Fraile, K. J., Vaikevicius, V. K., and Hilgers, R.: Mitomycin C and Bleomycin in the treatment of far-advanced cervical cancer: A southwest oncology group study. *Cancer Treat Rep, 64:*1139-1140, 1980.
161. Livingston, R. B., Einhorn, L. H., Bodey, G. P., Burgess, M. A., Freirich, E. J., and Gottlieb, J. A.: COMB (Cyclophosphamide, Oncovin, Methyl CCNU and Bleomycin): A four drug combination in solid tumors. *Cancer, 36:*327-332, 1975.
162. Paladine, W., Cunningham, T. J., and Sponzo, R.: Intracavity Bleomycin in the management of malignant effusions. *Cancer, 38:*1903-1908, 1976.
163. Samuels, M. L., Holeye, P. Y., and Johnson, D. E.: Bleomycin combination chemotherapy in the management of testicular neoplasm. *Cancer, 36:*318-326, 1975.
164. Spigel, S. C., and Coltman, C. A., Jr.: Therapy of mycosis fungoides with Bleomycin. *Cancer, 32:*767, 1973.
165. Tobey, R. A.: Arrest of Chinese hamster cells in G_2 following treatment with the antitumor drug Bleomycin. *J Cell Physiol, 79:*259-266, 1972.
166. Umezawa, H.: Chemistry and mechanism of action of Bleomycin. *Fed Proc, 33:*2296-2302, 1974.
167. Vugrin, D., Whitmore, W. F., Cvitkovic, E., Grabstald, H., Sogani, P., Barzell, W., and Golbey, R. B.: Adjuvant chemotherapy combination of Vinblastine, Actinomycin D, Bleomycin, and Chlorambucil following retroperitoneal lymph node dissection for stage II testis tumor. *Cancer, 47:*840-844, 1981.
168. Bakowski, M. T., Brearley, R. L., and Wrigley, P. F.: Treatment of blast cell crisis of chronic myeloid leukemia with ICRF-159 (Razoxane). *Cancer Treat Rep, 63:*2085-2087, 1979.
169. Creech, R. H., Engstrom, P. F., Harris, D. T., Catalano, R. B., and Bellet, R. E.: Phase

II study of ICRF-159 in refractory metastatic breast cancer. *Cancer Treat Rep, 63:*111-114, 1979.

170. Dyment, P. G., Starling, K. A., Land, V. J., Cangir, A., Komp, D. M., and Sexauer, C. L.: ICRF-159 (Razoxane) in the treatment of periatric solid tumors: A southwest oncology group study. *Cancer Treat Rep, 63:*1397-1398.
171. Flannery, E. P., Corder, M. P., Sheehan, W. W., Pajak, T. F., and Bateman, J. R.: Phase II study of ICRF-159 in non-Hodgkin's lymphomas. *Cancer Treat Rep, 62:*465-467, 1978.
172. Gilbert, J. M., Cassell, P., Ellis, H., Wastell, C., Hermon-Taylor, J., and Hellman, K.: Adjuvant treatment with Razoxane (ICRF-159) following resection of cancer of the stomach. *Recent Results Cancer Res, 68:*217-221, 1978.
173. Hellman, K., and Burrage, K.: Control of malignant metastases by ICRF-159. *Nature* (London), *224:*273-275, 1969.
174. Olweny, C. L., Sikyewunda. W., and Otim, D.: Further experience with Razoxane (ICRF-159;-NSC-129943) in treating Kaposi's sarcoma. *Oncolory, 37:*174-176, 1980.
175. Poster, D. S., Penta, J., Marsoni, S., Bruno, S., and MacDonald, J. S.: Bis-Diketopiperazine derivatives in clinical oncology: ICRF-159. *Cancer Clin Trials, 3:*315-320, 1980.
176. Salsburg, A. J., Burrage, K., and Hellman, K.: Inhibition of metastatic spread by ICRF-159: Selective delection of malignant characteristics. *Br Med J, 4:*344-346, 1970.
177. Sharpe, H. B. A., Field, E. O., and Hellman, K.: Mode of action of cytostatic agent "ICRF-159." *Nature* (London), *226:*524-526, 1970.
178. Venditti, J. M.: Treatment schedule dependency of experimentally active anti leukemic (L-1210) drugs. *Cancer Chemother Rep,* Part 3, *2:*35-59, 1971.
179. Vogl, S. E., Lanham, R., and Kaplan, B. H.: Combination chemotherapy of advanced colorectal cancer with Triazinate and ICRF-159 after failure of 5-Fluorouracil. *Oncology, 37:*314-315, 1980.
180. Wampler, G. L., Speckhard, V. J., and Regelson, W.: Phase I clinical study of Adriamycin-ICRF-159 combination and other ICRF-159 drug combinations. *Proc Am Soc Clin Oncol, 15:*189, 1974.
181. Wang, G. M., and Finch, M.: Studies on the mechanism of Razoxane induced reduction of Daunomycin toxicity. *Proc Am Assoc Cancer Res, 20:*23, 1979.
182. Alberts, D. S., Manning, M. R., Coulthard, S. W., Koopmann, C. F., Jr., and Herman, T. S.: Adriamycin/Cis-platinum/Cyclophosphamide combination chemotherapy for advanced carcinoma of the parotid gland. *Cancer, 47:*645-648, 1981.
183. Bagley, C. M., Bosllick, F. W., and DeVita, V. T.: Clinical pharmacology of Cyclophosphamide. *Cancer Res, 33:*226-233, 1973.
184. Carter, S. K., and Livingston, R. B.: Cyclophosphamide in solid tumors. *Cancer Treat Rev, 2:*295, 1975.
185. Cohen, J. L., Jao, J. Y., and Jusko, W. J.: Pharmacokinetics of Cyclophosphamide in man. *Br J Pharmacol, 43:*667-680, 1971.
186. Dalley, D. N., Levi, J. A., and Aroney, R. S.: Combination chemotherapy with Cyclophosphamide, Adriamycin, and 5-Fluorouracil (CAF) in advanced breast carcinoma. *Med J Aust, 1:*216-218, 1980.
187. Faber, O. K., and Mouridsen, H. T.: Cyclophosphamide activation and corticosteroids. *N Engl J Med, 291:*211, 1974.
188. Fairley, K. F., Barrie, J. U., and Johnson, W.: Sterility and testicular atrophy related by Cyclophosphamide therapy. *Lancet, 1:*568-569, 1972.
189. Hill, D. L.: *A Review of Cyclophosphamide.* Springfield, Charles C Thomas, 1975.

190. Hutter, A. M., Bauman, A. W., and Frank, I. N.: Cyclophosphamide and severe hemorrhagic cystitis. *N Y State J Med, 69:*305-509, 1969.
191. Jones, S. E., Durie, B. G. M., and Salmon, S. E.: Combination chemotherapy with Adriamycin and Cyclophosphamide for advanced breast carcinoma. *Cancer, 36:*90-97, 1975.
192. Levine, A. S., Appelbaum, F. R., Graw, R. G., Jr., Magrath, I. T., Pizzo, P. A., Poplack, D. G., and Ziegler, J. L.: Sequential combination chemotherapy (containing high-dose Cyclophosphamide) for metastatic osteogenic sarcoma. *Cancer Treat Rep, 62:*247-250, 1978.
193. Muggia, F. M., Chia, G., Reed, L. J., and Romney, S. L.: Doxorubicin-Cyclophosphamide. Effective chemotherapy for advanced endometrial Adenocarcinoma. *J Obstet Gynecol, 128:*314-319, 1977.
194. Mullins, G. M., and Colvin, M.: Intensive Cyclophosphamide (NSC-26271) therapy for solid tumors. *Cancer Chemother Rep, 59:*411-419, 1975.
195. Shepp, M., Necheles, T. F., Banks, H. H., Oh, W. H., and Iimbler, S.: Adjuvant treatment of osteogenic sarcoma with high-dose Cyclophosphamide. *Cancer Treat Rep, 62:*295-296, 1978.
196. Skarin, A. T., Rosenthal, D. S., Moloney, W. C., and Frei, E., III: Combination chemotherapy of advanced non-Hodgkin's lymphoma with Bleomycin, Adriamycin, Cyclophosphamide, Vincristine, and Prednisone (BACVP). *Blood, 49:*759-770, 1977.
197. Topelow, A. A., Rothenberg, S. P., and Cottrell, T. S.: Interstitial pneumonia after prolonged treatment with Cyclophosphamide. *Am Rev Respir Dis, 108:*114-117, 1973.
198. Wall, R. L., and Clausen, K. P.: Carcinoma of the urinary bladder in patients receiving Cyclophosphamide. *N Engl J Med, 293:*271-275, 1975.
199. Warne, G. L., Fairley, K. F., Hobbs, J. B., Martin, F. I. R.: Cyclophosphamide-induced ovarian failure. *N Engl J Med, 289:*1159-1162, 1963.
200. Cole, S. R., Myers, J. J., Klasky, A. U.: Pulmonary disease with Chlorambucil therapy. *Cancer, 41:*455-459, 1978.
201. Ezdinli, E. Z., and Stutzman, L.: Chlorambucil therapy for lymphomas and chronic lymphocytic leukemia. *JAMA, 191:*444-450, 1965.
202. Han, T., Ezdinli, E. Z., Shimaoka, K., and Desai, D. V.: Chlorambucil vs. combined Chlorambucil-corticosteroid therapy in chronic lymphocytic leukemia. *Cancer, 31:*502-512, 1973.
203. Knospe, W. H., Loeb, V., Jr., and Huguley, C. M., Jr.: Bi-weekly Chlorambucil treatment of chronic lymphocytic leukemia. *Cancer, 33:*555, 1974.
204. Lahey, M. E., Heyn, R. M., Newton, W. A., Jr., Shore, N., Smith, W. B., Leikins, S., and Hammond, D.: Histiocytosis X: Clinical trial of Chlorambucil: A report from childrens cancer study group. *Med Pediatr Oncol, 7:*197-203, 1979.
205. Lane, S. D., Besa, E. C., Justh, G., and Joseph, R. R.: Fatal interstitial pneumonitis following high-dose intermittent Chlorambucil therapy for chronic lymphocytic leukemia. *Cancer, 47:*32-36, 1981.
206. Lerner, H. J.: Acute myelogenous leukemia in students receiving Chlorambucil as long-term adjuvant chemotherapy for stage II breast cancer. *Cancer Treat Rep, 62:*1135-1138, 1978.
207. Mayr, A. C., Jungi, W. F., and Senn, H. J.: A well tolerated oral combination of Chlorambucil (Leukeran R), Methotrexate, Fluorouracil, Prednisone (LMFP) in disseminated breast cancer. *Cancer Treat Rev, 6(Suppl.):*115-120, 1979.
208. Miller, D. G., Diamond, H. D., and Carver, L. F.: The clinical use of Chlorambucil: A critical study. *N Engl J Med, 261:*525-528, 1959.

209. Moore, G., Bross, I. D. J., Ausman, R., Nadler, S., Jones, R., Slack, N., and Rimm, A. A.: Effects of Chlorambucil (NSC-3088) in 374 patients with advanced cancer. *Cancer Chemother Rep, 52:*661-666, 1968.
210. Reeves, B. R.: Chlorambucil and Chromosomal damage. *Br Med J, 4:*22-23, 1975.
211. Rose, M. S.: Busulphan toxicity syndrome caused by Chlorambucil. *Br Med J, 2:*123, 1975.
212. Sanitsky, A., Rai, K. R., Glidewell, O., and Silver, R. T.: (Cancer and leukemia group B). Comparison of daily versus intermittent Chlorambucil and Prednisone therapy in the treatment of patients with chronic lymphocytic leukemia. *Blood, 50:*1049-1059, 1977.
213. Alberts, D. S., Chang, S. Y., Chen, H. S. G., Evans, T. L., and Moon, T. E.: Variability of melphalan (M) absorption in man. *Proc Am Assoc Cancer Res, 19:*334, 1978.
214. Cooling, B. W., and Chakera, T. M.: Pulmonary fibrosis following therapy with melphalan for multiple myeloma. *J Clin Pathol, 25:*668-673, 1972.
215. Cornwell, G. G., Pajak, T. F., and McIntyre, O. R.: Hypersensitivity reactions to IV Melphalan during treatment of multiple myeloma: Cancer and leukemia Group B experience. *Cancer Treat Rep, 63:*399-403, 1979.
216. Einhorn, N.: Acute leukemia after chemotherapy (Melphalan). *Cancer, 44:*444-447, 1978.
217. Golomb, F. M., Bromberg, J., and Dubin, N.: A controlled study of isolated perfusion as an adjunct to surgical therapy for primary melanoma of the distal extremities. *Proc Am Assoc Cancer Res, 20:*313, 1979.
218. Koops, H. S., Oldhoff, T., Vanderploeg, E., Vermey, A., Eibergen, R., and Beekhuis, H.: Some aspects of the treatment of primary malignant melanoma of the extremities by isolated regional perfusion. *Cancer, 39:*27-33, 1977.
219. McArthur, J. R., Athens, J. W., and Wintrobe, M. M.: Melphalan and myeloma: Experience with a low-dose continuous regimen. *Ann Intern Med, 72:*665-670, 1970.
220. McIntyre, O. R., Leone, L., and Pajak, T. F.: The use of intravenous Melphalan (L-PAM) in the treatment of multiple myeloma. *Blood, 52:*274, 1978.
221. Rutledge, F.: Chemotherapy of ovarian cancer with Melphalan. *Clin Obstet Gynecol, 11:*354, 1968.
222. Taetle, R., Dickman, P. S., and Feldman, P. S.: Pulmonary histopathologic changes associated with Melphalan therapy. *Cancer, 42:*1239-1245, 1978.
223. Anderson, A. P., and Brincker, H.: Intracavity Thio-Tepa in malignant pleural and peritoneal effusions. *Acta Radiol, 7:*369-378, 1968.
224. Boyd, P. J. R., and Burnard, K. G.: Proceedings: Adjuvant intravesical Thio-Tepa and bladder tumor recurrence. *Br J Surg, 62:*162, 1975.
225. Bruce, D. W., and Edgcomb, J. H.: Pancytopenia and generalized sepsis following treatment of cancer of the bladder with instillations of Triethylene Thiophosphoramide. *J Urol, 97:*482-485, 1967.
226. Burnard, K. G., Boyd, P. J. R., Mayo, M. E., Shuttleworth, K. E. P., Lloyd-Davies, R. W.: Single dose intravesical Thio-Tepa as an adjuvant to cystodiathermy in the treatment of transitional cell bladder carcinoma. *Br J Urol, 48:*55-59, 1976.
227. Edwards, M. S., Levin, V. A., Seager, M. L., Pischer, T. L., and Wilson, C. B.: Phase II evaluation of Thio-Tepa for treatment of central nervous system tumors. *Cancer Treat Rep, 63:*1419-1421, 1973.
228. Gutin, P. H., Weiss, H. D., Wiernik, P. H., and Walker, M. D.: Intrathecal N, N'N''-Triethylene Thiophosphoramide [Thio-Tepa (NSCy396)] in the treatment of malignant meningeal disease: Phase I-II study. *Cancer, 38:*1471-1475, 1976.

229. Kardinal, C. G., and Donegan, W. L.: Second cancers after prolonged adjuvant Thio-Tepa for operable carcinoma of the breast. *Cancer, 45:*2042-2046, 1980.
230. Kottmeir, H. L.: Treatment of ovarian carcinomas with Thio-Tepa. *Clin Obstet Gynecol, 11:*428-438, 1968.
231. Nocks, B. N., Nieh, P. T., and Prout, G. R., Jr.: A longitudinal study of patients with superficial bladder carcinoma successfully treated with weekly intravesical Thio-Tepa. *J Urol, 122:*27-29, 1979.
232. Schellhammer, P. F.: Renal failure associated with the use of Thio-Tepa. *J Urol, 110:*498-501, 1973.
233. Ultmann, J. E., Hyman, G. A., Crandall, C., Naujoks, H., and Gellhorn, A.: Triethylenethiophosphoramide (Thio-Tepa) in the treatment of neoplastic disease. *Cancer, 10:*902-911, 1957.
234. Arduino, L. J., and Mellinger, G. T.: Clinical trial of Busulfan (NSC-750) in advanced carcinoma of prostate. *Cancer Chemother Rep, 51:*295-303, 1967.
235. Burns, W. A., McFarland, W., and Matthews, M. J.: Busulphan induced pulmonary disease: Report of a case and review of the literature. *Am Rev Respir Dis, 101:*408-413, 1970.
236. Diamond, I., Anderson, M. M., and McCreadie, S. R.: Transplacental transmission of Busulfan (Myleran) in a mother with leukemia. Production of fetal malformation and cytomegaly. *Pediatrics, 25:*85-90, 1960.
237. Feingold, M. L., and Koss, L. G.: Effects of long term administration of Busulfan. *Arch Intern Med, 124:*66-71, 1969.
238. Galton, D. A. G.: Myleran in chronic myeloid leukemia. *Lancet, 1:*208-213, 1953.
239. Heard, B. E., and Cooke, R. A.: Busulfan lung. *Thorax, 23:*187-193, 1968.
240. Hyman, G. A., and Gelhorn, A.: Myleran therapy in malignant neoplastic disease: Use of 1,4-Dimethane-sulfonoxybutane with emphasis on chronic granulocytic leukemia. *JAMA, 161:*994-997, 1956.
241. Min, K. W., and Gyorkey, F.: Interstitial pulmonary fibrous, atypical epithelial changes and bronchiolar cell carcinoma following Busulfan therapy. *Cancer, 22:*1027, 1032, 1968.
242. Pedersen-Bjergaard, J., Nissen, N. I., Sirensen, H. M., Hou-Jensen, K., Larsen, M. S., Ernst, P., Ersbil, J., Knudtzon, S., and Rose, C.: Acute non-lymphocytic leukemia in patients with ovarian carcinoma following long-term treatment with Treosulfan (Dihydroxybusulfan). *Cancer, 45:*19-29, 1980.
243. Stuart, J. J., Crocker, D. L., and Roberts, H. R.: Treatment of Busulfan-induced pancytopenia. *Arch Intern Med, 136:*1181-1183, 1976.
244. Altman, S. J., Fletcher, W. S., Andrews, N. C., Wilson, W. L., and Pisher, T.: Yoshi 864 (NSC-102627) 1-Propanol, 3, 3′-Iminodidimethanesulfonate (ester) Hydrochloride, a Phase I study. *Cancer, 35:*1145-1147, 1975.
245. Douglass, H. O., Kaufman, J., Engstrom, P. F., Klassen, D. J., and Carbone, P. P.: Single agent chemotherapy of advanced colorectal cancer with ICRF-159, Yoshi-864, Piperazinedione (PZD), CCNU, Actinomycin-D (DACT), L-PAM, or Methotrexate (MTX). *Proc Am Assoc Cancer Res, 20:*434, 1979.
246. EL-Merzabini, M. M., and Sakurai, Y.: Inhibition of tumor growth by new sulfonic acid esters of aminoglycols. *Gann, 56:*575-587, 1965.
247. Glasofer, E. D., Weiss, A. J., and Manthei, R. W.: Studies on the disposition of 1-propanol-3, 3′-iminodidimethanesulfonate. *Pharmacologist, 16:*262, 1974.
248. Hirano, M., Miura, M., Kakizawa, H., Morita, A., Uetani, T., and Ohno, R.: Effect of two new sulfonic acid esters of aminoglycols on chronic myelogenous leukemia. *Cancer Chemother Rep, 56:*47-52, 1972.
249. Glum, R. H., Corson, J. M., Wilson, R. E., Greenberger, J. S., Canellos, G. P., and Frei,

E., III: Successful treatment of metastatic sarcomas with cyclophosphamide, Adriamycin, and DTIC (CAD). *Cancer, 46:*1722-1726, 1980.

250. Carter, S. K., and Freidman, M. A.: 5-(3,3-Dimethyl-1-Triazeno)-Imidazole-4-Carboxamide (DTIC, DIC, NSC-45388) — A new antitumor agent with activity against malignant melanoma. *Eur J Cancer, 8:*85-92, 1972.
251. Comis, R. L.: DTIC (NSC-45388) in malignant melanoma: A perspective. *Cancer Treat Rep, 60:*165-176, 1976.
252. Gardere, S., Hussain, S., and Cowan, D. H.: Treatment of metastatic malignant melanoma with a combination of 5-(3,3-Dimethyl-1-Triazeno)-Imidazole-4-Carboxamide (NSC-45388), Cyclophosphamide (NSC-26271), and Vincristine (NSC-67574). *Cancer Chemother Rep, 56:*357-361, 1972.
253. Householder, G. E., and Loo, T. L.: Disposition of 5-(3,3-Dimethyl-1-Triazeno)-Imidazole-4-Carboxamide — A new antitumor agent. *J Pharmacol Exp Ther, 179:*386-395, 1971.
254. Luce, J. K., Torn, L. B., and Price, H.: Combination Dimethyl Triazeno Imidazole Carboxamide (NSC-45388:DIC) Vincristine (NSC67574) and 1,3-Bis(2-Chlorethyl)-1-Nitrosourea (NSC 409962:BCNU) chemotherapy of disseminated malignant melanoma. *Proc Am Assoc Cancer Res, 11:*50, 1970.
255. Presant, C. A., Lowenbraun, S., Bartolucci, A. A., Smalley, R. V., and The Southeastern Cancer Study Group: Metastatic sarcomas: Chemotherapy with Adriamycin, Cyclophosphamide, and Methotrexate alternating with actinomycin D, DTIC, and Vincristine. *Cancer, 47:*457-465, 1981.
256. Schwarz, M. A., Gutterman, J. U., Burgess, M. A., Heilbrun, L. K., Murphy, W. K., Bodey, G. P., Stone, E., Turner-Chism, V., and Hersh, E. M.: Chemoimmunotherapy of disseminated malignant melanoma with DTIC-BCG, transfer factor + Melphalan. *Cancer, 45:*2506-2515, 1980.
257. Yap, B. S., Baker, L. H., Sinkovics, J. G., Rivkins, S. E., Bottomley, R., Thigpen, T., Burgess, M. A., Benjamin, R. S., and Bodey, G. P.: Cyclophosphamide, Vincristine, Adriamycin, and DTIC (CYVADIC) combination chemotherapy for the treatment of advanced sarcomas. *Cancer Treat Rep, 64:*93-98, 1980.
258. Anderson, T., Devita, V. T., and Young, R. C.: BCNU (NSC-409962) in the treatment of advanced Hodgkin's Disease: Its role in remission introduction and maintenance. *Cancer Treat Rep, 60:*761-767, 1976.
259. Bennet, J. M., Bakemier, R. F., and Carme, P. P.: Clinical trials with BCNU (NSC-409962) in malignant lymphomas by Eastern Cooperative Oncology Group. *Cancer Treat Rep, 60:*739-745, 1976.
260. Durant, J. R., Norgard, M. J., Murad, T. M., and Bartolucci, A. A.: Pulmonary toxicity associated with Bis-Chloroethyl Nitrosourea (BCNU). *Ann Intern Med, 90:*191-194, 1979.
261. Ensminger, W. D., Thompson, M., and Come, S.: Hepatic arterial BCNU: A pilot pharmacologic study in patients with liver tumors. *Cancer Treat Rep, 62:*1509-1512, 1978.
262. Kann, H. E., Jr., Kohn, K. W., and Lyles, T. M.: Inhibition of DNA repair by the 1, 3-Bis (2-Chloroethyl)-1-Nitrosoureas. Breakdown product, 2-Chloroethyl Isocyanate. *Cancer Res, 34:*398-402, 1974.
263. Lokish, J. J., Drum, D. W., and Kaplan, W.: Hepatic toxicity of Nitrosourea analogues. *Clin Pharmacol Ther, 16:*363-367, 1974.
264. Madajewicz, S., West, C. R., Park, H. C., Ghoorah, J., Avellanosa, A. M., Takita, H., Karakousis, C., Vincent, R., Caracandas, J., and Jennings, E.: Phase II study — intra-arterial BCNU therapy for metastatic brain tumors. *Cancer, 47:*653-657, 1981.

265. Marsh, J. C., Deconti, R. C., and Hubbard, S. P.: Treatment of Hodgkin's Disease and other cancers with 1,3-Bis(2-Chloroethyl)-1-Nitrosourea (BCNU-NSC-409962). *Cancer Chemother Rep, 55:*599, 1971.
266. McLennan, R., and Taylor, H. R.: Optic neuroretinitis in association with BCNU and Procarbazine. *Med Pediatr Oncol, 4:*43-48, 1978.
267. Oliverio, V. T.: Toxicology and pharmacology of the nitrosoureas. *Cancer Chemother Rep, 4:*13-20, 1973.
268. Rege, V. B., and Owens, A. H.: BCNU (NSC-409962) in the treatment of advanced Hodgkin's Disease, lymphosarcoma and reticulum cell sarcoma. *Cancer Chemother Rep, 58:*383-393, 1974.
269. Salmon, S. E.: Nitrosoureas in multiple myeloma. *Cancer Treat Rep, 60:*789-794, 1976.
270. Tobey, R. A., and Crissman, H. A.: Comparative effects of three nitrosourea derivatives on mammalian cell cycle progression. *Cancer Res, 35:*460-470, 1975.
271. Walker, M. D.: Nitrosoureas in central nervous system tumors. *Cancer Chemother Rep, 4:*21-26, 1973.
272. Wheeler, G. P., and Alexander, J. A.: Duration of inhibition of synthesis of DNA in tumors and host tissues after single doses of nitrosoureas. *Cancer Res, 36:*1470-1474, 1976.
273. Wheeler, G. P., and Bowden, B. J.: Some effects of BCNU on synthesis of protein and nucleic acids. *Cancer Res, 25:*1770-1776, 1965.
274. Zackheim, H. S., and Epstein, E. H.: Treatment of mycosis fungoides with topical nitrosourea compounds. *Arch Dermatol, 111:*1564-1570, 1975.
275. Ahmann, D. L.: Nitrosoureas in the management of disseminated malignant melanoma. *Cancer Treat Rep, 60:*747-751, 1976.
276. Bray, D., Oliverio, V., Adamson, R., and Devita, F.: Cell cycle effects produced by 1-(2-Chloroethyl)-3-Cyclohexyl-1-Nitrosourea (CCNU) and its decomposition products. *S Proc Am Assoc Cancer Res, 11:*12, 1970.
277. Cheng, C. J., Fijimuar, S., Grunberger, D., and Weinstein, I. B.: Interaction of 1-(2-Chloroethyl)-3-Cyclohexyl-1-Nitrosourea (NSC-79037) with nucleic acids and proteins *in vivo* and *in vitro*. *Cancer Res, 32:*22-27, 1972.
278. Deconti, R. C., Hubbard, S. P., Pinch, P., and Bertino, J. R.: Treatment of advanced neoplastic disease with 1-(2-Chloroethyl)-3-Cyclohexyl-1-Nitrosourea (CCNU; NSC-79037). *Cancer Chemother Rep, 57:*201-207, 1973.
279. Fewer, D., Wilson, C. B., Boldrey, E. B., and Enot, J. K.: Phase II study of 1-(2-Chloroethyl)-3-Cyclohexyl-1-Nitrosourea (CCNU; NSC-79037) in the treatment of brain tumors. *Cancer Chemother Rep, 56:*421-427, 1972.
280. Hansen, H. H., Selawry, O. S., Pajak, T. F., Spurr, C. L., Falkson, G., Brunner, K., Cuttner, J., Nissen, N. I., and Holland, J. F.: The superiority of CCNU in the treatment of advanced Hodgkin's Disease: Cancer and leukemia group B study. *Cancer, 47:*14-18, 1981.
281. Hoogstraten, B., Gottlieb, J. A., Caoili, E., Tucker, W. G., Talley, R. W., and Haut, A.: CCNU(1-2-Chloroethyl-3-Cyclohexyl-1-Nitrosourea, NSC-79037) in the treatment of cancer. *Cancer, 32:*38-43, 1973.
282. Kann, H. E., Jr., Kohn, K. W., Wilderlite, L.: Effects of 1,3-Bis (2-Chloroethyl)-1-Nitrosourea and related compounds on nuclear RNA metabolism. *Cancer Res, 34:*1982-1988, 1974.
283. Klaassen, D., and Rapp, E.: Phase II study of CCNU in the treatment of advanced gastrointestinal malignancy. *Cancer Chemother Rep, 57:*112, 1973.
284. Oliverio, V. T.: Pharmacology of the nitrosoureas — an overview. *Cancer Treat Rep, 60:*703-707, 1976.
285. Rodgers, R. W., Gamble, J. F., Loh, K. K., and Shullenberger, C. C.: Adriamycin,

Bleomycin, DIC, CCNU; and Prednisone (ABDIC) chemotherapy in MOPP-resistant Hodgkin's Disease. *Cancer, 46:*2349-2355, 1980.

286. Rosenblum, M. L., Reynolds, A. F., Smith, K. A., Rumack, B. H., and Walker, M. D.: Chloroethyl-Cyclohexyl-Nitrosourea (CCNU) in the treatment of malignant brain tumors. *J Neurosurg, 39:*306-314, 1973.
287. Takita, H., and Brugarolas, A.: Effect of CCNU (NSC-79037) on bronchogenic carcinoma. *J Natl Cancer Inst, 50:*49-53, 1973.
288. Wasserman, T. H., Slavik, M., and Carter, S. K.: Review of CCNU in clinical cancer therapy. *Cancer Treat Rev, 1:*131-151, 1974.
289. Wheeler, G. P., and Bowden, B. J.: Effects of 1,3-Bis(2-Chloroethyl)-1-Nitrosurea and related compounds upon the synthesis of DNA by cell free systems. *Cancer Res, 35:*460-470, 1978.
290. Williams, S., and Einhorn, L.: Combination chemotherapy with Doxorubicin and lomustine. *JAMA, 238:*1659-1661, 1977.
291. Baker, L. H., and Vaitkevicius, E. G.: The gastrointestinal committee of the southwest oncology group: Randomized prospective trial comparing 5-Fluorouracil (NSC-19893) to 5-Fluorouracil and Methyl-CCNU (NSC-95441) in advanced gastrointestinal cancer. *Cancer Treat Rep, 60:*733-737, 1976.
292. Cohen, M. H., Schoenfeld, D., and Wolter, J.: Randomized trial of chlorpromazine, caffeine, and methyl-CCNU in disseminated melanoma. *Cancer Treat Rep, 64:*151-153, 1980.
293. Falkson, G., and Falkson, H. C.: Fluorouracil, Methyl-CCNU and Vincristine in cancer of the colon. *Cancer, 38:*1468-1470, 1976.
294. Kemeny, N., Yagoda, A., and Golbey, R.: Randomized study of 2 different schedules of methyl CCNU (ME CCNU), 5-Fluorouracil (5-FU) and Vincristine (VCR) for metastatic colorectal carcinoma. *Proc Am Assoc Cancer Res, 18:*336, 1977.
295. Schein, P. S.: 1-Methyl-1-Nitrosourea depression of Brain Nicotinamide Adenine Dinucleotide in the production of neurological toxicity. *Proc Soc Exp Biol Med, 131:*517-520, 1969.
296. Shaw, M. T., Bonnet, J. D., Wilson, H., and Heilbrun, L. K.: Baker's antifol in combination with 5-Fluorouracil and Methyl-CCNU in the treatment of metastatic colorectal cancer: A southwest oncology group study (protocol 7764). *Cancer Treat Rep, 64:*247-250, 1980.
297. Sieber, S. M., and Adamson, R. H.: Potential hazards associated with the use of 1-Methyl-1-Nitrosourea (NSC-23909). *Cancer Chemother Rep, 58:*617-618, 1974.
298. Wasserman, T. H., Slavik, M., and Carter, S. K.: Methy CCNU in clinical cancer therapy. *Cancer Treat Rev, 1:*251, 1974.
299. Young, R. C., Walker, M. D., Canellos, G. P., Schein, P. S., Chabner, B. A., and Devita, V. T.: Initial clinical trials with Methyl CCNU 1-(2-Chloroethyl)-3-(4-Methyl Cyclohexyl)-1-Nitrosourea (ME CCNU). *Cancer, 31:*1164-1169, 1973.
300. Bachur, N. R.: Adriamycin (NSC-123127) pharmacology. *Cancer Chemother Rep,* Part 3, *6:*153-158, 1975.
301. Banks, M. D., Pontes, J. E., Izbicki, R. M., and Pierce, J. M.: Topical instillation of Doxorubicin HCL in the treatment of superficial transition cell carcinoma of the bladder. *J Urol, 118:*757-760, 1977.
302. Benjamin, R. S.: Pharmacokinetics of Adriamycin (NSC-123127) in patients with sarcomas. *Cancer Chemother Rep, 58:*271-273, 1974.
303. Bern, M. M., McDermott, W., Cady, B., Oberfield, R. A., Trey, C., Clouse, M. E., Tullis, J. L., and Parker, L. M.: Intra-arterial hepatic infusion and intravenous Adriamycin for treatment of hepato cellular carcinoma. *Cancer, 42:*399-405, 1978.

304. Canceres, E., Zaharia, M., Moran, M., and Tejada, F.: Adjuvant whole-lung radiation with or without Adriamycin treatment in osteogenic sarcoma. *Cancer Treat Rep, 62:*297-299, 1978.
305. Cortes, E. P., Holland, J. F., Wany, J. J., Sink, L. F., Blom, J., Senn, H., Bank, A., and Glidewell, O.: Amputation and Adriamycin in primary osteosarcoma. *N Engl J Med, 291:*998-1000, 1974.
306. Creagan, E. T., Fleming, T. R., Edmonson, J. H., Ingle, J. N., and Woods, J. E.: Cyclophosphamide, Adriamycin, and Cis-Diammine Dichloroplatinum (II) in the treatment of patients with advanced head and neck cancer. *Cancer, 47:*240-244, 1981.
307. Davis, H. L., and Davis, T. E.: Daunorubicin and Adriamycin in cancer treatment: An analysis of their roles and limitations. *Cancer Treat Rep, 63:*809-815, 1979.
308. Ettinger, L. J., Douglass, H. O., Jr., Higby, D. J., Mindell, E. R., Nime, F., Ghoorah, J., and Freeman, A. I.: Adjuvant Adriamycin and Cis-Diammine Dichloroplatinum (Cis-platinum) in primary osteosarcoma. *Cancer, 47:*248-254, 1981.
309. Ferrans, V. J.: A review of cardiac pathology in relation to anthracycline cardiotoxicity. *Cancer Treat Rep, 62:*955-961, 1978.
310. Fossati-Bellani, F., Gasparini, M., and Bonadonna, G.: Adriamycin in the adjuvant treatment of operable oestosarcoma. *Recent Results Cancer Res, 68:*25-27, 1978.
311. Gottlieb, J. A., and Hill, C. S.: Chemotherapy of thyroid cancer with Adriamycin. *N Engl J Med, 290:*193-197, 1974.
312. Gottlieb, J. A., Rivkin, S. E., Spigel, S. C., Hoogstraten, B., O'Bryan, R. M., and Singhakowinta, A.: Superiority of Adriamycin over oral nitrosoureas in patients with advanced breast cancer. *Cancer, 33:*519-526, 1974.
313. Legha, S. S., Benjamin, R. S., Yayo, H. Y., and Freireich, E. J.: Augmentation of Adriamycin's therapeutic index by prolonged continuous IV infusion for advanced breast cancer. *Proc Am Assoc Cancer Res, 20:*261, 1979.
314. McCredie, K. B., Hewlett, J. S., and Kennedy, A.: Sequential Adriamycin-Arac(A-OAP) for remission induction (RI) of adult acute leukemia (AAL). *Proc Am Assoc Cancer Res, 17:*239, 1976.
315. McKelvey, E. M., Gottlieb, J. A., Wilson, H. E., Haut, A., Talley, R. W., Stephens, R., and Lane, M.: Hydroxyl Daunorubicin (Adriamycin) combination chemotherapy in malignant lymphoma. *Cancer, 38:*1484-1493, 1976.
316. Rivkin, S. E., Gottlieb, J. A., Thigpen, T., Elmawla, N. G., Saiki, J., and Dixon, D. O.: Methyl CCNU and Adriamycin for patients with metastatic sarcomas: A southwest oncology group study. *Cancer, 46:*446-451, 1980.
317. Salmon, S. E., and Jones, S. E.: Chemotherapy of advanced breast cancer with a combination of Adriamycin and Cyclophosphamide. *Proc Am Assoc Cancer Res, 15:*90, 1974.
318. Samuels, L., Newton, W. A., Jr., and Heyn, R.: Daunorubicin therapy in advanced neuroblastoma. *Cancer, 27:*831-834, 1971.
319. Alberts, D. S., Bachur, N. R., and Holtzman, J. L.: The pharmacokinetics of Daunomycin in man. *Clin Pharmacol Ther, 12:*96-104, 1971.
320. Holton, C. P., Vietti, T. J., and Atletal, N.: Clinical study of Daunomycin and Prednisone for induction of remission in children with advanced leukemia. *N Engl J Med, 280:*171-174, 1969.
321. Huffman, D. H., Benjamin, R. S., and Bachur, N. R.: Daunorubicin metabolism in acute non-lymphatic leukemia. *Clin Pharmacol Ther, 13:*895-905, 1972.
322. Jones, B.: Daunomycin in the treatment of resistant acute lymphoblastic leukemia. *Blood, 30:*890-891, 1967.

323. Theologides, A., Yarbro, J. W., and Kennedy, B. J.: Daunomycin inhibition of DNA and RNA synthesis. *Cancer, 21:*16-21, 1968.
324. Von Hoff, D. D., Rozencweig, M., Layard, M., Slavik, M., and Muggia, F. M.: Daunomycin-induced cardiotoxicity in children and adults. *Am J Med, 62:*200-208, 1977.
325. Wantzin, G. L., Karle, H., Philip, P., and Killman, S. A.: The effect of Daunomycin on cell proliferation and protein synthesis of human leukemic blast cells. *Eur J Cancer, 12:*291-298, 1976.
326. Weirnik, P. H., Glidewell, O. J., Hoagland, H. C., Brunner, K. W., Spurr, C. L., Cuttner, J., Silver, R. T., Carey, R. W., Delduca, V., Kung, F. H., and Holland, J. F.: A comparative trial of Daunorubicin, Cytosine Arabinoside, and Thioguanine, and a combination of the three agents for the treatment of acute myelocytic leukemia. *Med Pediatr Oncol, 6:*261-277, 1979.
327. Dangio, G. J., Farber, S., and Maddock, C. L.: Potentiation of x-ray effects by Actinomycin D. *Radiology, 73:*175-177, 1959.
328. Frei, E. III: The clinical use of Actinomycin. *Cancer Chemother Rep, 58:*49-54, 1947.
329. Green, D. M., Sallan, S. E., and Krishan, A.: Actinomycin D in childhood acute lymphocytic leukemia. *Cancer Treat Rep, 62:*829-831, 1978.
330. Philips, F. S., Schwartz, H. S., Sternberg, S. S., and Tan, C. T. C.: The toxicity of Actinomycin D. *Ann N Y Acad Sci, 89:*348-360, 1970.
331. Reich, E.: Biochemistry of Actinomycin. *Cancer Res, 28:*1428, 1963.
332. Samson, M. K., Baker, L. H., Talley, R. W., Fraile, R. J., McDonald, B.: Phase I-II study of intermittent bolus administration of DTIC and Actinomycin D in metastatic malignant melanoma. *Cancer Treat Rep, 62:*1223-1225, 1978.
333. Tatterall, M. H. N., Sodegren, J. E., Sergupta, S. K., Trites, D. H., Modest, E. J., and Frei, E.: Pharmacokinetics of Actinomycin D in patients with malignant melanoma. *Clin Pharmacol Ther, 17:*701-708, 1975.
334. Ahr, D. J., Scialla, S. J., and Kimball, D. B.: Acquired platelet dysfunction following Mithramycin therapy. *Cancer, 41:*448-454, 1978.
335. Curreri, A. R., and Ansfield, F. J.: Mithramycin — human toxicity and preliminary therapeutic investigation. *Cancer Chemother Rep, 8:*18-22, 1960.
336. Davies, J., Trask, C., and Souhami, R. L.: Effect of Mithramycin on widespread painful bone metastases in cancer of the breast. *Cancer Treat Rep, 63:*1835-1838, 1979.
337. Kennedy, B. J.: Metabolic and toxic effects of Mithramycin during tumor therapy. *Am J Med, 49:*494-503, 1970.
338. Kennedy, B. J., Griffin, W. O., and Lober, P.: The specific effect of Mithramycin on embryonal carcinoma of the testis. *Cancer, 18:*1631, 1965.
339. Kofman, S., and Eisenstein, R.: Mithramycin in the treatment of disseminated cancer. *Cancer Chemother Rep, 32:*77-81, 1963.
340. Parsons, V., Baum, M., Self, M.: Effect of Mithramycin on calcium and hydroxyproline metabolism in patients with malignant disease. *Br Med J, 1:*474-479, 1967.
341. Slayton, R. E., Shnider, B. L., Eliase, E., Horton, J., and Perlia, C. P.: New approach to the treatment of hypercalcemia: The effect of short term treatment with Mithramycin. *Clin Pharmacol Ther, 12:*833-837, 1971.
342. Yarbro, J. W., Wollheim, M., and Kennedy, B. J.: Differential inhibition of RNA synthesis by Mithramycin. *Clin Res, 13:*341, 1965.
343. Baker, L. H., Opipari, M. I., and Izbicki, R. M.: Phase II study of Mitomycin C, Vincristine, and Bleomycin in advanced squamous cell carcinoma of the uterine cervix. *Cancer, 38:*2222-2224, 1976.

344. Campos, L. T., Franti, V. P., Dossey, J. E., Khera, H. C., Boulefindis, D., and Arkus, R. L.: Adjuvant therapy by intra-arterial infusion and BCG for adenocarcinoma of the colon, Stage Duke's C. *Proc Am Assoc Cancer Res, 20:*351, 1979.
345. Fortuny, I. E., Theologides, A., and Kennedy, B. J.: Hepatic arterial infusion for liver metastases from colon cancer: Comparison of Mitomycin C (NSC-26980) and 5-Fluorouracil (NSC-19893). *Cancer Chemother Rep, 59:*401-404, 1975.
346. Iyer, V., and Szybalski, N.: Mitomycin and Porfiromycin: Chemical mechanism of activation and cross-linking of DNA. *Science, 145:*55-58, 1964.
347. Kato, T., Kumagni, I., Nemoto, R., Tamakawa, Y., and Harada, M.: Intra-arterial use of microencapsulated Mitomycin C(MMC-MC) in the treatment of advanced prostatic cancer: A preliminary report. *Proc Am Assoc Cancer Res, 20:*408, 1979.
348. Koyama, H., Wada, T., Takahaski, Y., Iwanga, T., Aoki, Y., and Wada, A.: Intraarterial infusion chemotherapy as a preoperative treatment of locally advanced breast cancer. *Cancer, 36:*1603-1612. 1973
349. Krebs, H. B., Girtanner, R. E., Nordquist, S. R., Mineau, I., Helmkamp, B. F., and Averette, H. E.: Treatment of advanced cervical cancer by combination of Bleumycin and Mitomycin-C. *Cancer, 46:*2159-2161, 1980.
350. Lawson, D., Moore, M., and Smalley, R.: An evaluation of Hexamethyl-Melamine, Cis-Diammine Dichloroplatinum, and Mitomycin-C in advanced breast cancer, a pilot study of the Southeastern Cancer Study Group. *Cancer Clin Trials, 3:*293-296, 1980.
351. Liu, K., Mittelman, A., Sproul, E. E., and Elias, E. C.: Renal toxicity in man treated with Mitomycin C. *Cancer, 28:*1314-1320, 1971.
352. Mishina, T., Oda, K., Muratha, S., Ooe, H., Muri, Y., and Takahashi, T.: Mitomycin C bladder instillation therapy for bladder tumor. *J Urol, 114:*217-219, 1974.
353. Moertel, C. G., Reitemier, R. J., and Hahn, R. G.: Mitomycin C therapy in advanced gastrointestinal cancer. *JAMA, 204:*1045-1048, 1968.
354. Orwoll, E. S., Kiessling, P. J., and Patterson, J. R.: Interstitial pneumonia from Mitomycin. *Ann Intern Med, 89:*352-355, 1978.
355. Patton, A. J., Knight, E. W., and Tennant, J. D.: Mitomycin C administered by high dose induction regimen in the treatment of cancer. *Proc Am Assoc Cancer Res, 20:*387, 1979.
356. Smith, F. P., Hoth, D. F., Levin, B., Karlin, D. A., MacDonald, J. S., Woolley, P. V., III, and Schein, P. S.: 5-Fluorouracil, Adriamycin, and Mitomycin-C (FAM) chemotherapy for advanced adenocarcinoma of the pancreas. *Cancer, 46:*2014-2018, 1980.
357. Wise, G. R., Kuhn, I. N., and Godfrey, T. E.: Mitomycin in large infrequent dosages in breast cancer. *Med Pediatr Oncol, 2:*55-60, 1976.
358. Zimmerman, S. E., Smith, F. P., and Schein, P. S.: Chemotherapy of pancreatic carcinoma. *Cancer, 47:*1724-1728, 1981.
359. Dentino, M., Luft, F. C., Yum, M. N., Williams, S., and Einhorn, L. H.: Longterm effect of Cis-Diammine Dichloride Platinum (CDDP) on renal function and structure in man. *Cancer, 41:*1274-1281, 1978.
360. Eagan, R. T., Fleming, T. R., Frytak, S., Creagan, E. T., Ingle, J. N., and Kvols, L. K.: The role of Cis-Dichlorodiammine Platinum (II) in squamous cell lung cancer. *Cancer Treat Rep, 64:*87-91, 1980.
361. Einhorn, L. H., and Donohue, J.: Cis-Diammine Dichloroplatinum, Vinblastine and Bleomycin combination chemotherapy in disseminated testicular cancer. *Ann Intern Med, 87:*293-298, 1977.

362. Einhorn, L. H., and Williams, S. D.: The role of Cis-Platinum in solid tumor therapy. *N Engl J Med, 300:*289-291, 1979.

363. Ettinger, L. J., Douglass, H. O., Jr., Higby, D. J., Mindell, E. R., Nime, F., Ghoorah, J., and Freeman, A. I.: Adjuvant adriamycin and Cis-Diammine Dichloroplatinum (Cis-Platinum) in primary osteosarcoma. *Cancer, 47:*248-254, 1981.

364. Frick, G. A., Ballentine, R., Driever, C. W., and Kramer, W. G.: Renal excretion kinetics of high-dose Cis-Dichlorodiammine Platinum (II) administered with hydration and Mannitol diuresis. *Cancer Treat Rep, 63:*13-16, 1979.

365. Gralla, R. J., Cvitkovic, E., and Golbey, R. B.: Cis-Dichlorodiammine Platinum (II) in non-small cell carcinoma of the lung. *Cancer Treat Rep, 63:*1585-1588, 1979.

366. Howle, J. A., and Gale, G. R.: Cis-Dichlorodiammine Platinum (II): Persistent and selective inhibition of DNA synthesis *in Vivo. Biochem Pharmacol, 19:*2757-2762, 1970.

367. Jacobs, C., Bertino, J. R., Goffinet, D. R., Fee, W. E., and Goode, R. L.: 24-hour infusion of Cis-Platinum in head and neck cancers. *Cancer, 42:*2135-2140, 1978.

368. Madias, N. E., and Harrington, J. T.: Platinum nephrotoxicity. *Am J Med, 65:*307-314, 1978.

369. Ochs, J. J., Freeman, A. I., Douglass, H. O., Jr., Higby, D. S., Mindell, E. R., and Sinks, L. F.: Cis-Dichlorodiammine Platinum (II) in advanced osteogenic sarcoma. *Cancer Treat Rep, 62:*239-245, 1978.

370. Ostrow, S., Hahn, D., Wiernik, P. H., and Richards, R. D.: Ophthalmologic toxicity after Cis-Dichlorodiammine Platinum (II) therapy. *Cancer Treat Rep, 62:*1591-1594, 1978.

371. Pesando, J. M., Come, S. E., Stark, J., Packer, L. M., Griffiths, C. T., and Canellos, G. P.: Cis-Diammine Dichloroplatinum (II) therapy for advanced ovarian cancer. *Cancer Treat Rep, 64:*1147-1148, 1980.

372. Roberts, J. J., and Pascoe, J. M.: Cross-linking of complementary strands of DNA in mammalian cells by antitumor platinum compounds. *Nature* (London), *235:*282-284, 1972.

373. Sarna, G., Skinner, D. G., Smith, R. B., Zighelboim, J., Goodnight, J. E., and Feig, S.: Cis-Diammine Dichloroplatinum (II) alone and in combination in the treatment of testicular and other malignancies. *Cancer Treat Rep, 64:*1077-1082, 1980.

374. Schaefer, S. D., Wright, C. G., Post, J. D., and Frenkel, E. P.: Cis-Platinum vestibular toxicity. *Cancer, 47:*857-859, 1981.

375. Soloway, M. S., Ikard, M., and Ford, K.: Cis-Diammine Chloroplatinum (II) in locally advanced and metastatic urothelial cancer. *Cancer, 47:*476-480, 1981.

376. Tattersall, M. H., Lander, H., Bain, R., Stocks, A. E., Woods, R. L., Fox, R. M., Byrne, E., Trotten, J. R., and Roos, I.: Cis-Platinum treatment of metastatic adrenal carcinoma. *Med J Aust, 1:*419-421, 1980.

377. Von Hoff, D. D., Schilsky, R., Reichert, C. M., Reddick, R. L., Rozencweig, M., Young, R. C., and Muggia, F. M.: Toxic effects of Cis-Dichlorodiammine Platinum (II) in man. *Cancer Treat Rep, 63:*1527-1531, 1979.

378. Wiesenfeld, M., Reinders, E., Corder, M., Yoo, T. J., Dietz, B., and Lovett, J.: Successful re-treatment with Cis-Dichlorodiammine Platinum (II) after allergic reactions. *Cancer Treat Rep, 63:*219-221, 1979.

379. Zwelling, L. A., and Kohn, K. W.: Mechanism of action of Cis-Dichlorodiammine Platinum (II). *Cancer Treat Rep, 63:*1439-1444, 1979.

380. Adolphe, A. B., Glasofer, E. D., Troetel, W. M., Ziegenfuss, J., Stambhugh, J. E., Weiss, A. J., and Manthei, R. W.: Fate of streptozotocin (NSC-85998) in patients with advanced cancer. *Cancer Chemother Rep, 59:*547-556, 1975.

381. Adolphe, A. B., Glasofer, E. D., Troetel, W. M., Weiss, A. J., and Manthei, R. W.: Preliminary pharmacokinetics of Streptozotocin and antineoplastic antibiotic. *J Clin Pharmacol, 17:*379-388, 1977.
382. Band, P. R., Canellos, G. P., Sears, M., Israel, L., and Pocock, S. J.: Phase II trial with Bleomycin, CCNU and Streptozoticin in patients with metastatic cancer of the breast. *Cancer Treat Rep, 61:*1365-1367, 1977.
383. Bhuyan, B. K., Scheidt, L. G., and Fraser, T. J.: Cell cycle specificity of several antitumor agents. *Proc Am Assoc Cancer Res, 11:*8, 1970.
384. Broder, L. E., and Carter, S. K.: Pancreatic islet cell carcinoma. II. Results of therapy with Streptozotocin in 52 patients. *Ann Intern Med, 79:*108-118, 1973.
385. Diggs, C. H., Wiernik, P. H., and Sutherland, J. C.: Treatment of advanced untreated Hodgkin's Disease with SCAB — an alternative to MOPP. *Cancer, 47:*224-228, 1981.
386. DuPriest, R. W., Huntington, M. C., Massay, W. H., Weiss, A. J., Wilson, W. L., and Fletcher, W. S.: Streptozotocin therapy in 22 cancer patients. *Cancer, 35:*358-376, 1975.
387. Feldman, J. M., Quickel, K. E., Jr., Mareck, R. L., and Lebovitz, H. E.: Streptozotocin treatment of metastatic carcinoid tumors. *South Med J, 65:*1325-1330, 1972.
388. Kane, R. C., Bernath, A. M., and Cashdollar, R. R.: Phase II trial of Streptozotocin for small cell anaplastic carcinoma of the lung. *Cancer Treat Rep, 62:*477-478, 1978.
389. Moertel, G. G., Hanley, J. A., and Johnson, L. A.: Streptozocin alone compared with Streptozocin plus Fluorouracil in the treatment of advanced islet-cell carcinoma. *N Engl J Med, 303:*1189-1194, 1980.
390. Moertel, G. G., Reitmeier, R. J., Schutt, A. J., and Hahn, R. G.: Phase II study of Streptozotocin (NSC-85998) in the treatment of advanced gastrointestinal cancer. *Cancer Chemother Rep, 55:*303-307, 1971.
391. Myerowitz, R. L., Sartiano, G. P., and Cavallo, T.: Nephrotoxic and cytoproliferative effects of Streptozotocin. *Cancer, 38:*1550-1555, 1978.
392. Schein, P. S., Cooney, D. A., and Kernon, M. C.: The use of Nicotinamide to modify the toxicity of Streptozotocin diabetes without loss of antitumor activity. *Cancer Res, 27:*2324-2332, 1967.
393. Seligman, M., Bukowski, R. M., Groppe, C. W., Weick, J. K., Hewlett, J. S., and Greenstreet, R. L.: Chemotherapy of metastatic gastrointestinal neoplasms with 5-Fluorouracil and Streptozotocin. *Cancer Treat Rep, 61:*1375-1377, 1977.
394. Sibay, T. M., and Hayes, J. A.: Potential carcinogenic effect of Streptozotocin. *Lancet, 2:*912, 1969.
395. Taylor, S., Belt, R. J., Haas, C. D., Stephens, R. L., and Hoogstraten, B.: Phase I evaluation of Chlorozotocin: Single dose every six weeks. *Cancer, 46:*2365-2368, 1980.
396. Chiuten, D. F., Rozencweig, M., Von Hoff, D. D., and Muggia, F. M.: Clinical trials with the hexitol derivatives in the U. S. *Cancer, 47:*442-451, 1981.
397. Creagan, E. T., Eagan, R. T., and Rubin, J.: Phase I evaluation of the combination 1,3-Bis(2-Chloroethyl)-1-Nitrosourea (BCNU; NSC-409962) and Dianhydrogalactitol (DAG; NSC-132313) in patients with advanced neoplastic diseases. *Med Pediatr Oncol, 7:*179-180, 1979.
398. DeJager, R., Brugarolas, A., Hansen, H., Cavalli, F., Ryssel, H., Siegenthaler, P., Clarysse, A., Renard, J., Kenis, Y., and Alberto, P.: Dianhydrogalactitol (NSC-132313): Phase II study in solin tumors. *Eur J Cancer, 15:*971-974, 1979.
399. Eagan, R. T., Frytar, S., and Rubin, J.: Dianhydrogalactitol (DAG) vs. polychemotherapy in non-small cell lung cancer. *Proc Am Assoc Cancer Res, 17:*21, 1976.

400. Elson, L. A., Jarman, M., and Ross, W. J.: Toxicity, hematological effects and antitumor activity of epoxides derived from disubstituted hexitols mode of action of Mannitol Myleran and Dibromomanitol. *Eur J Cancer, 4:*617-625, 1968.

401. Hahn, R. G., Bauer, M., Wolter, J., Creech, R., Bennett, J. M., and Wampler, G.: Phase II study of single-agent therapy with Megestrol Acetate, VP-16-213, Cyclophosphamide, and Dianhydrogalactitol in advanced renal cell cancer. *Cancer Treat Rep, 63:*513-515, 1979.

402. Otvos, L., Elekes, I., Kraicsovits, F., and Institoris, L.: Sterochemistry of the reactions of biopolymers. III. Alkylations of DNA with Dibromodulcitol and analogous sugars. *Chem Abs, 76:*109-327, 1972.

403. Espana, P., Wiernik, P. H., and Walker, M. D.: Phase II study of Dianhydrogalactitol in malignant glioma. *Cancer Treat Rep, 62:*1199-1200, 1978.

404. Brockman, R. W.: Biochemical aspects of drug combination *Cancer Chemother Rep,* Part 2, *4:*115, 1974.

405. Capizzi, R. L., Keiser, L. W., and Sartorelli, A. C.: Combination chemotherapy — theory and practice. *Semin Oncol, 4:*277, 1977.

406. DeVita, V. T., Jr., and Schein, P. S.: The use of drugs in combination for the treatment of cancer. *N Engl J Med, 288:*998-1006, 1973.

407. DeVita, V. T., Young, R. C., and Canellos, G. P.: Combination versus single agent chemotherapy: A review of the basis for selection of drug treatment of cancer. *Cancer, 35:*98-110, 1975.

408. Frei, E., III: Combination cancer therapy. *Cancer Res, 32:*2593-2607, 1972.

409. Madoc-Jones, H., and Mauro, F.: Site of action of cytotoxic agents in the cell life. In Sartorelli, A. C. and Johns, D. G. (Eds.): *Handbook of Experimental Pharmacology.* New York, Springer Verlag, 1974, pp. 205-219.

410. Skipper, H. E.: Combination therapy: Some concepts and results. *Cancer Chemother Rep,* Part 2, *4:*137, 1974.

411. Valeriote, F. A., and Edelstein, M. B.: The role of cell kinetics in cancer chemotherapy. *Semin Oncol, 4:*217-226, 1977.

412. Van Putten, L. M.: The kinetics of cell kill and cell proliferation in relation to curability and malignant disease. In Staquet, M.: *The Design of Clinical Trials in Cancer Therapy.* Scientifiques Europennes, Brussels, 1972, p. 116.

413. Brockman, R. W.: Mechanisms of resistance. In Sartorelli, A. C., and Johns, D. G. (Eds.): *Antineoplastic and Immunosuppressive Agents.* Part I. New York, Springer-Verlag, 1974, pp. 352-410.

414. Dedrick, R. L., Zaharko, D. S., and Bender, R. A.: Pharmacokinetic considerations on resistance to anticancer drugs. *Cancer Chemother Rep, 59:*795, 1975.

415. Hall, T. C.: Prediction of response to therapy and mechanisms of resistance. *Semin Oncol, 4:*193-202, 1977.

416. Schabel, F. M., Jr.: The use of tumor growth kinetics in planning "curative" chemotherapy of advanced solid tumors. *Cancer Res, 29:*3384-3389, 1969.

417. Skeel, R. T., and Lindquist, C. A.: Clinical aspects of resistance to antineoplastic agents. In Becker, F. F. (Ed.): *Cancer, A Comprehensive Treatise.* New York, Plenum Press, 1977, Vol. 5, pp. 113-143.

418. Skipper, H., Hutchison, D. J., Schabel, F., Schmidt, L. H., Goldin, A., Brockman, R. W., Venditti, J., and Wadonsky, I.: A quick reference chart on cross resistance between anticancer agents. *Cancer Chemother Rep,* Part I, *4:*493-498, 1972.

419. Welch, A. D.: The problem of drug resistance in cancer chemotherapy. *Cancer Res, 19:*359-371, 1959.

420. Cassady, J. R., and Jaffe, N.: Protection from chemotherapeutic epilation by prior irradiation. *Radiology, 112:*197, 1974.

421. Fairley, K. F., Barrie, J. U., and Johnson, W.: Sterility and testicular atrophy related to Cyclophosphamide therapy. *Lancet, 1:*568, 1972.
422. Marsh, J. C.: The effects of cancer chemotherapeutic agents on normal hematopoietic precursor cells: A review. *Cancer Res, 36:*1853, 1976.
423. Rose, D. P., and Davis, T. E.: Ovarian function in patients receiving adjuvant chemotherapy for breast cancer. *Lancet, 1:*1174, 1977.
424. Siris, E. S., Leventhal, G. G., and Vaitukaitis, J. L.: Effects of childhood leukemia and chemotherapy on puberty and reproductive function in girls. *N Engl J Med, 294:*1143, 1976.
425. Trainor, K. J., and Morley, A. A.: Screening of cytotoxic drugs for residual bone marrow damage. *J Natl Cancer Inst, 57:*1237, 1976.
426. Cadman, E.: Toxicity of chemotherapeutic agents. Sartorelli, A. C. and Johns, D. G. (Eds.): *Antineoplastic and Immunosuppressive Agents.* New York, Springer-Verlag, 1974, Part I, pp. 59-111.
427. Creaven, P. J., and Mihich, E.: The clinical toxicity of anti cancer drugs and its prediction. *Semin Oncol, 4:*147, 1977.
428. Harris, C. C.: The carcinogenicity of anticancer drugs: A hazard in man. *Cancer, 37:*1014, 1976.
429. Khandekar, J. D., Kurtides, E. S., and Stalzer, R. C.: Acute erythroleukemia complicating prolonged chemotherapy for ovarian carcinoma. *Arch Intern Med, 137:*355, 1977.
430. Schein, P. S., and Winokur, S. H.: Immunosuppressive and cytotoxic chemotherapy long term complications. *Ann Intern Med, 82:*84, 1975.
431. Sieber, S. M., and Adamson, R. H.: Toxicity of antineoplastic agents in man: Chromosomal aberrations, anti-fertility effects, congenital malformations, and carcinogenetic potential. *Adv Cancer Res, 22:*57, 1975.
432. Sostman, H. D., Matthay, R. A., and Putman, C. E.: Cytotoxic drug-induced lung disease. *Am J Med, 62:*608, 1977.
433. Toledo, T. M., Harper, R. C., and Moser, R. G.: Fetal effects during cyclophosphamide and irradiation therapy. *Ann Intern Med, 74:*87, 1971.
434. Weiss, H. D., Walker, M. D., and Wiernik, P. H.: Neurotoxicity of commonly used antineoplastic agents. *N Engl J Med, 291:*75, 1974.
435. Brodkey, J. S., Pearson, O. H., and Manni, A.: Hypophysectomy for relief of bone pain in breast cancer. *N Engl J Med, 299:*1016, 1978.
436. Devitt, J. E., and Hardwick, J. M.: Role of bilateral adrenalectomy (and oophorectomy) in the management of patients with metastatic breast cancer. *Am J Surg, 137:*629-633, 1979.
437. LaRossa, J. T., Strong, M. S., and Melby, J. C.: Endocrinologically incomplete transethmoidal transsphenoidal hypophysectomy with relief of bone pain in breast cancer. *N Engl J Med, 298:*1332-1335, 1978.
438. Levin, A. B., Benson, R. C., Jr., Kati, J., and Nilsson, T.: Chemical hypophysectomy for relief of bone pain in carcinoma of the prostate. *J Urol, 119:*517-521, 1978.
439. Friedman, M. A., Hoffman, P. G., Jr., Dandolos, E. M., Lagios, D., Johnston, W. H., and Siiteri, P. K.: Estrogen receptors in male breast cancer: Clinical and pathologic correlations. *Cancer, 47:*134-137, 1981.
440. Galli, M. C., DeGiovanni, C., Nicoletti, G., Grilli, S., Nanni, P., Prodi, G., Gola, G., Rocchetta, R., and Orlandi, C.: The occurrence of multiple steroid hormone receptors in disease-free and neoplastic human ovary. *Cancer, 47:*1297-1302, 1981.
441. Gambrell, R. D., Jr.: The role of hormones in endometrial cancer. *South Med J, 71:*1280-1286, 1978.

442. Gustafsson, J. A., Ekman, P., Snochowski, M., Zetterberg, A., Pousette, A., and Hogbeg, B.: Correlation between clinical response to hormonal therapy and steroid receptor content in prostatic cancer. *Cancer Res, 38:*4345-4358, 1978.
443. Hasson, J., Luthan, P. A., and Kohl, M. W.: Comparison of estrogen receptor levels in breast cancer samples from mastectomy and frozen section specimens. *Cancer, 47:*138-139, 1981.
444. Horwitz, K. B., and McGuire, W. L.: Studies on mechanisms of estrogen and anti-estrogen action in human breast cancer. *Recent Results Cancer Res, 71:*45-58, 1980.
445. Jensen, E. V., Smith, S., and Desombre, E. R.: Hormone dependency in breast cancer. *J Steroid Biochem, 7:*911-917, 1976.
446. Kiang, D. T., Frenning, D. H., Gay, J., Goldman, A. I., and Kennedy, B. J.: Combination therapy of hormone and cytotoxic agents in advanced breast cancer. *Cancer, 47:*452-456, 1981.
447. Kiang, D. T., Frenning, D. H., Goldman, A. I., Ascensao, V. F., and Kennedy, B. J.: Estrogen receptors and responses to chemotherapy and hormonal therapy in advanced breast cancer. *N Engl J Med, 299:*1330-1334, 1978.
448. Kontturi, M., and Sontaniemi, E.: Effect of estrogen in liver function of prostatic cancer patients. *Br Med J, 4:*204-205, 1969.
449. Kontturi, M., and Sontaniemi, E.: Estrogen-induced metabolic changes during treatment of prostatic cancer. *Scand J Clin Lab Invest, 25:*45, 1970.
450. Korenman, S. G.: Specific estrogen binding by the cytoplasm of human breast carcinoma. *J Elin Endocrinol, 30:*639-645, 1970.
451. Lemon, H. M.: Abnormal estrogen metabolism and tissue estrogen receptors in breast cancer. *Cancer, 25:*423, 1970.
452. Lemon, H. M.: Pathophysiologic considerations in the treatment of menopausal patients with oestrogens; the role of oestriol in the prevention of mammary carcinoma. *Acta Endocrinol Suppl, 233:*17-27, 1980.
453. Maass, H., and Jonat, W.: Endocrine treatment of advanced breast cancer. *Recent Results Cancer Res, 71:*102-111, 1980.
454. Reiner, W. G., Scott, W. W., Eggleston, J. C., and Walsh, P. C.: Long-term survival after hormonal therapy for stage D prostatic cancer. *J Urol, 122:*183-184, 1979.
455. Samaan, N. A., Buzdar, A. U., Aldinger, K. A., Schultz, P. A., Yang, K. P., Romsdahl, M. M., and Martin, R.: Estrogen receptor: A prognostic factor in breast cancer. *Cancer, 47:*554-560, 1981.
456. Segaloff, A.: Pharmacological receptor determination in endocrine therapy of breast cancer. *Ann Rev Pharmacol Toxicol, 20:*429-439, 1980.
457. Smith, P. H., Akdas, A., Mason, M. K., Richards, B., Robinson, M. R., DePauw, M., and Sylvester, R.: Hormone therapy in prostatic cancer. *Acta Urol Belg, 48:*98-105, 1980.
458. Taylor, J. R.: Intravenous and oral trial of Stilbestrol Diphosphate in prostatic cancer. *Can Med Assoc J, 80:*880-882, 1959.
459. Brodsky, I.: The role of androgens and anabolic steroids in the treatment of cancer. *Semin Drug Treat, 3:*15-25, 1973.
460. Fishman, J., and Hellman, L.: 7_B, 17_a-Dimethyltestosterone (Calusterone)-induced changes in the metabolism, production rate, and excretion of estrogens in women with breast cancer: A possible mechanism of action. *J Clin Endocrinol Metab, 42:*365-369, 1976.
461. Goldberg, I. S.: Testosterone propionate therapy in breast cancer — a cooperative study. *JAMA, 183:*1069, 1964.
462. Kennedy, B. J.: Fluoxymesterone therapy in advanced Breast cancer. *N Engl J Med, 259:*673-675, 1958.

463. Legha, S. S., Buzdar, A. U., Smith, T. L., Swenerton, K. D., Hortobagyi, G. N., and Blumenschein, G. R.: Response to hormonal therapy as a prognostic factor for metastatic breast cancer treated with combination chemotherapy. *Cancer, 46:*438-445, 1980.
464. Rigberg, S. V., and Brodsky, I.: Potential roles of androgens and the anabolic steroids in the treatment of cancer — a review. *J Med, 6:*271-290, 1975.
465. Segaloff, A.: Testosterone and miscellaneous steroids in the treatment of advanced mammary cancer. *Cancer, 10:*808-812, 1957.
466. Thomas, A. N., Gordan, G. S., Goldman, L., and Lowe, R.: Antitumor efficacy of 2_a-Methyl Dihydrotestosterone Propionate in advanced breast cancer. *Cancer, 15:*176-178, 1962.
467. Zava, D. T., and McGuire, W. L.: Estrogen receptors in androgen-induced breast tumor regression. *Cancer Res, 37:*1608-1610, 1977.
468. Cuna, G. R., Calciati, A., Strada, M. R., Bumma, C., and Campio, L.: High dose Medroxyprogesterone Acetate (MPA) treatment in metastatic carcinoma of the breast: A dose-response evaluation. *Tomori, 64:*143-149, 1978.
469. Delena, M., Brambilla, C., Valagussa, P., and Bona Dona, G.: High-dose Medroxyprogesterone Acetate in breast cancer resistant to endocrine and cytotoxic therapy. *Cancer Chemother Pharmacol, 2:*175-180, 1979.
470. Gambrell, R. D., Jr.: The prevention endometrial cancer in postmenopausal women with progestogens. *Maturitas, 1:*107-112, 1978.
471. Gambrell, R. D., Jr.: The role of hormones in endometrial cancer. *South Med J, 71:*1280-1286, 1978.
472. Hoffman, P. G., and Siiteri, P. K.: Sex steroid receptors in gynecologic cancer. *Obstet Gynecol, 55:*648-652, 1980.
473. Howitz, K. B., and McGuire, W. L.: Specific progesterone receptors in human breast cancer. *Steroids, 25:*497-505, 1975.
474. Kardinal, C. G., and Donegan, W. L.: Cancer of the breast, endocrine and hormonal therapy. *Major Probl Clin Surg, 5:*361-404, 1979.
475. Kennedy, B. J.: Progestogens in the treatment of carcinoma of the endometrium. *Surg Gynecol Obstet,* 1, *27:*103-114, 1968.
476. Kneale, B., Evans, J.: Progestogen therapy for advanced carcinoma of the endometrium. *Med J Aust, 2:*1101-1104, 1969.
477. Muggia, F. M., Cassileth, P. A., Ochoa, M., Jr., Flatow, F. A., Gellhorn, A., and Hyman, G. A.: Treatment of breast cancer with Medroxyprogesterone Acetate. *Ann Intern Med, 68:*328-337, 1971.
478. Reifenstein, E. C., Sr.: Hydroxyprogesterone Caproate therapy in advanced endometrial cancer. *Cancer, 27:*485-502, 1971.
479. Teulings, F. A., VanGilse, H. A., Henkelman, M. S., Portengen, H., and Alexieva-Figusch, J.: Estrogen, androgen, glucocorticoid, and progesterone receptors in progestin-induced regression of human breast cancer. *Cancer Res, 40:*2557-2561, 1980.
480. Waterman, E. A., and Benson, R. C.: Medrogestone therapy in advanced endometrial adenocarcinoma. *Obstet Gynecol, 30:*626-634, 1967.
481. Baxter, J. D., Harris, A. W., Tomkins, G. M., and Cohn, M.: Glucocorticoid receptors in lymphoma cells in culture: Relationship to glucocorticoid killing activity. *Science* (Washington, D. C.), *171:*189, 1971.
482. Ernst, P., and Killmann, S.: Perturbation of generation of human leukemic blast cells by cytostatic therapy *in vivo:* Effect of corticosteroids. *Blood, 36:*689, 1970.
483. Ezdinli, E. Z., Stutzman, L., Aungst, W. C., and Firat, D.: Corticosteroid therapy for lymphomas and chronic lymphocytic leukemia. *Cancer J Clin, 23:*900, 1969.

484. Hall, T. C., Choi, O. S., Abadi, A., and Krant, M. J.: High-dose corticoid therapy in Hodgkin's Disease and other lymphomas. *Ann Intern Med, 66:*1144, 1967.
485. Lippman, M. E., Perry, S., and Thompson, E. B.: Glucocorticoid binding proteins in myeloblasts of acute myelogenous leukemia. *Am J Med, 59:*224-227, 1975.
486. Lippman, M. E., Yarbro, G. K., and Leventhal, B. G.: Clinical implications of glucocorticoid receptors in human leukemia. *Cancer Res, 38:*4251-4256, 1978.
487. Marmont, A., and Fusco, F. A.: Massive doses of predni-steroids in the treatment of acute leukemia: Clinical experience and therapeutic considerations. *Minerva Med, 51:*3437-3450, 1960.
488. Bloom, H. J. G., and Boesen, E.: Antiestrogens in treatment of breast cancer: Value of Nafoxidine in 52 advanced cases. *Br Med J, 2:*7-10, 1974.
489. Butler, W. B., Kelsey, W. H., and Goran, N.: Role of insulin in modifying the response of the human breast cancer cell line MCF-7 to antiestrogens. *Proc Am Assoc Cancer Res, 20:*247, 1979.
490. Heuson, J. C., Coune, A., and Staguet, M.: Clinical trial of Nafoxidine, an antiestrogen in advanced breast cancer. *Eur J Cancer, 8:*387-389, 1972.
491. Paladine, W., Longacre, D., Hemmings, P., and Harper, G.: Nafoxidine, an antiestrogen in hypernephroma. *Proc Am Assoc Cancer Res, 20:*293, 1979.
492. Adam, H. K., Patterson, J. S., Kamp, J. F., Ribieo, G. G., and Wilkinson, P. M.: The metabolism of tamoxifen in man. *Proc Am Assoc Cancer Res, 20:*47, 1979.
493. Aisner, J., Ross, D. D., and Wiernik, P. H.: Tamoxifen in advanced male breast cancer. *Arch Intern Med, 139:*480-481, 1979.
494. Al-Sarraf, M.: The clinical trial of Tamoxifen in patients with advanced renal cell cancer: A Southwest Oncology Group Study. *Proc Am Assoc Cancer Res, 20:*378, 1979.
495. Cocconi, G., DeLisi, V., Boni, C., Amadori, D., Poletti, T., and Bertusi, M.: Chemotherapy (CMF) vs combination of hormonal and chemotherapy (CMF plus Tamoxifen) in metastatic breast cancer. *Proc Assoc Cancer Res, 20:*302, 1979.
496. Henningsen, B.: Clinical experience with Tamoxifen for estrogen receptor blocking therapy in metastatic breast cancer. *Prog Clin Biol Res, 12:*479-482, 1977.
497. Kiang, D. T., and Kennedy, B. J.: Tamoxifen (antioestrogen) therapy in advanced breast cancer. *Ann Intern Med, 87:*687-690, 1977.
498. Levin, J., Markham, M. J., Greenwald, E. S., Willner, D., Kream, J., Zumoff, B., and Fukushima, D. K.: Effect of Tamoxifen treatment on cortisol metabolism and the course of the disease in advanced breast cancer. *Cancer, 47:*1394-1397, 1981.
499. Manni, A., Arafah, B., and Pearson, O. H.: Estrogen and progesterone receptors in the prediction of response of breast cancer to endocrine therapy. *Cancer, 46:*2838-2841, 1980.
500. McGuire, W. L.: Current status of estrogen receptors in human breast cancer. *Cancer, 36:*638-644, 1975.
501. Mouridsen, H., Palshof, T., Patterson, J., and Battersby, L.: Tamoxifen in advanced breast cancer. *Cancer Treat Rev, 5:*131-141, 1978.
502. Orr, J. D., MacDonald, J. A., and Thomson, J. W.: Tamoxifen in the palliative treatment of advanced breast cancer. A clinical review. *J R Coll Surg Edinb, 24:*141-147, 1979.
503. Patterson, J. S., and Battersby, L. A.: Tamoxifen: An overview of recent studies in the field of oncology. *Cancer Treat Rep, 64:*775-778, 1980.
504. Rose, C., Thorpe, S. M., Liber, J., Daenfeldt, J. L., Palshof, T., and Mouridsen, H. T.: Therapeutic effect of Tamoxifen related to estrogen receptor level. *Recent Results Cancer Res, 71:*134-141, 1980.

505. Stoll, B. A.: Clinical experience with Tamoxifen in advanced breast cancer. *Recent Results Cancer Res, 71:*207-211, 1980.
506. Swenerton, K. D., White, G. W., and Boyes, D. A.: Treatment of advanced endometrial carcinoma with Tamoxifen. *N Engl J Med, 301:*105, 1979.
507. Ward, H. W., Arthur, K., Banks, A. J., Bond, W. H., Brown, I., Freeman, W. E., Holme, G. M., Jones, W. G., Newsholme, G. A., and Ostrowski, M. J.: Antioestrogen therapy for breast cancer — a report on 300 patients treated with Tamoxifen. *Clin Oncol, 4:*11-17, 1978.
508. Willis, K. J., London, D. R., Ward, H. W. C., Butt, W. L., Lynch, S. S., and Rudd, B. T.: Recurrent breast cancer treated with antioestrogen Tamoxifen: Correlation between hormonal changes and clinical course. *Br Med J, 1:*425-428, 1977.
509. Bergenstal, D. M., Hertz, R., Lipsett, M. D., and Moy, R. H.: Chemotherapy of adrenocortical cancer with O, P'-DDD. *Ann Intern Med, 53:*672-679, 1960.
510. Fang, V. S.: Cytotoxic activity of 1-(O-Chlorophenyl)-1-(P-Chlorophenyl)-2, 2-Dichloroethane (Mitotane) and its analogs on feminizing adrenal neoplastic cells in culture. *Cancer Res, 39:*135-145, 1979.
511. Helson, L., Wollner, N., Murphy, M. L., and Schwartz, M. K.: Metastatic adrenal cortical carcinoma: Biochemical changes accompanying clinical regression during therapy with O, P'-DDD. *Clin Chem, 17:*1191, 1971.
512. Kupfer, D., and Peets, L.: The effect of O, P'-DDD on cortisol and hexobarbital metabolism. *Biochem Pharmacol, 15:*573, 1966.
513. Lubitz, J. A., Freeman, L., and Okun, R.: Mitotane use in inoperable adrenal cortical carcinoma. *JAMA, 223:*1109, 1973.
514. Moy, R. H.: Studies of the pharmacology of O, P'-DDD in man. *J Lab Clin Med, 58:*296, 1961.
515. Zumoff, B.: The hypouricemic effect of O, P'-DDD. *Am J Med Sci, 278:*145-147, 1979.
516. Fishman, L. M., Liddle, G. W., Island, D. P., Fleischer, N., and Kuchel, O.: Effects of Amino-glutethimide on adrenal function in man. *J Clin Endocrinol Metab, 27:*481-490, 1968.
517. Friedlander, M. L.: Aminoglutethimide and prostatic cancer. *Lancet, 2:*1373, 1980.
518. Gamacho, A. M., Cash, R., Brough, A. J., and Wilroy, R. S.: Inhibition of adrenal steriodogenesis by Amino-glutethimide and the mechanism of action. *JAMA, 202:*20, 1967.
519. Harvey, H. A., Santen, R. J., Osterman, J., Samojlik, E., White, D. S., and Lipton, A.: A comparative trial of transsphensidal hypophysectomy and estrogen suppression with Aminoglutethimide in advanced breast cancer. *Cancer, 43:*2207-2214, 1979.
520. Koelmeyer, T. D., Stephens, E. J., and Wood, H. F.: Experience with 6-aminoglutethimide in the treatment of metastatic breast cancer. *Clin Oncol, 4:*323-327, 1978.
521. Lawrence, B. V., Lipton, A., Harvey, H. A., Santen, R. J., Wells, S. A., Jr., Cox, C. E., White, D. S., and Smart, E. K.: Influence of estrogen receptor status on response of metastatic breast cancer to Aminoglutethimide therapy. *Cancer, 45:*786-791, 1980.
522. Lawrence, B. V., Santen, R. J., Lipton, A., Harvey, H. A., Hamilton, R., and Mercurio, T.: Pancytopenia induced by Aminoglutethimide in the treatment of breast cancer. *Cancer Treat Rep, 62:*1581-1583, 1978.
523. Lipton, A., and Santen, R. J.: Medical adrenalectomy using Amino-glutethimide and Dexamethasone in advanced breast cancer. *Cancer, 33:*503-512, 1974.
524. Newsome, H. H., Brown, P. W., Terz, J. J., and Lawrence, W.: Medical and surgical

adrenalectomy in patients with advanced breast carcinoma. *Cancer, 39:*542-546, 1977.

525. Samojlik, E., Veldhuis, J. D., Wells, S. A., and Santen, R. J.: Preservation of androgen secretion during estrogen suppression with Aminoglutethimide in the treatment of metastatic breast carcinoma. *J Clin Invest, 65:*602-612, 1980.
526. Santen, R. J., Lipton, A., and Kendall, J.: Successful medical adrenalectomy with Amino-glutethimide. *JAMA, 230:*1661-1665, 1974.
527. Wells, S. A., Jr., Santen, R. J., Lipton, A., Haagensen, D. E., Jr., Ruby, E. J., Harvey, H., and Dilley, W. G.: Medical adrenalectomy with Aminoglutethimide: Clinical studies in post menopausal patients with metastatic breast carcinoma. *Ann Surg, 187:*475-484, 1978.
528. Barnes, P. A., and Rees, D. J.: *A Concise Textbook of Radiotherapy.* London, Faber & Faber, 1972.
529. Fletcher, G. H.: *Textbook of Radiotherapy.* Philadelphia, Lea & Febiger, 1980.
530. Halnan, K. E.: *Recent Advances in Cancer and Radiotherapeutics:* Clinical Oncology. London, Churchill Livingston, 1972.
531. Moss, W. T., Brand, W. N., and Battifura, H.: *Radiation Oncology: Rationale, Technique, Results.* St. Louis, C. V. Mosby, 1979.
532. Paterson, R.: *The Treatment of Malignant Disease by Radiotherapy,* ed. 2. Baltimore, Williams & Wilkins, 1963.
533. Selman, J.: *The Fundamentals of X-ray and Radium Physics,* ed. 6. Springfield, Charles C Thomas, 1977.
534. Van Roosenbeek, E., and Delclos, L.: *The Radioactive Patient: Care, Precautions, and Procedures in Diagnosis and Therapy.* Flushing, N. Y., Medical Examination Pub. Co., 1975.
535. Andrews, J. R.: Dose-time relationships in cancer radiotherapy: A clinical radiobiology study of extremes of dose and time. *Am J Roentgenol, 93:*56, 1965.
536. Andrews, J. R.: *The Radiobiology of Human Cancer Radiotherapy.* Philadelphia, W. B. Saunders, 1968.
537. D'Angio, G. J., Farber, S., and Maddock, C. L.: Potentiation of x-ray effects by Actinomycin D. *Radiology, 73:*175-177, 1959.
538. Deschner, E. E., and Gray, L. H.: Influence of oxygen tension on x-ray induced chromosomal damage in Ehrlich ascites tumor cells irradiated *in vitro* and *in vivo. Radiat Res, 11:*115, 1959.
539. Elkind, M. M.: Fractionated dose radiotherapy and its relationship to survival curve shape. *Cancer Treat Rev, 3:*1, 1976.
540. Elkind, M. M., and Sutton, H.: X-ray damage and recovery in mammalian cells in culture. *Nature, 184:*1293-1295, 1959.
541. Ellis, F.: Dose, time and fractionation: A clinical hypothesis. *Clin Radiol, 20:*1-7, 1969.
542. Glassburn, J. R., Brady, L. W., and Plenk, H. P.: Hyperbaric oxygen in radiation therapy. *Cancer, 39:*751, 1977.
543. Gray, L. H.: Comparative studies of the biological effects of x-rays, neutrons and other ionizing radiations. *Br Med Bull, 4:*11-18, 1946.
544. Gray, L. H.: Radiobiologic basis of oxygen as a modifying factor in radiation therapy. *Am J Roentgenol Radium Ther Nucl Med, 85:*803-815, 1961.
545. Hall, E. J.: Radiation dose-rate: A factor of importance in radiobiology and radiotherapy. *Br J Radiol, 45:*81, 1972.
546. Hall, E. J., Bedford, J. S., and Oliver, R.: Extreme hypoxia; its effect on the survival of mammalian cells irradiated at high and low dose-rates. *Br J Radiol, 39:*302, 1966.
547. Howard, A., and Pelc, S. R.: Synthesis of deoxyribonucleic acid in normal and irradiated cells and its relation to chromosome breakage. *Heredity, 6:*261, 1952.

548. Lea, D.: *Actions of Radiations on Living Cells.* New York, The MacMillan Co., 1947.
549. Painter, R. B., and Young, B. R.: X-ray-induced inhibition of DNA synthesis in Chinese hamster ovary, human hela, and mouse L cells. *Radiat Res, 64:*648, 1975.
550. Puck, T. T.: Action of radiation on mammalian cells. III. Relationship between reproductive death and induction of chromosome anomalies by X-irradiation of Euploid human cells *in vitro. Proc Natl Acad Sci, 44:*772-780, 1958.
551. Puck, T. T., and Marcus, P. I.: Action of x-rays on mammalian cells. *J Exp Med, 103:*653-666, 1956.
552. Sinclair, W. K., and Kohn, H. I.: The relative biological effectiveness of high-energy photons and electrons. *Radiology, 82:*800, 1964.
553. Tolmach, L. J., and Jones, R. W.: Dependence of the rate of DNA synthesis in X-irradiated hela S_3 cells on dose and time after exposure. *Radiat Res, 69:*117, 1977.
554. Withers, H. R.: Response of tissues to multiple small dose fractions radiat. *Res, 71:*24, 1977.
555. Baglan, R. J., and Marks, J. E.: Comparison of symptomatic and prophylactic irradiation of brain metastases from oat cell carcinoma of the lung. *Cancer, 47:*41-45, 1981.
556. Cantril, S. T., and Buschke, F.: The clinical usefulness and limitations of supervoltage roentgen therapy. *Radiology, 53:*313-328, 1949.
557. Dobelbower, R. R., Jr.: Current radiotherapeutic approaches to pancreatic cancer. *Cancer, 47:*1729-1733, 1981.
558. Maheshwari, Y. K., Hill, C. S., Jr., Haynie, T. P., III, Hickey, R. C., and Samaan, N. A.: I^{131} therapy in differentiated thyroid carcinoma: M. D. Anderson Hospital experience. *Cancer, 47:*664-671, 1981.
559. Matsumoto, K., Kakizoe, T., Mikuriya, S., Tanaka, T., Kondo, I., and Umegaki, Y.: Clinical evaluation of intraoperative radiotherapy for carcinoma of the urinary bladder. *Cancer, 47:*509-513, 1981.
560. Nisce, L. Z., Safai, B., and Kim, J. H.: Effectiveness of once weekly total skin electron beam therapy in mycosis fungoides. *Cancer, 47:*870-876, 1981.
561. Nisce, L. Z., Safai, B., and Poussin-Rosillo, H.: Once weekly total and subtotal skin electron beam therapy for Kaposi's sarcoma. *47:*640-644, 1981.
562. Parker, R. G.: Palliative radiation therapy. *JAMA, 190:*1000-1002, 1964.
563. Paterson, R.: The use and abuse of palliative radiotherapy. *J Fac Radiol, 8:*235-238, 1957.
564. Strauss, A., Dritschilo, A., Nathanson, L., and Piro, A. L.: Radiation therapy of malignant melanomas: An evaluation of clinically used fractionation schemes. *Cancer, 47:*1262-1266, 1981.
565. Tapley, N. Duv.: *Clinical Applications of the Electron Beam.* New York, John Wiley & Sons, 1976.
566. Baserga, R., Yokoo, H., and Henegar, G. C.: Thorotrast-induced cancer in man. *Cancer, 13:*1021-1031, 1960.
567. Bisgard, J. D., and Hunt, H. B.: Influence of roentgen rays and radium in epiphyseal growth of long bones. *Radiology, 26:*56-64, 1936.
568. Bizzozero, O. J., Johnson, K. G., and Ciocco, A.: Radiation-related leukemia in Hiroshima and Nagasaki, 1946-1964. *N Engl J Med, 274:*1095-1101, 1966.
569. Boden, G.: Radiation myelitis of the cervical spinal cord. *Br J Radiol, 21:*464-469, 1948.
570. Boice, J. D.: Cancer following medical irradiation. *Cancer, 47:*1081-1090, 1981.
571. Brill, A. B., and Forgotson, E. H.: Radiation and congenital malformations. *Am J Obstet Gynecol, 90:*1149-1168, 1964.

572. Bruce, A.: Radiation as a carcinogenic agent. *Radiat Res, 3:*272-280, 1955.
573. Cahan, W. G., Woodard, H. Q., Higinbotham, N. L., Stewart, F. W., and Coley, B. L.: Sarcoma arising in irradiated bone. *Cancer, 1:*3-29, 1948.
574. Castro, L., Choi, S. H., and Sheehan, F. R.: Radiation induced bone sarcomas; report of five cases. *Am J Roentgenol Radium Ther Nucl Med, 100:*924-930, 1967.
575. Court-Brown, W. M., Doll, R., and Hill, A. B.: Incidence of leukemia after exposure to diagnostic irradiation in utero. *Br Med J, 2:*1539-1545, 1960.
576. Crompton, M. R., and Layton, D. D.: Delayed radionecrosis of the brain following therapeutic x-radiation of the pituitary. *Brain, 84:*85-91, 1961.
577. Hempelmann, L. H., Pifer, J. W., Burke, G. J., Terry, R., and Ames, W. R.: Neoplasms in persons treated with x-rays in infancy for thymic enlargement; a report of the third follow-up survey. *J Natl Cancer Inst, 38:*317-341, 1967.
578. Janower, M. L., and Miettinen, O. S.: Neoplasms after childhood irradiation of the thymus gland. *JAMA, 215:*753-756, 1971.
579. Kaplan, I. I.: Genetic effects in children and grandchildren of women treated for infertility and sterility by roentgen therapy; report of a study of thirty-three years. *Radiology, 72:*518-521, 1959.
580. Lamerton, L. F.: Radiation carcinogenesis. *Br Med Bull, 20:*134-138, 1964.
581. Luxton, R. W.: Radiation nephritis. *Q J Med, 22:*215-292, 1953.
582. Maier, J. G., Perry, R. H., Saylor, W., and Sulak, M. H.: Radiation myelitis of the dorsolumbar spinal cord. *Radiology, 93:*153-160, 1969.
583. March, H. C.: Leukemia in radiologists in a 20 year period. *Am J Med Sci, 200:*282-286, 1950.
584. Martland, H. S.: The occurrence of malignancy in radioactive person; a general review of the data gathered in the study of radium dial painters with special reference to the occurrence of osteogenic sarcoma and interrelationship of certain blood diseases. *Am J Cancer, 15:*2435-2516, 1931.
585. Mason, G. R., Guernsey, J. M., Hanks, G. E., and Nelsen, T.S.: Surgical therapy for radiation enteritis. *Oncology, 22:*241-257, 1968.
586. McMahon, H. E., Murphy, A. S., and Bates, M. I.: Endothelial cell sarcomas in liver following thoratrast injections. *Am J Pathol, 23:*585-611, 1947.
587. Palmer, E. D.: The gastroscopic picture of postirradiation gastritis. *Am J Roentgenol Radium Ther, 60:*360-367, 1948.
588. Pettit, V. D., Chamness, J. T., and Ackerman, L. V.: Fibromatosis and fibrosarcoma following irradiation therapy. *Cancer, 7:*149-158, 1954.
589. Pohle, E. A., and Frank, R. C.: Radiation osteitis of the ribs. *J Bone & Joint Surg, 31-A:*654-657, 1949.
590. Pool, T. L.: Irradiation cystitis. *JAMA, 168:*854-856, 1958.
591. Reed, G. B., and Cox, A. J., Jr.: The human liver after radiation injury. *Am J Pathol, 48:*597-611, 1966.
592. Rubin, P., Duthie, R. B., and Young, L. W.: The significance of scoliosis in postirradiated Wilms' tumor and neuroblastoma. *Radiology, 79:*539-559, 1962.
593. Sambrook, D. K.: Split-course radiation therapy in malignant tumors. *Am J Roentgen Radium Ther Nucl Med, 91:*34-45, 1964.
594. Schull, W. J.: A geneticist looks at the radiation hazard. *Radiology, 72:*522-528, 1959.
595. Shellabarger, C. J.: Radiation carcinogenesis. *Cancer, 37:*1090, 1976.
596. Sinclair, W. K.: X-ray induced heritable damage (small colony formation) in cultured mammalian cells. *Radiat Res, 21:*584, 1964.
597. Soloway, H. B.: Radiation-induced neoplasms following curative therapy for retinoblastoma. *Cancer, 19:*1984-1988, 1966.

598. Vaeth, J. M., Feigenbaum, L. Z., and Merrill, M. D.: Effects of intensive radiation on the human heart. *Radiology, 76:*755-762, 1961.
599. Warren, S., and Gates, O.: Radiation pneumonitis; experimental and pathologic observations. *Arch Pathol, 30:*440-460, 1940.
600. Wharton, J. T., Delclos, L., Gallagher, S., and Smith, J. P.: Radiation hepatitis induced by abdominal irradiation with the Cobalt-60 moving strip technique. *Am J Roentgenol Radium Ther Nucl Med, 117:*73-80, 1973.
601. Ficker, S.: *Compendium of Tumor Immunotherapy Protocols,* No. 6. Springfield, Va., National Technical Information Service, 1978.
602. Goodnight, J. E., Jr., and Morton, D. L.: Immunotherapy for malignant disease. *Ann Rev Med, 29:*231, 1978.
603. Harris, J. E., and Sinkovics, J. G.: *The Immunology of Malignant Disease.* Ed 3. St. Louis, C. V. Mosby, 1976.
604. Haskell, C. M.: Immunologic aspects of cancer chemotherapy. *Ann Rev Pharmacol Toxicol, 17:*179, 1977.
605. Terry, W. D., and Windhorst, D. (Eds.): *Immunotherapy of Cancer: Present Status of Trials in Man. Progress in Cancer Research and Therapy,* Vol. 6. New York, Raven Press, 1978.
606. Everall, K. D., Dowd, P., Davies, D. A., O'Neill, G. T., and Rowland, G. F.: Treatment of melanoma by passive humeral immunotherapy using antibody drug synergism. *Lancet, 1:*1105-1106, 1977.
07. Rosenberg, S. A., and Terry, W. D.: Passive immunotherapy of cancer in animals and man. *Adv Cancer Res, 25:*323-388, 1977.
08. Blume, M. R., Rosenbaum, E. H., Cohen, R. J., Gershon, J., Glassberg, A. B., and Shepley, E.: Adjuvant immunotherapy in high risk stage I melanoma with transfer factor. *Cancer, 47:*882-888, 1981.
09. Seigler, H., Buckley, C. E., Sheppard, L. B., Horne, B. J., and Shingleton, W. W.: Adoptive transfer and specific active immunization of patients with malignant melanoma. *Ann N Y Acad Sci, 277:*522-532, 1976.
10. Symes, M. O., Eckert, H., Feneley, R. C., Lai, T., Mitchell, J. P., Roberts, J. B., and Tribe, C. R.: Adoptive immunotherapy and radiotherapy in the treatment of urinary bladder cancer. *Br J Urol, 50:*328-331, 1978.
11. Symes, M. O., Mitchell, J. P., Eckert, H., Roberts, J. B., Feneley, R. C., Tribe, C. R., and Lai, T.: Transfer of adoptive immunity by intra-arterial injection of tumor-immune pig lymph node cells: Treatment of recurrent urinary bladder carcinoma after radical radiotherapy. *Urology, 12:*398-401, 1978.
12. Waldman, S. R., and Pilch, Y. H.: Leukopheresis of cancer patients for adoptive immunotherapy. In: Ascher, M. S. (Ed.): *Transfer Factor: Basic Properties and Clinical Applications.* New York, Academic Press, 1979, pp. 675-782.
13. Yonemoto, R. H.: Adoptive immunotherapy utilizing thoracic duct lymphocytes. *Ann N Y Acad Sci, 277:*7-19, 1976.
14. Baker, M. A., Falk, J. A., and Taub, R. N.: Immunotherapy of human acute leukemia: Antibody response to leukemia-associated antigens. *Blood, 52:*469-480, 1978.
5. Billings, R., and Terasaki, P. I.: Human leukemia antigen. 1. Production and characterization of antisera. *J Natl Cancer Inst, 53:*1635, 1638, 1974.
16. Biza, D., and Davies, D. A. L.: Solubilization and partial purification of human leukemic specific antigens. *Nature, 227:*1249-1251, 1970.
7. Chapuis, B. J., Powles, R., and Alexander, P.: Inability to demonstrate lytic antibodies to autologous leukemic cells in the sera from remission patients with acute

myelogenous leukemia treated with active specific immunotherapy. *Clin Ex Immunol, 32:*253-258, 1978.

618. Freireich, E. J., and Hersh, E. M.: Autoimmunization with acute leukemia cell Demonstration of increased lymphocyte responsiveness. *Int J Cancer, 11:*521-52 1973.
619. Friedman, W. H., and Kourilisky, F. M.: Stimulation of lymphocytes by autologo leukemia cells in acute leukemia. *Nature, 224:*227-279, 1969.
620. Granatek, C. H., Ezaki, K., Hersh, E. M., Keating, M. J., and Rasmussen, S.: Antibo responses of remission leukemia patients receiving active specific and non-speci immunotherapy. *Cancer, 47:*272-279, 1981.
621. Holland, J. F., and Bekesi, J. G.: Immunotherapy of human leukemia with neur minidase modified cells. *Med Clin North Am, 60:*539-549, 1976.
622. Leventhal, B. G., Halterman, R. H., Rosenberg, E. B., and Herberman, R. Immune reactivity of leukemia patients to autologous blast cells. *Cancer R 32:*1820-1825, 1972.
623. Mathe, G., Amiel, J. L., Schwarzenberg, L., Schneider, M., Cattan, A., Schlumbey J. R., Hayat, M., and DeVassal, F.: Active immunotherapy for acute lymphoblas leukemia. *Lancet, 1:*697-699, 1969.
624. McCredie, K. B., Bodey, G. P., Freireich, E. J., Hester, J. P., Rodriguez, V., a Keating, J. J.: Chemoimmunotherapy of adult acute leukemia. *Cancer, 47:*12 1261, 1981.
625. Meltier, M. S., Leonard, E. J., Rapp, H. J., and Boros, T.: Tumor specific antig solubilized by hypertonic potassium chloride. *J Natl Cancer Inst, 47:*703-709, 19
626. Poweles, R. L.: Immunotherapy for acute myelogenous leukemia using irradiat and unirradiated leukemia cells. *Cancer, 34:*1588-1562, 1974.
627. Poweles, R. L., Balchin, L. A., Hamilton-Fairley, G., and Alexander, P.: Recogniti of leukemia cells as foreign before and after autoimmunization. *Br Med J, 1:*4 489, 191.
628. Taylor, G. M., Freeman, C. B., and Harris, R.: Response of remission lymphocyte autochthonous leukemic myeloblast. *Br J Cancer, 33:*501-511, 1976.
629. Vanky, F., Klein, E., Stjernsward, J., and Tremple, G.: Lymphocyte stimulation autologous tumor cells in the presence of serum from the same patient or fr healthy donors. *Int J Cancer, 16:*850-860, 1975.
630. Bast, R. C., Jr., Zbar, B., Borsos, T., and Rapp, H. J.: BCG and cancer (Parts I and *N Engl J Med, 290:*1458-1469, 1974.
631. Garner, F. B., Meyer, C. A., White, D. S., and Lipton, A.: Immunotherapy employ aerosol BCG. *Proc Am Cos Clin Oncol Abstr, 729:*166, 1974.
632. Hawrylko, E., and Mackaness, G. B.: Immunopotentiation with BCG. IV. Fact affecting the magnitude of an antitumor response. *J Natl Cancer Inst, 51:*16 1688, 1973.
633. Hoover, R. N.: Bacillus Calmette-Guerin vacination and cancer prevention: A crit review of the human experience. *Cancer Res, 36:*452-654, 1976.
634. Hortobagyi, G. N., Gutterman, J. U., Blumenschein, G. R., Yap, H. Y., Buzdar, A. Tashima, C. K., Burgess, M. A., and Hersh, E. M.: Combined chemoimmunot apy for advanced breast cancer: A comparison of BCG and Levamisole. *Can 43:*1112-1122, 1979.
635. Hortobagyi, G. N., Richman, S. P., Dandridge, K., Gutterman, J. H., Blumensch G. R., and Hersh, E. M.: Immunotherapy with BCG administered by scarificat *Cancer, 42:*2293-2303, 1978.
636. Louie, A. C., Rozencweig, M., VonHoff, D. D., and Muggia, F. M.: Effective adju

treatments. A brief review of U. S. clinical trials. *Arch. Geschwulstforsch., 48:*563-658, 1978.

7. MacKaness, G. B., Audir, D. J., and Langrange, P. H.: Immunopotentiation with BCG: Immune response to different strains of preparations. *J Natl Cancer Inst., 51:*1655-1664, 1973.

8. Mathe, G., Halle-Panneko, O., and Bourut, C.: BCG in cancer immunotherapy. The results obtained with various BCG preparations in a screening study for systemic adjuvants applicable to cancer immunoprophylaxis or immunotherapy. *Natl Cancer Inst Monogr, 39:*107-112, 1973.

9. McKann, C. F., Hendrickson, C. G., Spitler, L. E., Gunnarsson, A., Banerjee, C., and Nelson, N. R.: Immunotherapy of melanoma with BCG: Two fatalities following intra-lesional injection. *Cancer, 35:*514-520, 1975.

0. McKneally, M. F., Maver, C. K., and Kausel, H. W.: Regional immunotherapy of lung cancer with intrapleural BCG. *Lancet, 1:*377-379, 1976.

1. Nathanson, L.: Use of BCG in the treatment of human neoplasms: A review. *Semin Oncol, 1:*337-350, 1974.

2. Richman, S. P., Gutterman, J. U., and Hersh, E. M.: Cancer immunotherapy. *Can Med Assoc J, 120:*322-324, 1979.

3. Ritch, P. S., McCredie, K. B., Gutterman, J. U., and Hersh, E. M.: Disseminated BCG disease associated with immunotherapy by scarification in acute leukemia. *Cancer, 42:*167-170, 1978.

4. Sparks, F. C.: Hazards and complications of BCG immunotherapy. *Med Clin North Am, 60:*499, 1976.

5. Spitler, L. E.: BCG, Levamisole and transfer factor in the treatment of cancer. *Prog Exp Tumor Res, 25:*178-192, 1980.

6. Bedikian, A. Y., Valvivieso, M., Maroun, J., Gutterman, J. U., Hersh, E. M., and Bodey, G. P.: Evaluation of Vindesine and MER in colorectal cancer. *Cancer, 46:*463-467, 1980.

7. Blumenschein, G. R., Hortobagyi, G. N., Richman, S. P., Gutterman, J. U., Tashima, C. K., Buzdar, A. U., Burgess, M. A., Livingston, R. B., and Hersh, E. M.: Alternating noncross-resistant combination chemotherapy and active nonspecific immunotherapy with BCG or MER-BCG for advanced breast carcinoma. *Cancer, 45:*742-749, 1980.

8. Britell, J. C., Ahmann, D. L., Bisel, H. F., Frytak, S., Ingle, J. N., Rubin, J., and O'Fallon, J. R.: Treatment of advanced breast cancer with Cyclophosphamide 5-Fluorouracil and Prednisone with and without Methanol-extracted residue of BCG. *Cancer Clin Trials, 2:*345-350, 1979.

Cuttner, J., Bedesi, J. G., and Holland, J. F.: Chemoimmunotherapy of acute leukemia using MER. *Proc Am Assoc Cancer Res, 17:*196, 1976.

0. Denefrio, J.: Systemic epitheloid granulomata following immunotherapy with methanol extraction residue of Bacillus Calmette-Guerin (MER). *Proc Am Assoc Cancer Res, 20:*386, 1979.

Krown, S. E., Hilal, E. Y., Pinsky, C. M., Hirshaut, Y., Wanebo, H. J., Hansen, J. A., Huvos, A. G., and Oettgen, H. F.: Intralesional injection of the methanol extraction residue of Bacillus Calmette-Guerin (MER) into cutaneous metastases of malignant melanoma. *Cancer, 42:*2648-2660, 1978.

Lokish, J. J., Garnick, M. B., and Legg, M.: Intralesional immunotherapy: Methanol extraction residue of BCG or purified protein derivative. *Oncology, 36:*236-241, 1979.

O'Connell, M. J., Moertel, C. G., Ritts, R. E., Jr., Frytak, S., and Reitemeier, R. J.: A comparative clinical and immunological assessment of methanol extraction residue of Bacillus Calmette-Guerin versus placebo in patients with advanced cancer. *Cancer Res, 39:*3720-3724, 1979.

654. Robinson, E., Bartal, A., Cohen, Y., and Mekori, T.: Adjuvant therapy in colorectal cancer (A randomized trial comparing radio-chemotherapy and radio-chemotherapy combined with the methanol extraction residue of BCG, MER). *Proc Am Assoc Cancer Res, 20:*408, 1979.
655. Robinson, E., Bartal, A., Cohen, Y., Milstein, D., and Mekori, T.: Adjuvant therapy in colorectal cancer (a randomized trial comparing radio-chemotherapy and radio-chemotherapy combined with methanol extraction residue of BDG, MER). *Biomedicine Express, 31:*8-10, 1979.
656. Vogl, S. E., Lumb, G., Bekes, J. G., and Holland, J. F.: Preclinical study of IV administration of MER-Methanol extraction residue of Bacillus Calmette-Guerin. *Cancer Treat Rep, 61:*901-903, 1977.
657. Voith, M. A., Lichtenfeld, K. M., Schimpff, S. C., and Wiernik, P. H.: Systemic complications of MER immunotherapy of cancer: Pulmonary granulomatosis and rash. *Cancer, 43:*500-504, 1979.
658. Weiss, D. W.: MER and other mycobacterial fractions in the immunotherapy of cancer. *Med Clin N Am, 60:*473-497, 1976.
659. Yamamura, Y., Sakatani, M., Ogura, T., and Azuma, I.: Adjuvant immunotherapy of lung cancer with BCG cell wall skeleton (BCG-CWS). *Cancer, 43:*1314-1319, 1979.
660. Zbar, B., Canti, G., Rapp, H. J., Bier, J., and Borsos, T.: Regression of established oral tumors after intralesional injection of living BCG or BCG cell walls. *Cancer 43:*1304-1307, 1979.
661. Adlam, C., Scott, M. T.: Lympho-reticular stimulatory properties of Corynebacterium Parvum and related bacteria. *J Med Microbiol, 6:*261-274, 1973.
662. Band, P. R., Jao-King, C., Urtasun, R. C., and Haraphingse, M.: Phase I study of Corynebacterium Parvum in patients with solid tumors. *Cancer Chemother Rep 59:*1139-1145, 1975.
663. Bartlett, G. L., Kreider, J. W., and Purnell, D. M.: Treatment of cancer using Corynebacterium Parvum: Similarity of two preparations in four animal tumor models. *Cancer, 46:*685-691, 1980.
664. Baum, M., and Breese, M.: Antitumor effect of Corynebacterium Parvum possible mode of action. *Br J Cancer, 33:*468-473, 1976.
665. Cheng, V. S. T., Suit, H. D., Wang, C. C., and Cummings, C.: Nonspecific immunotherapy by Corynebacterium Parvum: Phase I toxicity study in 12 patient with advanced cancer. *Cancer, 37:*1687-1695, 1976.
666. Fisher, B., Rubin, H., Sartiano, G., Ennis, L., and Wolmark, N.: Observations following Corynebacterium Parvum administration to patients with advanced malignancy: A Phase I study. *Cancer, 38:*119-130, 1976.
667. Fisher, B., Wolmark, N., Saffer, E., and Fisher, E. R.: Inhibitory effect of prolonged Corynebacterium Parvum and Cyclophosphamide administration on the growth of established tumors. *Cancer, 35:*135-143, 1975.
668. Israel, L., Edelstein, R., Depierre, A., and Dimitrov, N.: Daily intravenous infusion with Corynebacterium Parvum in twenty patients with disseminated cancer: A preliminary report of clinical and biologic findings. *J Natl Cancer Inst, 55:*29-3[illegible] 1975.
669. Kim, D. K., and Pfeifer, J.: Measurement of phagocytic activity of reticuloendothelial system (RES) by intralipid: Effect of C. Parvum treatment. *Surg Forum, 28:*85-8[illegible] 1977.
670. Oettgen, H. E., Pinsky, C. M., and Delmonte, L.: Treatment of cancer with immune

modulators Corynebacterium Parvum and Levamisole. *Med Clin N Am, 60:*511-537, 1976.

671. Patt, Y. Z., Wallace, S., Hersh, E. M., Hall, S. W., Menachem, Y. B., Granmayeh, M., McBride, C. M., Benjamin, R. S., and Mavligit, G. M.: Hepatic arterial infusion of Corynebacterium Parvum and chemotherapy. *Surg Gynecol Obstet, 147:*897-902, 1978.
672. Purves, E. C., Snell, M., Cope, W. A., Addison, I. E., Copland, R. F., and Berenbaum, M. C.: Subcutaneous Corynebacterium Parvum in bladder cancer: A controlled study of its immunological effects. *Br J Urol, 51:*278-282, 1979.
673. Royle, G., and Gill, P. G.: Metabolic changes following the intravenous infusion of Corynebacterium Parvum in man. *Cancer, 43:*1328-1330, 1979.
674. Scott, M. T.: Biological effects of the adjuvant Corynebacterium Parvum. II. Evidence for macrophage-T-cell interaction. *Cell Immunol, 5:*459-468, 1972.
675. Scott, M. T.: Corynebacterium Parvum as an immunotherapeutic anticancer agent. *Semin Oncol, 1:*367, 1974.
676. Scott, M. T., and Warner, S. L.: The accumulated effects of repeated systemic or local injections of low doses of Corynebacterium Parvum. *Cancer Res, 36:*1335-1338, 1976.
677. Sexhauer, C. L., Wells, J. R., Oleinick, S., Nitschke, B., Lankford, J., and Humphrey, G. B.: Non-specific immunostimulation with Corynebacterium Parvum in children with acute leukemia. *Clin Res, 24:*75, 1976.
678. Thatcher, N., Lamb, B., Swindell, R., and Crowther, D.: Effect of Corynebacterium Parvum on cellular immunity of cancer patients assayed sequentially over 63 days. *Cancer, 47:*285-290, 1981.
679. Yadeau, R., Bates, H. A., and Fortuny, I.: Lung cancer patients treated with Corynebacterium Parvum. Phase I toxicity study. *Minn Med, 62:*673-675, 1979.
680. Amery, W. K.: Final results of a multicenter placebo controlled Levamisole study of resectable lung cancer. *Cancer Treat Rep, 62:*1677-1683, 1978.
681. Amery, W. K.: Adjuvant Levamisole (LMS) in resectable lung cancer (RLC): A randomized double-blind study. *Proc Am Assoc Cancer Res, 20:*418, 1979.
682. Amery, W. K.: Adjuvant Levamisole in the treatment of patients with resectable lung cancer. *Ann Clin Res, 12:*1-83, 1980.
683. Amery, W. K., and Verhaegen, H.: Effects of Levamisole treatment in cancer patients. *J Rheumatol, 5:*123-135, 1978.
684. Chirigos, M. A., and Amery, W. K.: Combined Levamisole therapy: An overview of its protective effects. In *Immunotherapy of Human Cancer.* New York, Raven Press, 1978.
685. Churchill, W. H., Jr., and David, J. R.: Levamisole and cell-mediated immunity. *N Engl J Med, 289:*375-376, 1973.
686. Copeland, D., Stewart, T., and Harris, J.: Effect of Levamisole (NSC-177023) on *in vitro* human lymphocyte transformation. *Cancer Chemother Rep, 58:*167, 1974.
687. Gonzalez, R. L., Spitler, L. E., and Sagabiel, R. W.: Effect of Levamisole as a surgical adjuvant therapy for malignant melanoma. *Cancer Treat Rep, 62:*1703-1709, 1978.
688. Goyanes-Villaescusa, V.: Mitogenic stimulation by Levamisole on normal human lymphocytes and leukemic lymphoblasts. *Lancet, 1:*370, 1976.
689. Nemo, T., Dadey, B., and Han, T.: Non-T suppressor cell-mediated depression of T-lymphocyte response in breast cancer patients: Reversal effect of suppressor cells by Levamisole. *Proc Am Assoc Cancer Res, 20:*387, 1979.
690. Paterson, A. H. G.: A controlled trial of chemotherapy with or without Levamisole in patients with metastatic carcinoma of breast. *Proc Am Assoc Cancer Res, 20:*391, 1979.

691. Rosenthal, M., Trabert, U., and Muller, W.: Leucocytoxic effect of Levamisole. *Lancet, 1:*369, 1976.

692. Silverman, M., Thompson, J., Miller, A., Mansell, P., Sugarbaker, E., McKinney, C., and Vogel, C.: Mechanism of Levamisole (L) granulopenia (GP) in adjuvant chemoimmunotherapy programs for operable breast cancer. *Proc Am Assoc Cancer Res, 20:*381, 1979.

693. Smith, R. B., Dekernion, J., Lincoln, B., Skinner, D. G., and Kaufman, J. J.: Preliminary report of the use of Levamisole in the treatment of bladder cancer. *Cancer Treat Rep, 62:*1709-1714, 1978.

694. Spitler, L. E.: BCG, Levamisole and transfer factor in the treatment of cancer. *Prog Exp Tumor Res, 25:*178-192, 1980.

695. Spreafico, F.: Use of Levamisole in cancer patients. *Drugs, 20:*105-116, 1980.

696. Symoens, J., Veys, E., Mielants, M., and Pinals, R.: Adverse reactions to Levamisole. *Cancer Treat Rep, 62:*1721-1730, 1978.

697. Van Holder, R., and Van Hove, W.: Recurrent agranulocytosis after Levamisole. *Lancet, 1:*100, 1977.

698. Vogel, C. L., Lipscomb, D. L., Silverman, M. A., Kerns, A. L., Mansell, P. W., and Sugarbaker, E. V.: Levamisole granulocytopenia in patients receiving an adjuvant chemoimmunotherapy program after surgery for breast carcinoma with axillary lymph node involvement. *Cancer Treat Rep, 62:*1587-1589, 1978.

699. Wanebo, H. J., Hilal, E. X., Pinsky, C. M., Strong, E. W., Mile, V., Hirshout, Y., and Oettgen, H. F.: Randomized trial of Levamisole in patients with squamous cancer of the head and neck: A preliminary report. *Cancer Treat Rep, 62:*1663-1669, 1978.

700. Willoughby, M. L. N.: Levamisole and neutropenia. *Lancet, 1:*657, 1977.

701. Chretien, P. B., Lipson, S. D., Makuch, R. W., Kenady, D. E., Cohen, M. H.: Effects of Thymosin *in vitro* in cancer patients and correlation with clinical course after Thymosin immunotherapy. *Ann N Y Acad Sci, 332:*135-147, 1979.

702. Chretien, P. B., Lipson, S. D., Makuch, R. W., Kenady, D. E., Cohen, M. H., and Minna, J. D.: Thymosin in cancer patients: *In vitro* effects and correlations with clinical response to Thymosin immunotherapy. *Cancer Treat Rep, 62:*1787-1790, 1978.

703. Cohen, M. H., Chretien, P. B., Ihde, D. C., Fossieck, B. E., Jr., Makuch, R., Bunn, P. A., Jr., Johnston, A. V., Shackney, S. E., Matthews, M. J., Lipson, S. D., Kenady, D. E., and Minna, J. D.: Thymosin Fraction V and intensive combination chemotherapy, prolonging the survival of patients with small-cell lung cancer. *JAMA, 241:*1813-1815, 1979.

704. Constanzi, J., Daniels, J., Thurman, G., Goldstein, A., and Hokanson, J.: Clinical trials with Thymosin. *Ann N Y Acad Sci, 332:*148-159, 1979.

705. Goldberg, N. H., Lipson, S. D., Kenady, D. E., Simon, R. M., Cohen, M. H., and Chretien, P. B.: T-cell levels and response to Thymosin *in vitro* during intensive chemotherapy in cancer patients receiving Thymosin. *Surg Forum, 28:*151-152, 1977.

706. Goldstein, A. L., Marshall, G. D., Jr., and Rossio, J. L.: Thymosin Therapy: Approach to immunoconstitution in immunodeficiency disease and cancer. In: *Immunotherapy of Human Cancer.* New York, Raven Press, 1978, pp. 173-179.

707. Low, T. L., Thurman, G. B., Chincarini, C., McClure, J. E., Marshall, G. D., Hu, S. K., and Goldstein, A. L.: Current status of Thymosin research: Evidence for the existence of a family of thymic factors that control T-cell maturation. *Ann N Y Acad Sci, 332:*33-48, 1979.

708. Marshall, G. D., Jr., Low, T. L., Thurman, G. B., Hu, S. K., Rossio, J. L., Trivers, G., and Goldstein, A. L.: Overview of Thymosin activity. *Cancer Treat Rep, 62:*1731-1737, 1978.
709. Wara, W. M., Ammann, A. J., and Wara, D. W.: Effect of Thymosin and irradiation on immune modulation in head and neck and esophageal cancer patients. *Cancer Treat Rep, 62:*1775-1778, 1978.
710. Wolf, G. T., Kerney, S. E., and Chretien, P. B.: Improvement of impaired leukocyte migration inhibition by Thymosin in patients with head and neck squamous carcinoma. *Am J Surg, 140:*531-537, 1980.
711. Carter, N. A., and Horoszewicz, J. S.: Human interferon and its inducers: Clinical program overview at Roswell Park Memorial Institute. *Cancer Treat Rep, 62:*1897-1898, 1978.
712. Christopherson, I. S., Jordal, R., Osther, K., Lindenberg, J., Pedersen, P. H., and Berg, K.: Interferon therapy in neoplastic disease. A preliminary report. *Acta Med Scand, 204:*471-476, 1978.
713. Feinerman, B.: Tumor immunology and interferon. *South Med J, 71:*1409-1411, 1978.
714. Herberman, R. B., Djeu, J. Y., or Taldo, J. R., Holden, H. T., West, W. H., Bonnard, G. D.: Role of interferon in augmentation of natural and antibody-dependent cell-mediated cytotoxicity. *Cancer Treat Rep, 62:*1893-1896, 1978.
715. Matsubara, S., Suzuki, M., Nakamura, M., Edo, K., and Ishida, N.: Isolation of an inhibitor of Type II Interferon induction from tumor ascitic fluids. *Cancer Res, 40:*2534-2538, 1980.
716. Niblack, J. F.: Studies with low molecular weight inducers of Interferon in man. *Tex Rep Biol Med, 35:*528-534, 1977.
717. Puccetti, P., and Giampietri, A.: Immunopharmacology of pyran copolymer. *Pharmacol Res Commun, 10:*489-501, 1978.
718. Weissman, R. M., and Droller, M. J.: Interferon: A perspective. *Invest Urol, 18:*189-196, 1980.
719. Aranha, G. V., McKhann, C. F., Grage, T. B., Gunnarsson, A., and Simmons, R. L.: Adjuvant immunotherapy of malignant melanoma. *Cancer, 43:*1297-1303, 1979.
720. Helms, R. A., and Bull, D. M.: Natural killer activity of human lymphocytes against colon cancer. *Gastroenterology, 78:*738-744, 1980.
721. Pimm, M. V., Cook, A. J., and Baldwin, R. W.: Failure of Neuraminidase treatment to influence tumorigenicity or immunogenicity of syngenetically transplanted rat tumour cells. *Eur J Cancer, 14:*869-878, 1978.
722. Schulof, R. S., Fernandes, G., Good, R. A., and Gupta, S.: Neuraminidase treatment of human T lymphocytes: Effect of FC receptor phenotype and function. *Clin Exp Immunol, 40:*611-619, 1980.
723. Cooper, I. S.: Cryogenic surgery: A new method of destruction or extirpation of benign or malignant tissues. *N Engl J Med, 268:*244, 1963.
724. Cooper, I. S.: Cryobiology as viewed by the surgeon. *Cryobiology, 1:*44, 1964.
725. Cooper, I. S.: Cryosurgery for cancer. *Fed Proc, 24:*237-240, 1965.
726. Gage, A. A.: Cryosurgery for cancer: An evaluation. *Cryobiology, 5:*241, 1969.
727. Von Leden, H., and Cahan, W. G. (Eds.): *Cryogenics in Surgery.* Flushing, New York, Medical Examination Publishing Company, 1971.
728. Allington, H. V.: Liquid Nitrogen in the treatment of skin diseases. *California Med, 72:*153, 1950.
729. Barron, R. F.: *Cryogenic Systems.* New York, McGraw-Hill, 1966, pp. 3-12.
730. Cooper, I. S., Grissman, F., and Johnston, R.: A complete system for cryogenic surgery. *St. Barnabas Hospital Medical Bulletin, 1:*11-16, 1962.

731. Crump, R. E.: Cryo instruments: Thermoelectric and freon systems. *International Ophthalmology Clinics, 7:*309-323, 1967.
732. Jagodzinski, R. V., Soanes, W. A., and Gonder, M. J.: A multisensor temperature probe for cryosurgery. *J Cryosurgery, 1:*221-223, 1968.
733. Rinfret, A. P.: Cryobiology. In Vance, R. W. (Ed.): *Cryogenic Technology.* New York, Wiley, 1963, pp. 528-577.
734. Rowbotham, G. F., Haigh, A. L., and Leslie, W. G.: Cooling Cannula for use in the treatment of cerebral neoplasm. *Lancet, 1:*12-15, 1959.
735. Turtz, A. I.: Cryosurgery instrumentation. *J Cryosurgery, 1:*202-209, 1968.
736. Vance, R. W., and Duke, W. M.: *Applied Cryogenic Engineering.* New York, John Wiley and Sons, Inc., 1962, pp. 63-103.
737. White, A. C.: Liquid air in medicine and surgery. *Med Rec, 56:*109, 1899.
738. White, A. C.: Possibilities of liquid air to the physician. *JAMA, 36:*426, 1901.
739. Whitehouse, H. H.: Liquid air in dermatology: Its indications and limitations. *JAMA, 49:*371, 1907.
740. Asahina, A., and Emura, M.: Types of cell freezing and post thawing: Survival of mammalian ascites sarcoma cells. *Cryobiology, 2:*256-262, 1966.
741. Cahan, W. G.: Cryosurgery of malignant and benign tumors. *Fed Proc, 24:*241-248 1965.
742. Chambers, R., and Hale, H. P.: The formation of ice in protoplasm. *Proc Royal Soc Biol, 110:*336-352, 1932.
743. Farrant, J.: Mechanism of cell damage during freezing and thawing and its prevention. *Nature, 205:*1284-1289, 1965.
744. Gehenio, P. M., Rapatz, G. L., and Luyet, B. J.: Effects of freezing velocities in causing or preventing hemolysis. *Biodynasica, 9:*77, 1963.
745. Heard, B. E.: The histiological appearance of some normal tissues at low temperatures. *Brit J Surg, 42:*430-437, 1955.
746. Karow, A. M., Jr., and Webb, W. R.: Tissue freezing. *Cryobiology, 2:*49-108, 1965.
747. Lovelock, J. E.: The haemolysis of human red blood cells by freezing and thawing *Biochem Biophys Acta, 10:*414, 1953.
748. Mazur, P.: Kinetics of water loss from cells at sub-zero temperatures and the likelihood of intracellular freezing. *J Gen Physiol, 47:*347, 1963.
749. Mazur, P.: Factors affecting cell injury in cryosurgical freezing. *Bull Millar Fillmor Hosp, 14:*123-128, 1967.
750. Mazur, P.: Physical-chemical factors underlying cell injury in cryosurgical freezing In Rand, R. W., et al.: *Cryosurgery.* Springfield, Thomas, 1968, pp. 32-51.
751. Melnick, P. J.: Effect of freezing rates on the histochemical identification of enzym activity. *Fed Proc, 24, Suppl. 15:*S-259-A-267, 1965.
752. Meryman, H. T.: Mechanics of freezing in living cells and tissues. *Science, 124:*124-129, 1956.
753. Rapatz, G.: Cellular Structural and Ultrastructural Modifications Associated wit Cooling. In Musacchia, S. J. and Saunders, J. F. (Eds.): *Depressed Metabolism.* New York, Am. Elsevier, 1969, pp. 3-38.
754. Rinfret, A. P.: Factors affecting the erythrocyte during rapid freezing and thawing *Ann N Y Acad Sci, 85:*576-594, 1960.
755. Sherman, J. K., and Kim, R. S.: Freeze-thaw induced ultrastructural alterations of chromosomes following intracellular ice formation. *Cryobiology, 3:*367-368, 196[illegible]
756. Shikama, K.: Effect of freezing and thawing on the stability of double helix of DNA *Nature, 207:*529-530, 1965.
757. Smith, A. U.: *Biological Effects of Freezing and Supercooling.* Baltimore, Williams Wilkins, 1961, p. 217.

758. Smith, A. U., Polge, C., and Smiles, J.: Microscopic observations of living cells during freezing and thawing. *J Roy Micro Soc, 71:*186-195, 1951.
759. Smith, A. U., and Smiles, J.: Microscopic studies of mammalian tissues during cooling to and rewarming from −79 degrees C. *J Roy Micro Soc, 73:*134-139, 1953.
760. Stephenson, J. L.: Ice crystal growth during the rapid freezing of tissues. *J Biophys Bioch Cytol, 2:*45-52, 1956.
761. Stowell, R. E., Young, D. E., Arnold, E. A., and Trump, B. F.: Structural chemical and physical and functional alterations in mammalian nucleus following different conditions of freezing, storage and thawing. *Fed Proc, 24:*115-142, 1965.
762. Chilson, O. L., Costello, L., and Kaplan, N.: Effects of freezing on enzymes. *Fed Proc, 24:*55-65, 1965.
763. Fishbein, W. N., and Stowell, R. E.: Studies on the mechanism of freezing damage to mouse liver using a mitochondrial enzyme assay. I. Temporal localization of the injury phase during slow freezing. *Cryobiology, 4:*283-289, 1968.
764. Heber, U.: Freezing injury in relation to loss of enzyme activities and protection against freezing. *Cryobiology, 5:*188-201, 1968.
765. Lehmann, H.: Changes in enzymes at low temperatures, long-term preservation of blood. *Fed Proc, 24: Suppl. 15:*66-S-69, 1965.
766. Lovelock, J. E.: The denaturation of lipid-protein complexes as a cause of damage by freezing. *Proc R Soc B, 147:*427-433, 1957.
767. Mazur, P.: Physical and chemical changes during freezing and thawing of cell with special reference to blood cells. *Proc 11th Congr Int Soc Blood Trans,* Sydney, *No. 29,* 1966, pp. 764-777.
768. Mazur, P.: Physical-chemical factors underlying cell injury in cryosurgical freezing. In Rand, R. W., Rinfret, A. P., and Leden, H. (Eds.): *Cryosurgery.* Springfield, C. C Thomas, 1968, p. 32.
769. Smith, A. U.: *Biological Effects of Freezing and Supercooling.* London, Arnold, 1961.
770. Trump, B. F., Young, D. E., Arnold, E. A., and Stowell, R. E.: Effects of freezing and thawing on the structure, chemical constitution and functions of cytoplasmic structures. *Fed Proc, 24:*144-169, 1965.
771. Lovelock, J. E.: Hemolysis of thermal shock. *Brit J Haemat, 1:*117-129, 1955.
772. Lovelock, J. E.: Physical instability in thermal shock in red cells. *Nature, 173:*659-661, 1954.
773. Farrant, J.: Is there a common mechanism of protection of living cells by polyvinyl pyrrolidone and glycerol during freezing? *Nature* (London), *222:*1175, 1969.
774. Leibo, S. P., Farrant, J., Mazur, P., Hanna, M. G., and Smith, L. H.: Effects of freezing on marrow stem cell suspensions: Interactions of cooling and warming rates in the presence of PVP, sucrose or glycerol. *Cryobiology, 6:*315, 1970.
775. Lovelock, J. E.: The mechanism of the protective action of glycerol against haemolysis by freezing and thawing. *Biochem Biophys Acta, 11:*28, 1953.
776. Lovelock, J. E., and Bishop, M. W. H.: Prevention of freezing damage to living cells by dimethyl sulphoxide. *Nature* (London), *183:*1394, 1959.
777. Mazur, P., Leibo, S. P., Farrant, J., Chu, E. H. Y., Hanna, M. G., and Smith, L. H.: Interactions of cooling rate, warming rate and protective additive on the survival of frozen mammalian cells. In Wolstenholme, G. E. W. and O'Connor, M. (Eds.): *The Frozen Cell.* CIBA Foundation Symposium, Churchill, London, 1970, p. 69.
778. Persidsky, M., and Richards, V.: Mode of protection with polyvinyl Pyrrolidone in freezing of bone marrow. *Nature* (London), *196:*585, 1962.
779. Rapatz, G., and Luyet, B.: Effects of cooling rates on the preservation of erythrocytes in frozen blood containing various protective agents. *Biodynamica, 9:*333, 1965.
780. Rapatz, G., Sullivan, J. J., and Luyet, B.: Preservation of erythrocytes in blood

containing various protective agents, frozen at various rates and brought to a given final temperature. *Cryobiology, 5:*18, 1968.
781. Cahan, W. G.: Cryosurgery of malignant and benign tumors. *J St Barnabas Med Cent, 4:*285-294, 1967.
782. Kreyberg, L.: Local freezing. *Proc Roy Soc Biol, 147:*546-547, 1957.
783. Kreyberg, L.: Stasis and necrosis. *Scand J Clin Lab Invest, 15:*1-26, 1963.
784. Reite, O. B.: Functional qualities of small blood vessels in tissue injured by freezing and thawing. *Acta Physiol Scand, 63:*111-120, 1965.
785. Ablin, R. J., and Fontant, G.: Cryoimmunotherapy: Continuing studies toward determining a rational approach for assessing the candidacy of the prostatic cancer patient for cryoimmunotherapy and postoperative responsiveness. An interim report. *Cryobiology, 17:*170-177, 1980.
786. Ablin, R. J., Soanes, W. A., and Gonder, M. J.: Immunologic studies of the prostate: A review. *Internat Surg, 52:*8-21, 1969.
787. Bagley, D. H., and Faraci, R. P.: Tumor immunity following cryosurgery or electrocauterization. *Natl Cancer Inst Monogr, 49:*371-373, 1978.
788. Bonney, W. W., Henstorf, J. E., Emaus, S. P., Lubaroff, D. M., and Feldbush, T. L. Immunostimulation by cryosurgery: An orthotopic model of prostate and bladder cancer in the rat. *Natl Cancer Inst Monogr, 49:*375-381, 1978.
789. Bronson, P., Yantorno, C., Riera, C., and Shulman, S.: Cryo-immunology: The molecular classes in the antibody response. *Cryobiology, 3:*382, 1967.
790. Ghayasuddin, M., Zappi, E., and Shulman, S.: Cryoimmunization: Antibody response after sequential tissue freezing and injection of rabbit thyroid gland. *Cryobiology, 6:*262, 1969.
791. Gonder, M. J., Pfeiffer, L., Soanes, W. A., and Albin, R. J.: Prospects for cryoimmunotherapy in cases of metastasizing carcinoma of the prostate. *Cryobiology, 6:*26[illegible] 1969.
792. Menninger, F., Jr., Soanes, W. A., and Shulman, S.: Cryo-immunology: The antigen release following freezing. *Cryobiology, 3:*385, 1967.
793. Shulman, S.: Cryosurgery and autoimmunization: A critique. *J Cryosurg, 2:*84-8[illegible] 1969.
794. Shulman, S.: Cryo-immunology. Vance, R. W. and Weinstock, H. (Eds.): *Applications of Cryogenic Technology*. Los Angeles, Tinnon-Brown, Inc., 1969, pp. 130-131.
795. Shulman, S., Yantorno, C., and Bronson, P.: Cryoimmunology: A method of immunization to autologous tissue. *Proc Soc Exp Biol Med, 124:*658-661, 1967.
796. Yantorno, C., Gonder, M. J., Soanes, W. A., and Shulman, S.: The freezing of tissue during surgery and production of antibodies. *Fed Proc, 25:*731, 1966.
797. Conway, L. W., and Garcia, J. H.: Cryohypophysectomy. Postmortem findings in cases. *J Neurosurg, 32:*435-442, 1970.
798. Cooper, I. S.: Application of cryogenics to brain tumor surgery. Proceedings, 3 International Congress on Neurological Surgery, Copenhagen, 1965, pp. 7[illegible] 733.
799. Cooper, I. S., and Lee, A. S. J.: Cryothalamectomy-hypothermic congelation: technical advance in basal ganglia surgery. *J Amer Geriat Soc, 9:*714-718, 196[illegible]
800. Cooper, I. S., and Stellar, S.: Cryogenic freezing of brain tumors for excision destruction in situ. *J Neurosurg, 20:*921-930, 1963.
801. Dashe, A. M., Solomon, D. H., Rand, R. W., Frasier, S. D., Brown, J., and Spears, Stereotaxic hypophyseal cryosurgery in acromegaly and other disorders. *JAM[illegible] 198:*591-596, 1966.
802. Gye, R. S., Stanworth, P. A., Stewart, J. A., and Adams, C. B.: Cryohypophysecto[illegible] for bone pain of metastatic breast cancer. *Pain, 6:*201-206, 1979.

303. Rand, R. W.: Cryohypophysectomy in pituitary tumors with comments on radical pituitary tumor excision using microneurosurgical technique. Proc. III Internat. Cong. of Neurol. Surg. Copenhagen, August 23-28, 1965. *Excerpta International Congress Series, 110:*783-793, 1965.
304. Barton, T.: Cryosurgical treatment of nasopharyngeal neoplasm. *Am Surg, 32:*744, 1966.
305. Barton, T.: Cryosurgery in nose and throat tumors. *JAMA, 204:*570, 1968.
306. Cutt, R. A., Wolfson, R. J., Ishiyama, E., Rothwarf, F., and Myers: Preliminary results with experimental cryosurgery of the labyrinth. *Arch Otolaryng, 82:*147-155, 1965.
307. Hill, C. L.: Preliminary report on cryosurgery in otolaryngology. *Laryngoscope, 76:*109, 1966.
308. Hill, C. L.: Cryosurgical tonsillectomy, an evaluation. *Arch Otolaryng, 87:*434, 1968.
309. Lewis, J. S., and Cahan, W. G.: Cryosurgical management of glomus jugulare tumors. *Laryngoscope, 77:*912-917, 1967.
310. Manigera, A. J., Mazzarella, L. A., Minkowitz, S., and Moskowitz, H.: Maxillary sinus angiofibroma treated with cryosurgery. *Arch Otolaryng, 89:*527, 1969.
311. Miller, D.: Three years experience with cryosurgery in head and neck tumors. *Ann Otol Rhinol & Laryng, 78:*786, 1969.
312. Neel, H. B., 3rd: Cryosurgery for the treatment of cancer. *Laryngoscope, 90:*1-48, 1980.
313. Von Leden, H., and Rand, R. W.: Cryosurgery of the mouth, nose and throat. *Trans Amer Acad Ophthalm & Otolaryng, 70:*890, 1966.
314. Weaver, W. W., and Smith, D. B.: Selection of patients for cryosurgical treatment of oral pharyngeal cancer. *J Cryosurgery, 2:*53, 1969.
315. Zacarian, S. A.: Cryotherapy for head and neck tumors. *Compr Ther, 5:*48-54, 1979.
316. Wolfson, R. J., Cutt, R. A., Ishiyama, E., and Myers, D.: Cryosurgery of the labyrinth-preliminary report of a new surgical procedure. *Laryngoscope, 76:*733-757, 1966.
317. Hansen, R. I., and Lund, F. I.: Cryosurgery of the prostate. *Urol Int, 24:*160-165, 1969.
318. Jordan, W. P., Walker, D., Miller, G. H., and Drylie, D. M.: Cryotherapy of benign and neoplastic tumors of the prostate. *Surg Gynec Obstet, 125:*1265-1267, 1967.
319. Kaplan, J. H., and Kaplan, I.: Cryogenic, electro coagulative and spontaneous necrosis of a bladder neoplasma: A preliminary comparative study. *J Urol, 95:*531-535, 1966.
320. McDonald, J. H., Taylor, C. B., and Heckel, N. J.: Rapid freezing of the bladder. *J Urol, 64:*326, 1950.
321. Soanes, W. A., and Gonder, M. J.: Use of cryosurgery in prostatic cancer. *J Urol, 99:*793-797, 1968.
322. Abadir, D. M.: Combined curettage and cryosurgery for treatment of epithelial cancers of the skin. *J Dermatol Surg Oncol, 6:*633-635, 1980.
323. Grimmett, H.: Liquid nitrogen therapy: Histological observations. *Arch Derm, 83:*563-567, 1961.
324. Irvine, H. G., and Turnacliff, D. D.: Liquid oxygen in dermatology. *Arch Derm, 19:*270, 1929.
325. Martins, O., Oliveira, A. D. S., Picoto, A. D. S., and Verde, S. F.: Cryosurgery of large tumors on the dorsa of hands. *J Dermatol Surg Oncol, 6:*568-570, 1980.
326. Torre, D.: Cutaneous cryosurgery. *J Cryosurgery, 1:*202-209, 1968.
327. Zacarian, S. A., and Adham, M. I.: Cryotherapy of cutaneous malignancy. *Cryobiology, 2:*212-218, 1966.
328. Allen, E. E., McGill, J. I., Hall, V. L., Bodkin, R. E., MacDonald, H., Buchanan, R. B.,

White, J. E., Leppard, B. J., Goodwin, P. S., and Fraser, J.: Cryotherapy of basal cell lesions. *Trans Ophthalmol Soc U K, 99:*264-268, 1979.

829. Bellows, J. G.: *Cryotherapy of Ocular Diseases.* Philadelphia, J. B. Lippincott Co., 1966.
830. Bellows, J. G.: Cryotherapy of herpes virus keratitis in 1242 cases. *Int Surg, 50:*489-494, 1968.
831. Bellows, J. G.: Cryoextraction of cataracts in 800 consecutive cases. *Cryobiology, 6:*259-260, 1969.
832. Fraunfelder, F. T., Zacarian, S. A., Limmer, B. L., and Windfield, D.: Cryosurgery for malignancies of the eyelid. *Ophthalmology, 87:*461-465, 1980.
833. Kellman, C. D., and Cooper, I. S.: Cryogenic ophthalmic surgery. *Am J Ophth, 56:*737, 1963.
834. Krwawicz, T.: Intracapsular extraction of intumescent cataract by application of low temperature. *Brit J Ophth, 45:*279, 1961.
835. Norton, W. D.: *Cryotherapy in Retinal Detachment Surgery.* Symposium on Retina and Retinal Surgery. Trans New Orleans Academy of Ophth. St. Louis, C. V. Mosby Co., 1969.
836. Polack, F. M., and DeRoeth, A., Jr.: Effects of freezing on the ciliary body (cyclocryotherapy). *Invest Ophth, 3:*164, 1964.
837. Soll, D. B., and Harrison, S. E.: Basic concepts and an overview of cryosurgery in ophthalmic plastic surgery. *Ophthalmic Surg, 10:*31-36, 1979.
838. Uhlschmid, G., Kolb, E., and Largiader, F.: Cryosurgery of pulmonary metastases. *Cryobiology, 16:*171-178, 1979.
839. Cahan, W. G.: Cryosurgery of the uterus: Description of technique and potential applications. *Am J Obstet Gynecol, 88:*410-414, 1964.
840. Cahan, W. G., and Brouckunier, A., Jr.: Cryosurgery of the uterine cavity. *Am J Obst & Gynec, 99:*138-153, 1967.
841. Crisp, E. E., Asadourian, L., and Romberger, W.: Application of cryosurgery to gynecologic malignancy. *Obst & Gynec, 30:*668-753, 1967.
842. Hemmingsson, E., Stendahl, U., and Stenson, S.: Cryosurgical treatment of cervical intraepithelial neoplasia with follow-up of five to eight years. *Am J Obstet Gynecol, 139:*144-147, 1981.
843. Ostergard, D. R., Townsend, D. E., and Hirose, F. M.: The treatment of chronic cervicitis by cryotherapy. *Am J Obst & Gynec, 103:*426, 1968.
844. Ostergard, D. R., and Townsend, E.: The treatment of vulvar condyloma acuminata by cryosurgery. *Cryobiology, 5:*340-342, 1969.
845. Richart, R. M., Townsend, D. E., Crisp, W., Depetrillo, A., Ferenczy, A., Johnson, G., Lickrich, G., Roy, M., and Villasanta, U.: Cervical intraepithelial neoplasia treated by cryotherapy. *Am J Obstet Gynecol, 137:*823-826, 1980.
846. Tronstad, S. E., and Kirschner, R.: Treatment of cervical intraepithelial neoplasia with local excisional biopsy and cryosurgery. *Acta Obstet Gynecol Scand, 59:*349-353, 1980.
847. Weitzner, K.: The treatment of endocervicitis with carbon dioxide snow (dry ice). *Am J Surg, 48:*620-624, 1940.
848. Emmings, F. G., Koepf, S. W., and Gage, A. A.: Cryotherapy for benign lesions of the oral cavity. *J Oral Surg, 25:*320, 1967.
849. Emmings, F. G., Neider, M. E., and Green, G. W., Jr.: Freezing the mandible without excision. *J Oral Surg, 24:*145-155, 1966.
850. Gage, A. A.: Cryosurgery for oral cancer. *JAMA, 204:*565-569, 1968.
851. Gage, A. A., Koepf, S. W., Wehrle, D., and Emmings, F. G.: Cryotherapy for cancer of the lip and oral cavity. *Cancer, 18:*1646, 1965.

852. Sako, K., Marchetta, F. C., and Hayes, R. L.: Evaluation of cryosurgery in the treatment of intraoral leukoplakia. *J Cryosurgery, 2:*239, 1969.

853. Gage, A. A., and Erickson, R. B.: Cryotherapy and curettage for bone tumors. *J Cryosurg, 1:*60-66, 1968.

854. Hoekstra, H. J., Schraffordt, K. H., Oeseburg, H. B., and Oldhoff, J.: Two extensive giant cell tumours of the proximal humerus treated by resection-reconstruction or excochleation;cryosurgery. *Arch Chir Neerl, 31:*49-55, 1979.

855. Marcove, R. C., Lyden, J. P., Huvos, A. G., and Bullough, P. G.: Giant cell tumors treated by cryosurgery. *J Bone & Joint Surg, 55-A:*1633, 1973.

856. Marcove, R. C., and Miller, T. R.: Treatment of primary and metastatic bone tumors by cryosurgery. *JAMA, 207:*1890, 1969.

857. Marcove, R. C., and Miller, T. R.: The treatment of primary and metastatic localized bone tumors by cryosurgery. *Surg Clin No Amer, 49:*2, 1969.

858. Marcove, R. C., Miller, T. R., and Cahen, W. C.: The treatment of primary and metastatic bone tumors by repetitive freezing. *Bull N Y Acad Med, 44:*532, 1968.

859. Marcove, R. C., Stovell, P. B., Huvos, A. G., and Bullough, P. B.: The use of cryosurgery in the treatment of low and medium grade chondrosarcoma — A preliminary report. *Clin Orthop, 122:*147, 1977.

860. Marcove, R. C., Weis, L. D., Vaghaiwalla, M. R., and Pearson, R.: Cryosurgery in the treatment of giant cell tumors of bone: A report of 52 consecutive cases. *Clin Orthop, 134:*275-289, 1978.

861. Artz, C. P., McFarland, J. B., and Barnett, W. O.: Clinical evaluation of gastric freezing for peptic ulcer. *Ann Surg, 159:*758-764, 1964.

862. Cooper, I. S., and Hirose, T.: Cryogenic hepatic surgery. *J Cryosurg, 1:*116-122, 1968.

863. Gage, A. A.: Cryotherapy for inoperable rectal cancer. *Dis Colon Rectum, 11:*36-44, 1968.

864. Lewis, M. T., DeLacruz, T., Gazzaniga, D. A., and Ball, T.: Cryosurgical hemorrhoidectomy: Preliminary report. *Dis Colon Rectum, 12:*371-378, 1969.

865. Myers, R. S., Hammond, W. G., and Ketchem, A. S.: Cryosurgical necrosis of the head of the pancreas. *Ann Surg, 171:*413-418, 1970.

866. Ruffin, J. M.: Gastric "freezing": The life and death of a myth. *Hospital Practice,* pp. 57-63, 1970.

867. Sobel, S., Kaplitt, M. J., Halligan, J. C., and Sawyer, P. N.: Development of cryosurgical instrument for removal of obstructive atherosclerotic cores. *J Cryosurgery, 1:* 295-298, 1968.

868. Busch, W.: Uber den einfluss welchen heftigere erysipels zu weilen auf organistierte neubildungen ausueben. *Verhandl Naturh Preuss Thein Westphal, 23:*28-30, 1866.

869. Bruns, P.: Die Heilwirung des Erysipels auf geschwulste. *Beitr Klin Chir, 3:*443-466, 1887.

870. Coley, W. B.: The treatment of malignant tumors by repeated inoculations of erysipelas with a report of original cases. *Am J Med Sci, 105:*487-512, 1893.

871. Westermark, F.: Uber die Behandlung des ulcerirended cerix Carcinomas. Mittle Konstanter Warme. *Zbl Gynak, 20:*1335-1339, 1898.

872. Warren, S. L.: Preliminary study of the effect of artificial fever upon hopeless tumor cases. *Am J Roentgen, 33:*75-87, 1935.

873. Suer, R. P., Fisher, W. B., Pearson, R. W., and Triplett, D. A.: Burkitt's lymphoma: Tumor lysis following malignant hyperthermia. *Cancer Treat Rep, 64:*327-330, 1980.

874. Hornback, N. B., Shupe, R. E., Shidnia, H., Joe, B. T., Sayoc, E., Marshall, C.: Preliminary clinical results of combined 433 megahertz microwave therapy on patients with advanced cancer. *Cancer, 40:*2854-2863, 1977.

875. Kopecky, W. J., and Perez, C. A.: A microwave hyperthermia treatment and thermometry system. *Int J Radiat Oncol Biol Phys, 5:*2113-2115, 1979.
876. Luk, K. H.: Microwave hyperthermia at 2450 and 915 megahertz frequencies. *Henry Ford Hospital Med J, 29:*28-31, 1981.
877. Mendecki, J., Friedenthal, E., Botstein, C., Sterzer, F., Paglione, R., Nowogrodzki, M., and Beck, E.: Microwave-induced hyperthermia in cancer treatment: Apparatus and preliminary results. *Int J Radiat Oncol Biol Phys, 4:*1095-1103, 1978.
878. Noell, K. T., Woodward, K. T., Worde, B. T., Fishburn, R. I., and Miller, L. S.: Microwave-induced local hyperthermia in combination with radiotherapy of human malignant tumors. *Cancer, 45:*638-646, 1980.
879. Perez, C. A., Kopecky, W., Baglan, R., Rao, D. V., and Johnson, R.: Local microwave hyperthermia in cancer therapy. *Henry Ford Hospital Med J, 29:*16-23, 1981.
880. Sandhu, T. S., Kowal, H., and Johnson, R. J.: The development of microwave hyperthermia applicators. *Int J Radiat Oncol Biol Phys, 4:*515-519, 1978.
881. Holt, J. A. G.: The use of V.H.F. radiowaves in cancer therapy. *Austral Radiol, 19:*223-241, 1975.
882. Ishda, T., Kato, H., Miyakoshi, J., Furukawa, M., Ohsaki, S., and Kano, E.: Physical basis of RF hyperthermia for cancer therapy. 1. Measurement for distribution in absorbed power from radiofrequency exposure in Agar Phantom. *J Radiat Res* (Tokyo), *21:*180-189, 1980.
883. Leveen, H. H., Wapnick, S., Piccone, V., Falk, G., and Ahmed, N.: Tumor eradication by radiofrequency therapy. Response in 21 patients. *JAMA, 235:*2198-2200, 1976.
884. Sternhagen, C. J., Doss, J. D., Day, P. W., Edwards, W. S., Doberneck, R. C., Herzon, F. S., Powell, T. D., O'Brien, G. F., and Larkin, J. J.: Clinical radiofrequency current in oral cavity carcinomas and metastatic malignancies with continuous temperature control and monitoring. In Strefter, C. (Ed.): *Proceedings of Second Annual International Symposium on Cancer Therapy by Hyperthermia and Radiation.* Baltimore, Urban & Schwarzenberg, Inc., 1978, pp. 331-334.
885. Storm, F. K., Harrison, W. H., Elliott, R. S., Hatziethefilou, C., and Morton, D. L.: Human hyperthermic therapy: Relationship between tumor type and capacity to induce hyperthermia by radiofrequency. *Am J Surg, 138:*170-174, 1979.
886. Har-Kedar, I., and Bleehen, N. M.: Experimental and clinical aspects of hyperthermia applied to the treatment of cancer with special reference to the role of ultrasonic and microwave heating. Lett, J. T., Adler, H., and Felle, M. (Eds.): *Advances in Radiation Biology,* Vol. VI. New York, Academic Press, 1976, pp. 228-266.
887. Lele, P. P.: Induction of deep, local hyperthermia by ultrasound and electromagnetic fields: Problems and choices. *Radiat Environ Biophys, 17:*205-217, 1980.
888. Marmor, J. B., and Hahn, G. M.: Ultrasound heating in previously irradiated sites. *Int J Radiat Oncol Biol Phys, 4:*1029-1032, 1978.
889. Marmor, J. B., Pounds, D., Postic, T. B., and Hahn, G. M.: Treatment of superficial human neoplasms by local hyperthermia induced by ultrasound. *Cancer, 43:*188-197, 1979.
890. Schwan, H. P.: Electromagnetic and ultrasonic induction of hyperthermia in tissue-like substances. *Radiat Environ Biophys, 17:*189-203, 1980.
891. Ter Haar, G., Stratford, I. J., and Hill, C. R.: Ultrasonic irradiation of mammalian cells *in vitro* at hyperthermic temperatures. *Br J Radiol, 53:*784-789, 1980.
892. Cavaliere, R., Moricca, G., DiFilippo, F., Aloe, L., Monticelli, G., and Santori, F. S.: Hyperthermic perfusion 16 years after its clinical applications. *Henry Ford Hospital Med J, 29:*32-36, 1981.

893. Cavaliere, R., Moricca, G., DiFilippo, F., Caputo, A., Santori, F. S., and Monticelli, G.: Heat transfer problems during local perfusion in cancer treatment. *Ann N Y Acad Sci, 335:*311, 1980.
894. Englund, N. E., Hallbrook, T., and Leng, L.: Skin and muscle blood flow during regional perfusion with hyperthermal perfusate. *Scand J Thorac Cardiovasc Surg, 8:*77-79, 1974.
895. Spratt, J. S., Adcock, R. A., Sherrill, W., and Travathen, S.: Hyperthermic peritoneal perfusion system in canines. *Cancer Res, 40:*253-255, 1980.
896. Bull, J. M., Lees, D., Schuette, W., Whang-Peng, J., Smith, R., Bynum, G., Atkinson, E. R., Gottdiener, J. S., Gralnick, H. R., Shawker, T. H., and DeVita, V. T., Jr.: Whole body hyperthermia: A phase-I trial of a potential adjuvant to chemotherapy. *Ann Intern Med, 90:*317-323, 1979.
897. Cole, D. R., Pung, J., Kim, Y. D., Berman, R. A., and Cole, D. F.: Systemic thermotherapy (whole body hyperthermia). *Int J Clin Pharmacol Biopharm, 17:*329-333, 1979.
898. DuBois, M., Sato, S., Lees, D. E., Bull, J. M., Smith, R., White, B. G., Moore, H., and Macnamara, T. E.: Electroencephalographic changes during whole body hyperthermia in humans. *Electroencephalogr Clin Neurophysiol, 50:*486-495, 1980.
899. Grogan, J. B., Parks, L. C., and Minaberry, D.: Polymorphonuclear leukocyte function in cancer patients treated with total body hyperthermia. *Cancer, 45:*2611-2615, 1980.
900. Larkin, J. M., Edwards, W. S., and Smith, D. E.: Total body hyperthermia and preliminary results in human neoplasms. *Surg. Forum, 27:*121-122, 1976.
901. Lees, D. E., Kim, Y. D., Bull, J. M., Whang-Peng, J., Schuette, W., Smith, R., and MacNamara, T. E.: Anesthetic management of whole-body hyperthermia for the treatment of cancer. *Anesthesiology, 52:*418-428, 1980.
902. Pettigrew, R. T., Galt, J. M., Ludgate, C. M., and Smith, A. N.: Clinical effects of whole body hyperthermia in advanced malignancy. *Br Med J, 4:*679-682, 1974.
903. Bicher, H. I., Hetzel, F. W., Sandhu, T. S., Frinak, S., Vaupel, P., O'Hara, M. D., and O'Brien, T.: Effects of hyperthermia on normal and tumor microenvironment. *Radiology, 137:*523-530, 1980.
904. Cavaliere, R., Ciocatto, E. C., Giovanella, B. C., Heidelberger, C., Johnson, R. O., Margottini, M., Mondovi, B., Moricca, G., and Rossi-Fanelli, A.: Selective heat sensitivity for cancer cells. *Cancer Philad, 20:*1351-1381, 1967.
905. Dickson, J. A.: Hyperthermia in the treatment of cancer. *Lancet, 1:*202-205, 1979.
906. Field, S. B., and Bleehen, N. M.: Hyperthermia in the treatment of cancer. *Cancer Treat Rev, 6:*63-94, 1979.
907. Giovanella, B. C., Mosti, R., and Heidelberger, C.: Biochemical and biological effects of heat on normal and neoplastic cells. *Proc Ann Assoc Cancer Res, 10:*28, 1969.
908. Hartman, J. R., and Crile, G., Jr.: Heat treatment of osteogenic sarcoma. Report of 5 cases. *Clin Orthop, 61:*269-276, 1968.
909. Henle, K. J., and Dethlefsen, L. A.: Heat fractination and thermotolerance: A review. *Cancer Res, 38:*1843, 1978.
910. Hidvegi, E. J., Yatvin, M. B., Dennis, W. H., and Hidvegi, E.: Effect of altered membrane lipid composition and procaine on hyperthermic killing of ascites tumor cells. *Oncology, 37:*360-363, 1980.
911. Kim, S. H., Kim, J. H., and Hahn, E. W.: The radiosensitization of hypoxic tumor cells by hyperthermia. *Radiology, 114:*727-728, 1975.
912. Mondovi, B., Finaizi, A. A., Rotilio, G., Strom, R., Moricca, G., Rossi-Fanelli, A.: The biochemical mechanism of selective heat sensitivity of cancer cells. II. Studies of nucleic acids and protein synthesis. *Europ J Cancer, 5:*137-146, 1969.

913. Muckle, D. S., and Dickson, J. A.: The selective inhibitory effect of hyperthermia on the metabolism and growth of malignant cells. *Br J Cancer, 15:*771-778, 1978.
914. Nielsen, O. S., and Overgaard, J.: Hyperthermic radiosensitization of thermotolerant tumor cells *in vitro. Int J Radiat Biol, 35:*171-176, 1979.
915. Schrek, R.: Sensitivity of normal and leukemic lymphocytes and leukemic myeloblasts to heat. *J Nat Cancer Inst, 37:*649-654, 1966.
916. Shibata, H. R., and MacLean, L. D.: Blood flow to tumors. *Prog Clin Cancer, 2:*33-47, 1966.
917. Stewart, F., and Denekamp, J.: Tumour responses to hyperthermia and the therapeutic ratio. *Br J Radiol, 51:*73, 1977.
918. Strom, R., Scioscia, Santoro A., Grifo, C., Bozzi, A., Mondovi, B., and Rossi-Fanelli, A.: The biochemical mechanism of selective heat sensitivity of cancer cells. IV. Inhibition of RNA synthesis. *Europ J Cancer, 9:*103-112, 1973.
919. Suit, H. D.: Hyperthermic effects on animal tissues. *Radiology, 123:*483, 1977.
920. Wallach, D. F. H.: Basic mechanisms in tumor thermotherapy. *J Molec Med, 2:*381, 1971.
921. Willnow, V.: Autoradiographic study on the effect of hyperthermia (42.5 degrees C) on the proliferation kinetics of solid tumors in children. *Neoplasma, 27:*47-53, 1980.
922. Eden, M., Haines, B., and Kahler, H.: The pH of rat tumors measured *in vivo. J Natl Cancer Inst, 16:*541-556, 1955.
923. Meyer, K. A., Kammerling, E. M., Amtman, L., Koller, M., and Hoffman, S. J.: pH studies of malignant tissues in human beings. *Cancer Res, 8:*513-518, 1948.
924. Gerweck, L. E.: Modification of cell lethality at elevated temperatures. The pH effect. *Radiat Res, 70:*224-235, 1977.
925. Gerweck, L. E., and Rottinger, E.: Enhancement of mammalian cell sensitivity to hyperthermia by pH alteration. *Radiat Res, 67:*508-511, 1976.
926. Gullino, P. M., Grantham, F. H., Smith, S. H., and Haggerty, A. C.: Modifications of the acid-base status of the internal milieu of tumors. *J Nat Cancer Inst, 34:*857-860, 1965.
927. Nawslund, J., and Swenson, K. E.: Investigations on the pH of malignant tumours in mice and humans after administration of glucose. *Acta Obstet Gynecol Scand, 32:*359-367, 1953.
928. Overgaard, J.: Influence of extracellular pH on the viability and morphology of tumor cells exposed to hyperthermia. *J Natl Cancer Inst, 56:*1243-1250, 1976.
929. Streffer, C., Hengstebeck, S., and Tamulevicus, P.: Glucose metabolism in mouse tumor and liver with or without hyperthermia. *Henry Ford Hospital Med J, 29:*41-44, 1981.
930. Arcangeli, G., and Cividalli, A.: Local hyperthermia and radiation: A biologically-oriented clinical scheduling. *Henry Ford Hosp Med J, 29:*37-40, 1981.
931. Bicher, H. I., Sandhu, T. S., and Hetzel, F. W.: Hyperthermia and radiation in combination. A clinical fractionation regime. *Int J Radiat Oncol Biol Phys, 6:*867-870, 1980.
932. Bicher, H. I., Sandhu, T. S., and Hetzel, F. W.: Clinical thermoradiotherapy. *Henry Ford Hosp Med J, 29:*10-15, 1981.
933. Brenner, H. J., and Yerushalmi, A.: Combined local hyperthermia and x-irradiation in the treatment of metastatic tumors. *Br J Cancer, 33:*91-95, 1975.
934. Bruckner, V.: Combination of radiosensitizers and hyperthermia in tumour radiotherapy. *S Afr Med J, 59:*116-117, 1981.
935. Dewey, W. C., Hopowood, L. E., Sapareto, S. A., and Gerweck, L. E.: Cellular

responses to combinations of hyperthermia and radiation. *Radiology, 123:*463-474, 1977.

936. Hymmen, U., and Wieland, C.: Combined treatment of radioresistant malignant tumors with high frequency hyperthermia and gamma-rays therapy — recent results. *J Microwave Power, 14:*173-180, 1979.
937. Kim, J. H., Hahn, E. W., and Benjamin, F. J.: Treatment of superficial cancers by combination hyperthermia and radiation therapy. *Clin Bull, 9:*13-16, 1979.
938. Johnson, R. J. R., Sandhu, T. S., Hetzel, F. W., Kowal, H. S., Bicher, H. I., and Song, S.: A pilot study to investigate the therapeutic ratio of hyperthermia 41.5 degrees — 42.0 degrees C. and radiation. *Int. J Radiat Oncol Biol Phys, 5:*947-954, 1979.
939. Lunec, J., and Parker, R.: The influence of pH on the enhancement of radiation damage by hyperthermia. *Int J Radiat Biol, 38:*567-574, 1980.
940. Robinson, J. E., Eizenberg, M. J., and McCready, W. A.: Radiation and hyperthermia response of normal tissue in situ. *Radiology, 113:*195-198, 1974.
941. Saparreto, S. A., Raaphorst, P. G., and Dewey, W. C.: Cell killing and the sequencing of hyperthermia and radiation. *Int J Radiol Oncol Biol Phys, 5:*343-347, 1979.
942. Thrall, D. E., Gerweck, L. E., Gilette, E. L., and Dewey, W. C.: Effects of hyperthermia on the x-ray response of cells and tissues *in vivo* and *in vitro.* Lett, J., Adler, H., and Zelle, M. R. (Eds.): *Advances in Radiation Biology.* New York, Academic Press, 1976, Vol. VI, pp. 211-227.
943. Streffer, C. (Ed.): *Cancer Therapy by Hyperthermia and Radiation.* Baltimore, Urban & Schwarzenberg, 1978.
944. Westra, A., and Dewey, W. C.: Variation in sensitivity to heat shock during the cell cycle of Chinese hamster cells *in vitro. Int J Radiat Biol, 19:*467-477, 1971.
945. Barlogie, B., Corry, P. M., and Drewinko, B.: *In vitro* thermochemotherapy of human colon cancer cells with Cis-Dichlorodiammine platinum (II) and Mitomycin C. *Cancer Res, 40:*1165-1168, 1980.
946. Barlogie, B., Corry, P. M., Yip, E., Lippman, L., Johnston, D. A., Khalil, K., Tenczynski, T. F., Reilly, E., Lawson, R., Dosik, G., Rigor, B., Hawkenson, R., and Freireich, E. J.: Total-body hyperthermia with and without chemotherapy for advanced human neoplasms. *Cancer Res, 39:*1481-1485, 1979.
947. Hahn, G. M.: Potential for therapy of drugs and hyperthermia. *Cancer Res, 39:*2264-2268, 1979.
948. Hahn, G. M., Braun, J., and Har-Kedar, I.: Thermochemotherapy: Synergy between hyperthermia (42-43 degrees C.) and Adriamycin (or Bleomycin) in mammalian cell inactivation. *Proc Natl Acad Sci, 72:*937-940, 1975.
949. Kim, Y. D., Lees, D. E., Lake, C. R., Whang-Peng, J., Schuette, W., Smith, R., and Bull, J.: Hyperthermia potentiates Doxorubicin-related cardiotoxic effects. *JAMA, 241:*1816-1817, 1979.
950. Kowal, C. D., and Bertino, J. R.: Possible benefits of hyperthermia to chemotherapy. *Cancer Res, 39:*2285-2289, 1979.
951. Palzer, R. J., and Heidelberger, C.: Influence of drugs and synchrony on the hyperthermic killing of hela cells. *Cancer Res, 33:*422-427, 1973.
952. Goldenberg, D. M., and Langner, M.: Direct and abscopal antitumor action of local hyperthermia. *Z Naturforsch, 266:*359-361, 1971.

Chapter 2

Metastasis

INCIDENCE

METASTATIC TUMORS are undoubtedly the most frequently occurring malignant tumors of the spine. The great majority of them are comprised of carcinomas instead of sarcomas.[1-33] According to several relatively large autopsy series,[34-40] the overall incidence of spinal metastasis ranges from 15.6 percent to 41 percent. The studies also show that the most common metastatic tumor of the spine is breast carcinoma, which is closely trailed by prostatic carcinoma. Carcinomas from lung, colon, kidney, stomach, bladder, uterus, thyroid, etc., show less tendency to metastasize to the spine than breast and prostatic carcinomas. The ratio of bone metastases to primary bone tumors throughout the body is about twenty-five to one.

Metastatic tumors can reach the spine by three routes, namely, the vertebral venous system, the systemic circulation and direct extension. By means of intravascular injection technique, Batson (1940 and 1942)[41-42] and Codman and DeLong (1951)[43] had shown that in both human cadavers and experimental animals the vertebral venous system is a network of valveless veins around the spinal dura mater and vertebrae. This network has direct connections with the major portion of the body and provides bypasses for the caval, azygos, portal, and pulmonary venous systems. Increased intrathoracic or intrabdominal pressure, for example, can force the blood to flow from the superior and inferior vena cava into the vertebral venous system where the sluggish blood flow in the many venous pools makes it easy for tumor cells to take root and multiply in the spinal column. In addition, owing to the fact that the spinal column is composed of vertebrae with red bone marrow in which a rich sinusoid system is present, the endothelium of these sinusoids have larger than normal openings to facilitate the entrance of blood cells produced in the marrow space to enter the systemic circulation, but also encourage the influx of circulating tumor cells into the spinal intraosseous space.

The tumor cells that spread via the systemic circulation must first pass through the pulmonary artery and vein and undoubtedly contribute to the high incidence of pulmonary metastases and eventually settle in the spine through the nutrient arteries and haversian and Volkmann blood vessels.

The lack of direct communication between Batson's plexus and the portions of upper and lower extremities distal to the elbow and knee joints accounts for the infrequent occurrence of metastases to these regions. However, eleven cases of metastatic tumors to the hand and the foot have been seen at Henry Ford Hospital and were reported in three separate articles.[44-46] Furthermore, tumors arising from soft tissues adjacent to the spine can invade the spine by direct extension. For examples, we had encountered a large embryonal rhabdomyosarcoma of the erector spinae muscle which invaded the lumbar spinal canal through one of the lumbar intervertebral foramina. Scott (1952)[47] reported a pancreatic carcinoma with direct involvement of the spine, and Jarvis (1960)[48] described a case of sacral destruction caused by a recurrent rectal carcinoma.

On a statistical basis, different metastatic tumors predilect different age groups. For instances, under the age of five, neuroblastoma accounts for the majority of metastatic bone lesions. From age five to young adulthood, leukemia, osteosarcoma, malignant lymphomas, and Ewing's sarcoma are frequently the causes of metastatic bone diseases. However, after the age of forty, metastatic carcinomas and multiple myeloma are usually responsible for producing malignant bone lesions.

CLINICAL SYMPTOMS AND SIGNS

In the diagnosis of metastatic spinal tumors, a careful history taking is of the utmost importance because recent past history of cancer surgery plus the presence of constitutional symptoms such as weight loss, fever of unknown origin, malaise, night sweats, generalized weakness, anorexia, ease of fatigue, etc., strongly suggest the possible presence of widespread metastases. The most common complaint of spinal metastasis is back pain, which is often present in the thoracolumbar region and much less frequently in the cervical area.

Spinal cord or nerve compression can be caused by pathologic fracture of the tumor-riddled vertebral bodies or by epidural, subdural, or intramedullary metastatic involvements[49-68] which can produce hypesthesia, paresthesia, paresis, paralysis, muscle atrophy, muscle fasciculation, abnormal relfexes, clonus, kyphosis of the spine with gibbus formation, scoliosis, palpable paraspinal tumor mass, loss of coordination of upper and lower extremities, bowel and bladder disturbances, etc. The onset of these clinical symptoms can be gradual or abrupt and their progression likewise can be slow or rapid, depending on the nature of the tumor, its growth rate and the effectiveness of the patient's intrinsic defense mechanisms. As a general rule, metastatic tumors that produce osteolytic spinal lesions are more capable of bringing about vertebral collapse than the comparable tumors with osteoblastic spinal metastasis. Hypercalcemia caused by extensive skeletal metastases can produce polyuria, polydipsia, anorexia, depression, and even coma.

LABORATORY STUDIES

Anemia caused by bleedings and depressed hematopoiesis is probably the most common laboratory finding in widespread metastases. Leukocytosis, hyperuricemia, and elevated erythrocyte sedimentation rate can be brought about by tissue destruction by the primary tumors, their metastases, and the tumor-related infections. Extensive bone metastases, especially the osteolytic variety, can produce hypercalcemia,[69-81] hypercalciuria, hyperhydroxyprolinuria,[82-92] and elevated serum alkaline phosphatase[93-97] due to dissolution of the inorganic and organic matrix of bone. Impaired kidney function manifested in elevated serum BUN, creatinine and abnormal urinalysis can be caused by primary and metastatic neoplastic diseases of the kidney,[98-102] or by nephrocalcinosis secondary to metastasis-induced hypercalcemia. Sometimes, renal adenocarcinoma can produce a parathyroid hormone-like substance which is capable of producing hypercalcemia and metabolic alkalosis.[103-104] In addition, elevation of serum transaminases, hypoglycemia, and hyperbilirubinema in association with primary or metastatic pancreatic malignancies;[105-114] elevated liver enzymes, hypoglycemia, and hyperbilirubinemia in primary carcinoma of liver and liver metastases;[115-121] rise in serum acid phosphatase in primary and metastatic prostatic carcinoma;[122-128] increased serum and urinary catecholamines in primary and metastatic neuroblastoma, pheochromocytoma, paraganglioma, etc.,[129-137] are some of the other abnormal laboratory findings. When leptomeningeal metastasis is present, cerebrospinal fluid analysis may reveal the presence of carcinoma or sarcoma cells in addition to elevated CSF protein content below the level of myelographic block due to CSF stasis or secretion of protein by the tumor cells.

ROENTGENOGRAPHIC MANIFESTATIONS

Generally speaking, metastatic spinal tumors tend to be multifocal, but some of them such as renal and thyroid carcinomas often appear as solitary metastases prior to the discovery of their primary sites. Spinal metastases can have either an osteolytic or osteoblastic appearance or a mixture of both. In spite of the fact that the general appearance of bone metastases from a particular metastatic tumor is usually fairly uniform throughout the skeleton, e.g. generalized osteoblastic or osteolytic metastases, the same metastases may sometimes appear to be osteolytic in one or more bones and osteoblastic or mixed in the other parts of the same skeleton.

As a rule of thumb, the majority of metastatic tumors of mammary, pulmonary, renal, thyroid, colonic, and uterine origin tend to be osteolytic in nature (Figures 2-1 to 2-7). On the other hand, metastatic prostatic, gastric and pancreatic carcinomas, medulloblastoma, carcinoid tumors, osteoblastic osteogenic sarcoma, parosteal osteosarcoma, etc., are frequently osteoblastic in appearance[138-148] (Figures 2-8 to 2-10). However,

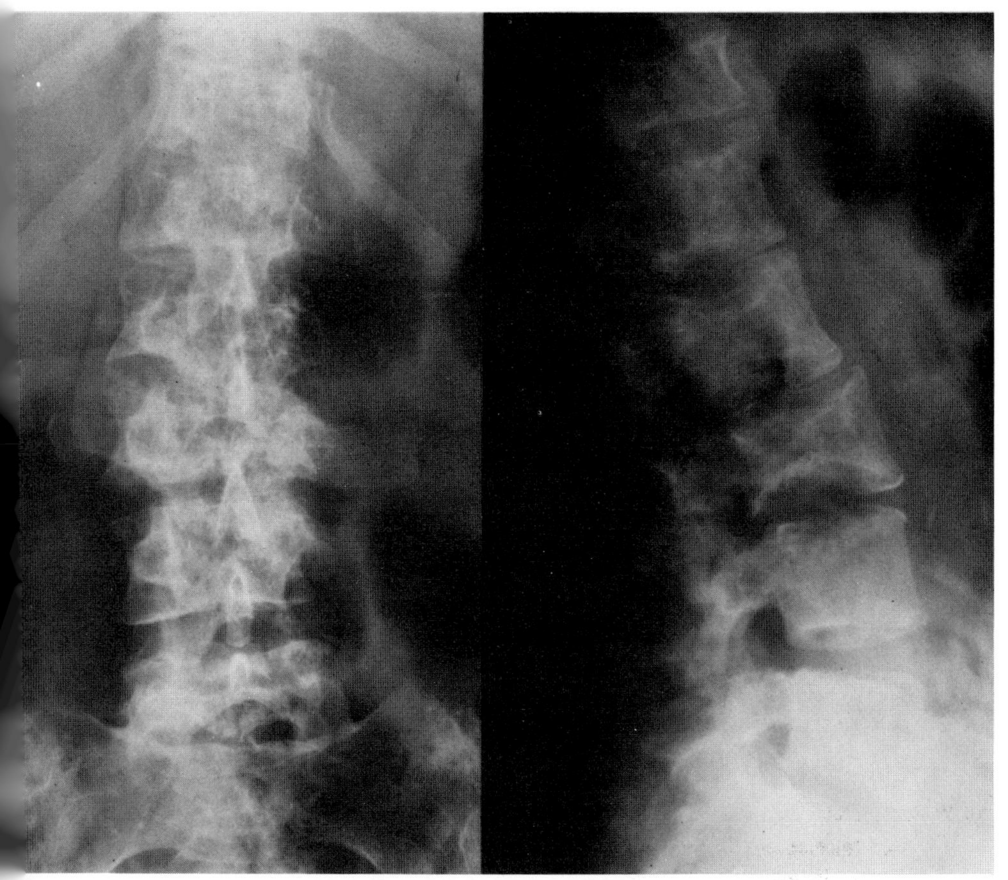

Figure 2-1. X-rays of lumbar spine showing extensive destruction of the vertebral bodies by metastatic breast carcinoma in a fifty-three-year-old female patient.

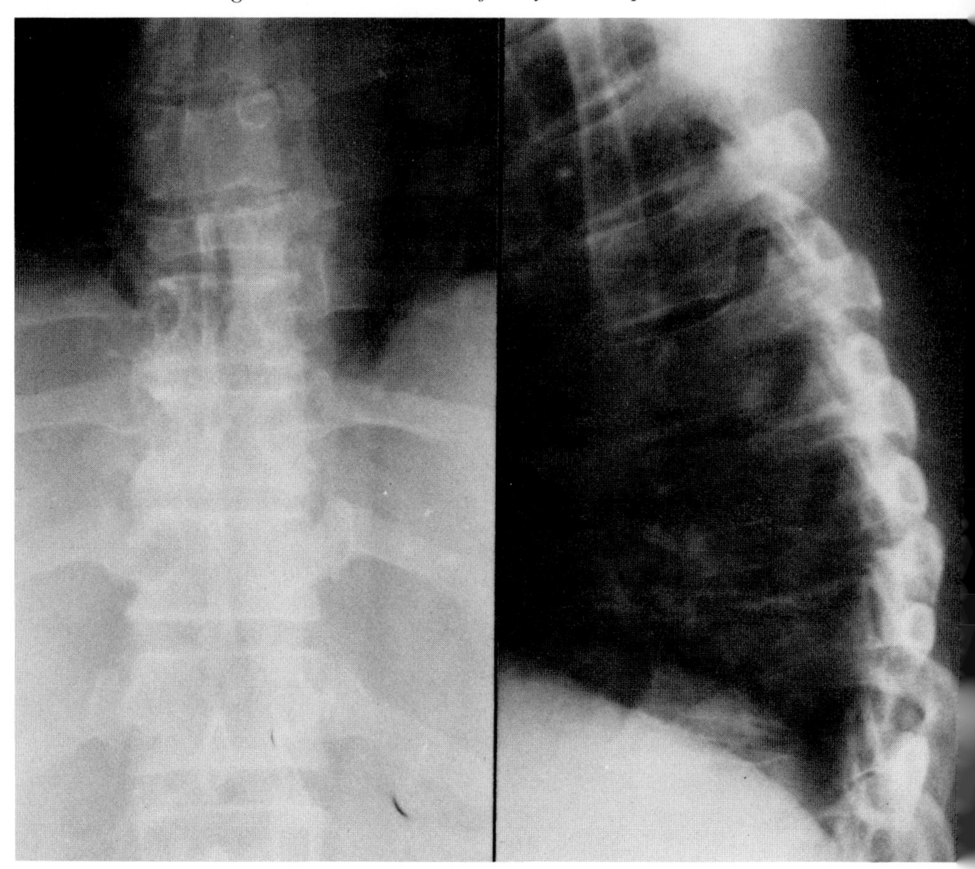

Figure 2-2. Roentgenograms of the lower thoracic region showing a severely compressed T8 vertebral body caused by a metastatic melanoma from the skin of a fifty-four-year-old man's back.

these typically osteolytic and osteoblastic carcinomas can also produce osteoblastic and osteolytic lesions, respectively, in a small percentage of cases[149-154] (Figures 2-11 to 2-14).

Although vertebral bodies are the favorite sites for metastases, the pedicles, laminae, and transverse and spinous processes can also be invaded by the metastatic tumors. Owing to the fact that osteolytic spinal lesions have a greater degree of trabecular destruction, compression fracture of the vertebrae is much more common in osteolytic lesions than in comparable osteoblastic lesions. Clinical experience shows that there is a direct relationship between the relative length of vertebral segment and its predilection for metastases that may explain why the thoracic spine is the most common site of metastases followed by lumbar spine and lastly by cervical spine. When extensive spinal metastases have taken place, para-

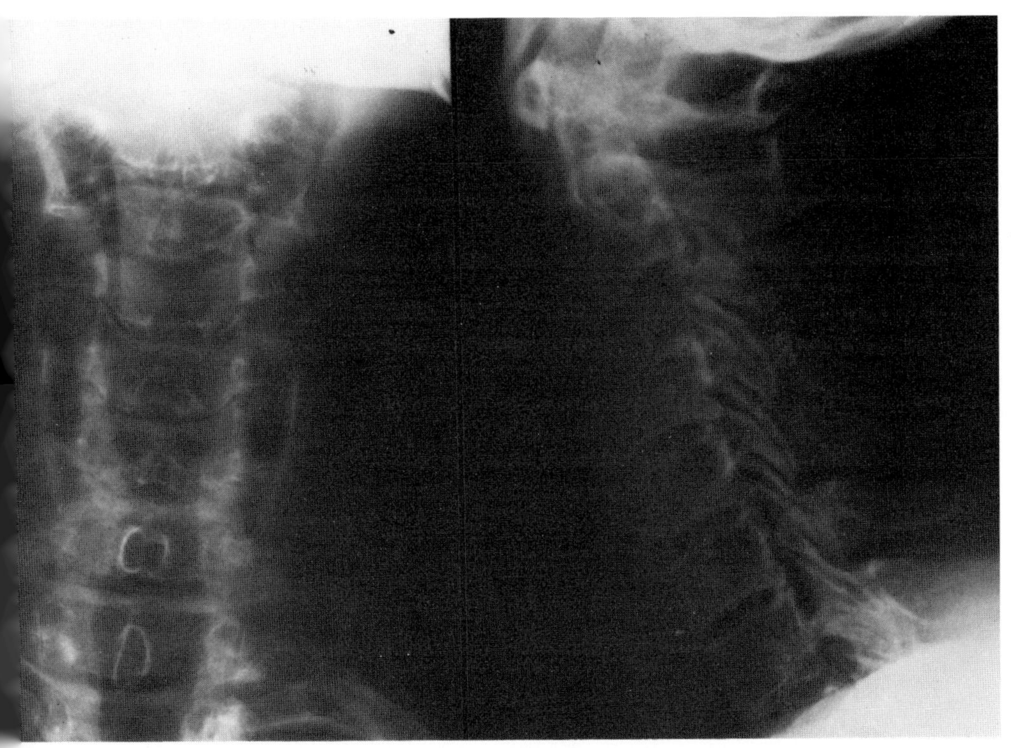

Figure 2-3. This sixty-six-year-old man had carcinoma of his lung that had completely destroyed the third cervical vertebral body by metastasis.

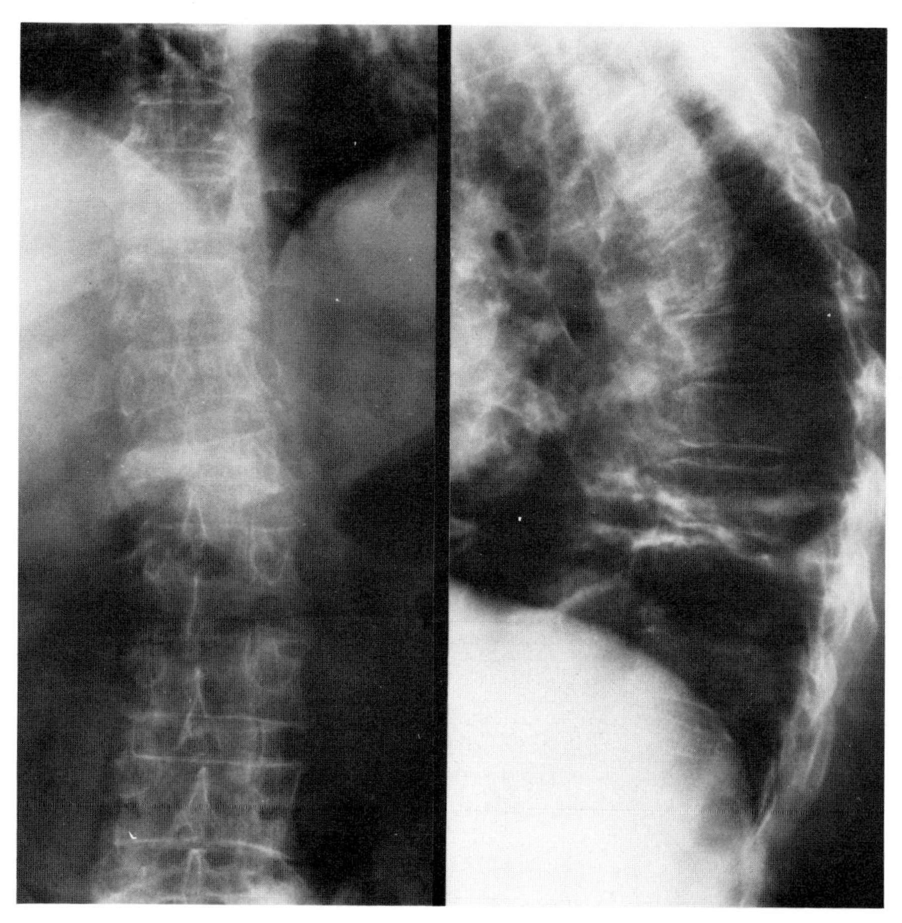

Figure 2-4. This set of x-rays belonged to a sixty-eight-year-old female with extensive spinal metastases from a colonic carcinoma. Note the marked osteoporosis throughout the thoracolumbar spine and several compression fractures, especially the L1 vertebra. The transverse radiopaque line through the first lumbar vertebral body is caused by compressed cortical and trabecular bone plus possible reparative new bone formation brought about by the compression fracture.

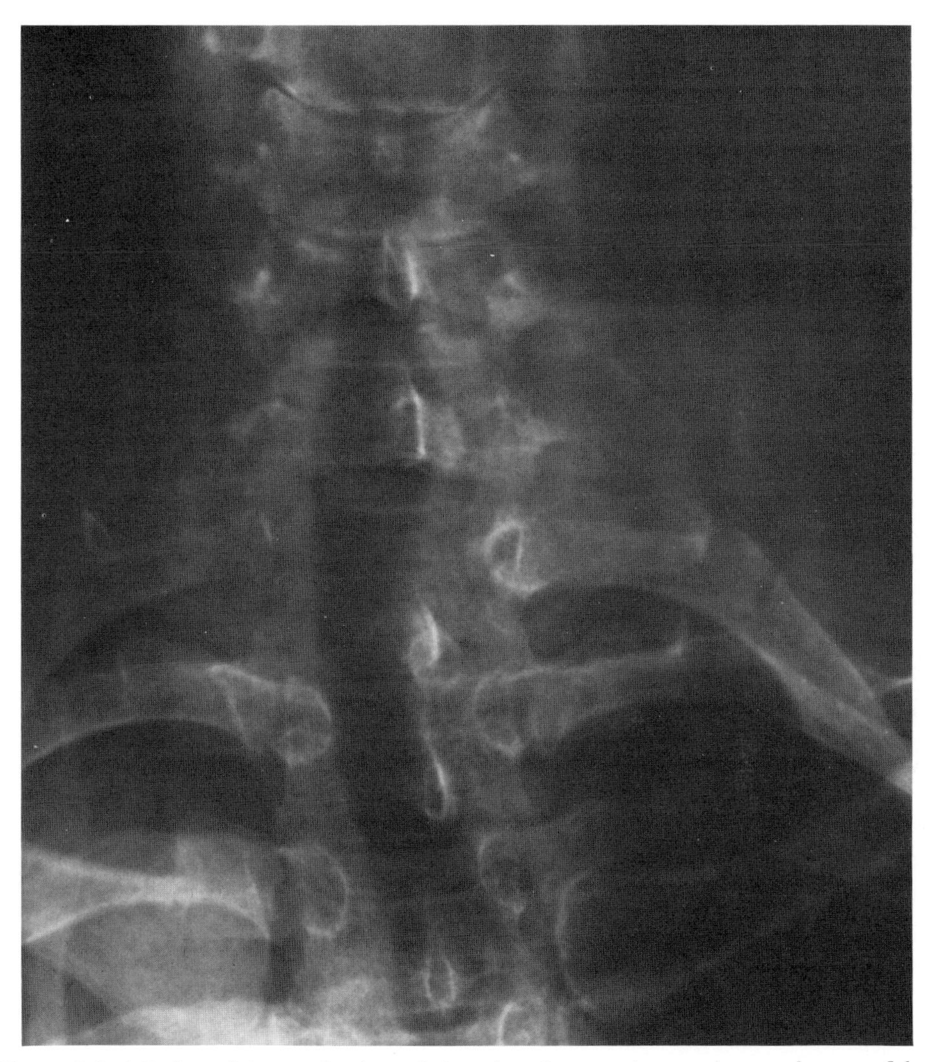

Figure 2-5. A-P view of the cervicothoracic junction shows an inconspicuous absence of the right pedicle of the first thoracic vertebra that can be easily missed by a casual observer. This patient was a fifty-nine-year-old woman who had carcinoma of her lung with spinal metastasis.

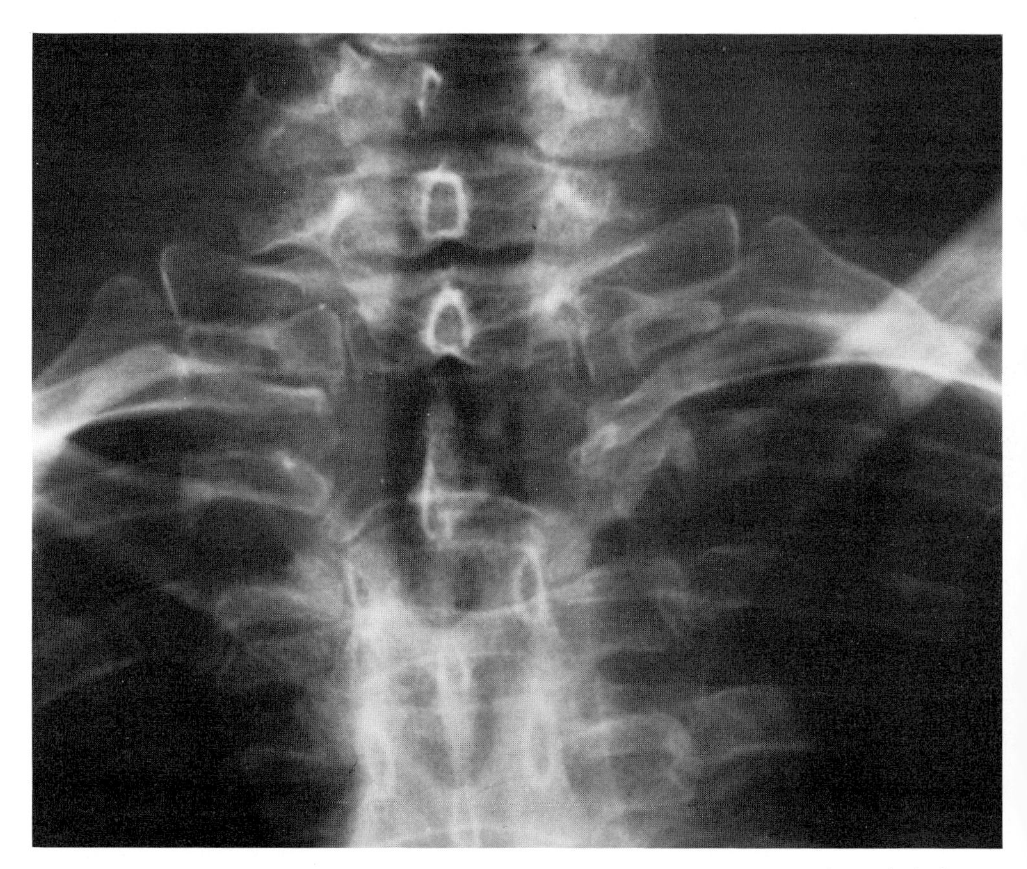

Figure 2-6. This forty-eight-year-old white female had severe and progressive pain in her upper chest and shoulders due to complete destruction of her second and third thoracic vertebrae by a metastatic breast carcinoma. Note the right and left second and third ribs no longer articulate with any bony elements.

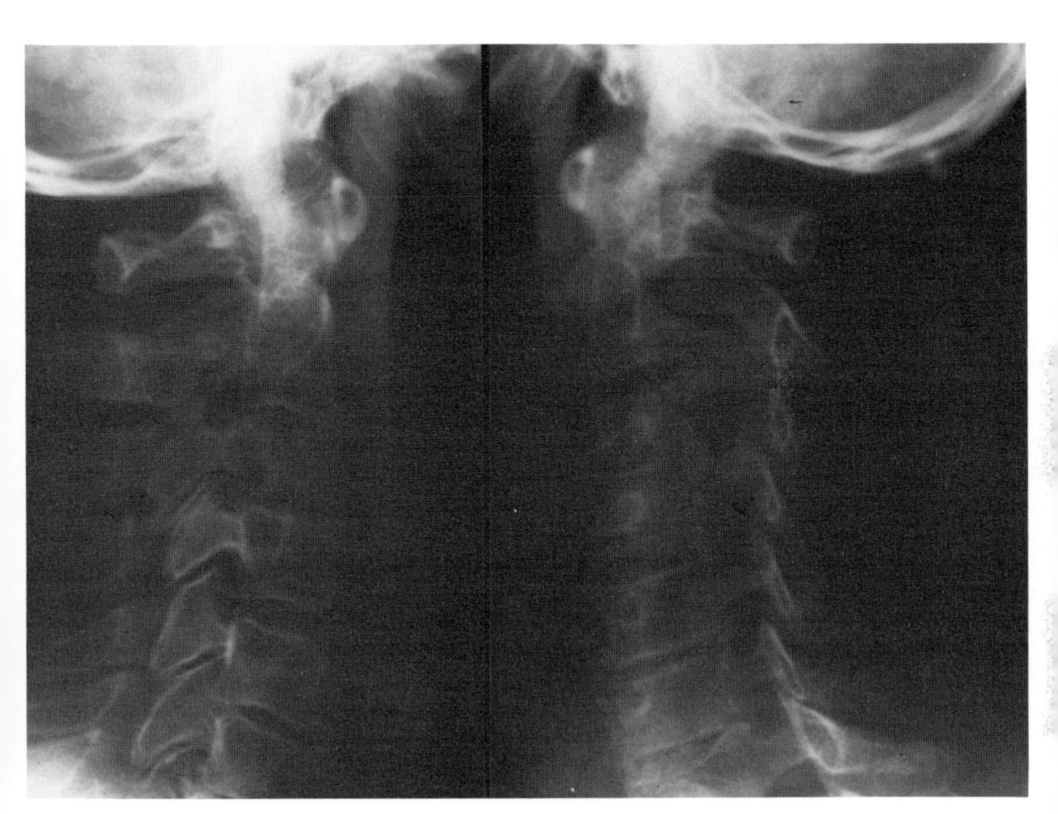

Figure 2-7. This fifty-five-year-old white male with constant neck pain was found to have a compression fracture of the third cervical vertebral body caused by a metastatic carcinoma of his lung. Trauma and primary bone tumors of the spine can also produce similar radiological appearance.

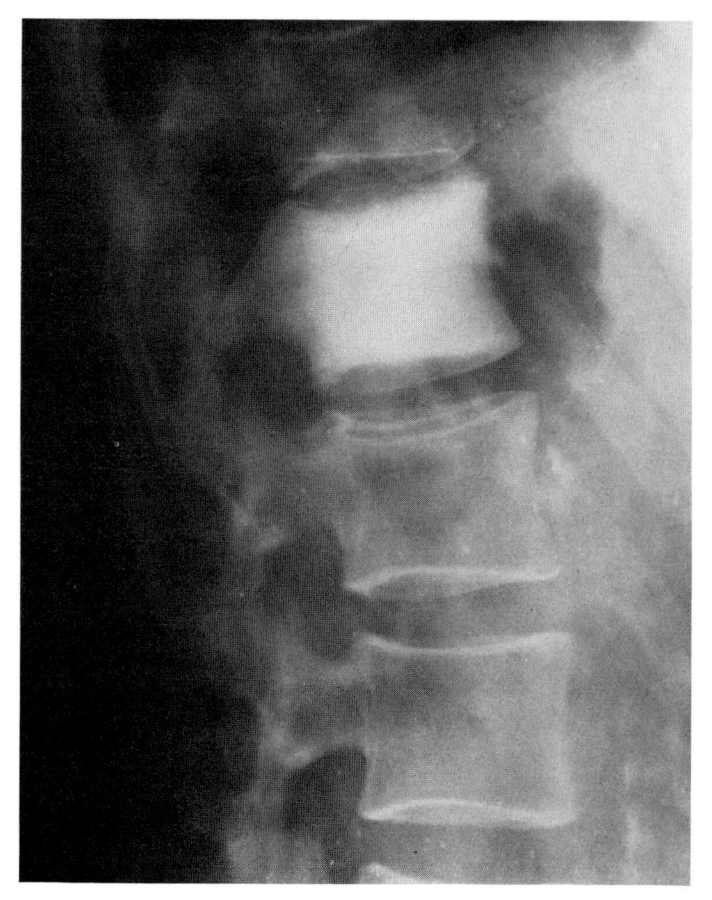

Figure 2-8. This sixty-eight-year-old man with prostatic carcinoma had a so-called ivory-vertebra of his first lumbar vertebra caused by prostatic metastasis. Hodgkin's disease can produce the same x-ray appearance.

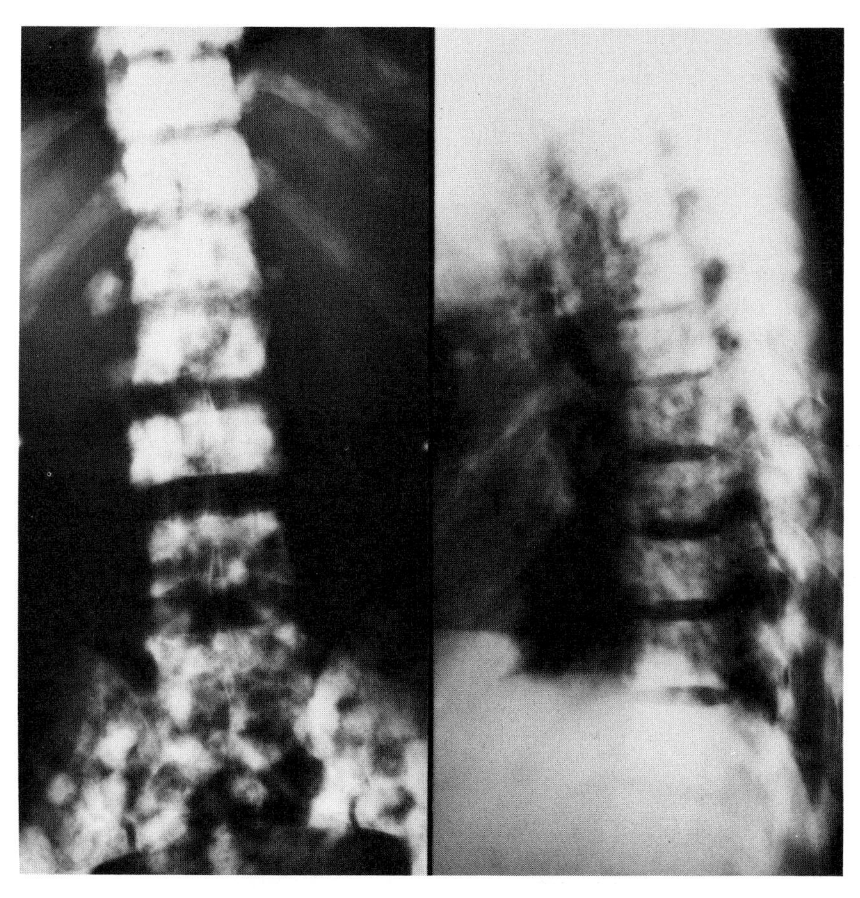

Figure 2-9. X-rays of the thoracic and lumbar spine showing extensive osteoblastic metastasis from a humeral osteogenic sarcoma of a fifty-four-year-old man who died only four weeks after this set of x-rays was taken.

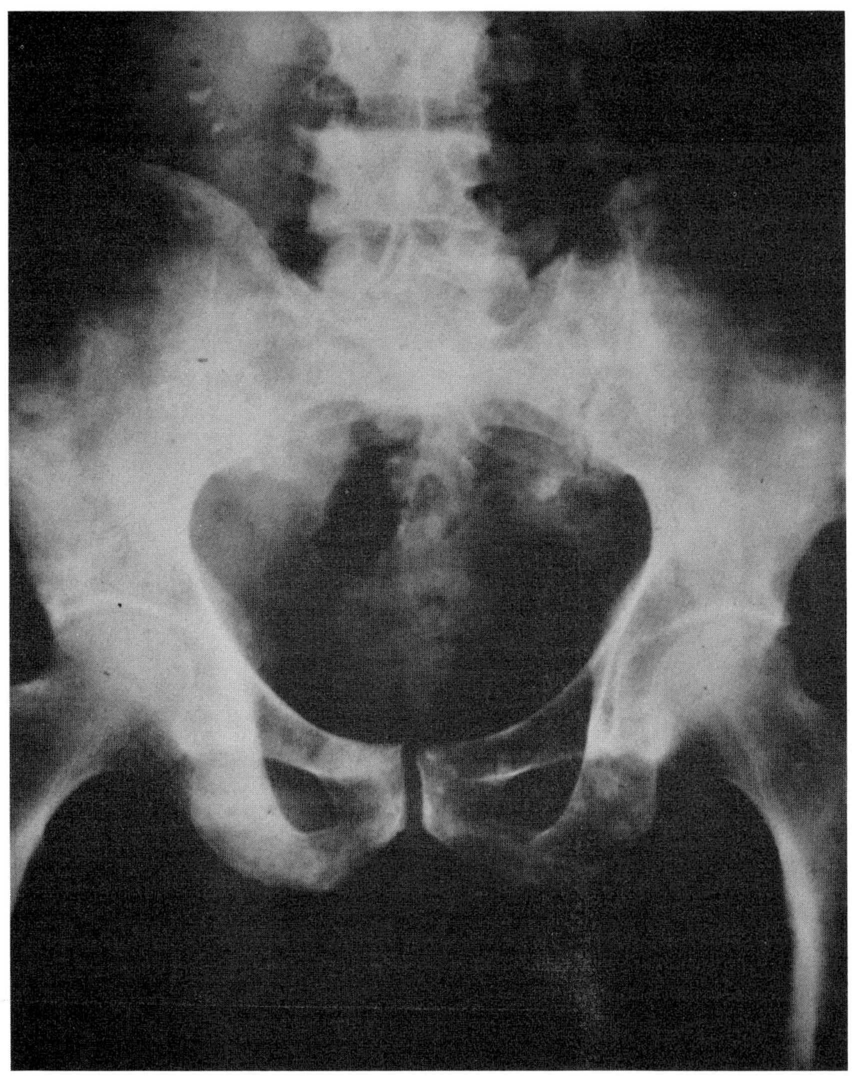

Figure 2-10. This sixty-two-year-old man with prostatic carcinoma had intensely osteoblastic metastasis throughout the pelvic bones and lumbar spine.

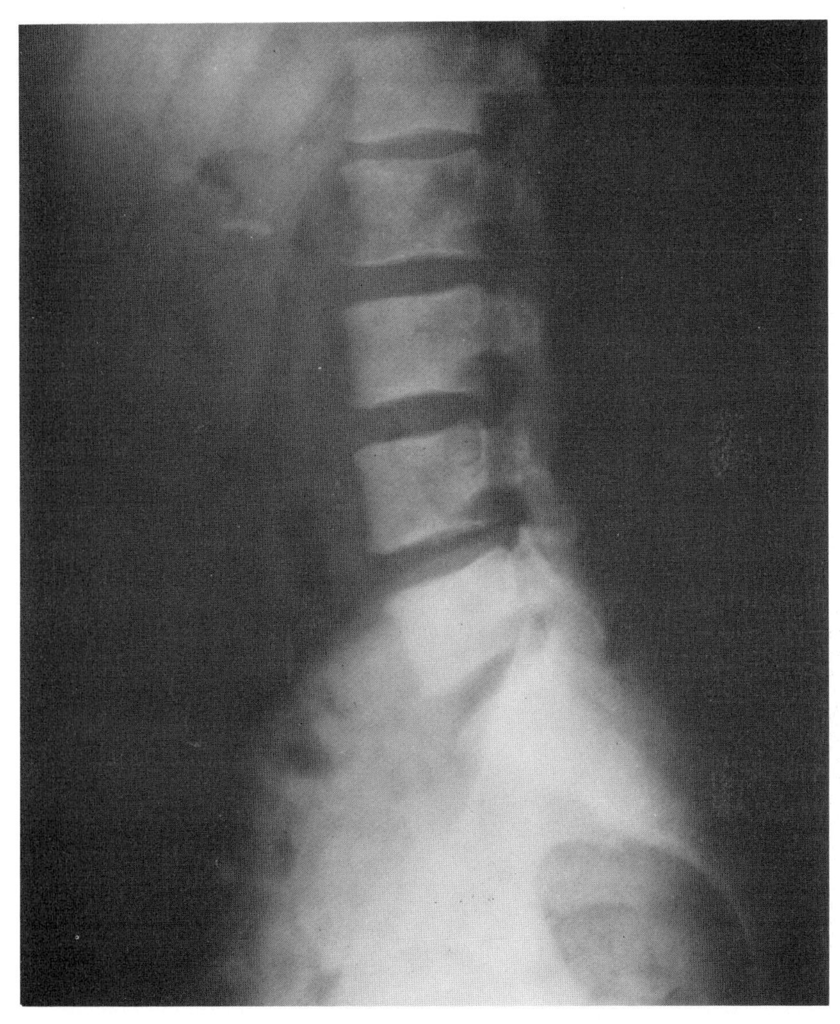

Figure 2-11. Lateral view of the lumbar spine showing uniformly osteoblastic metastasis throughout the lumbar spine and the sacrum of a thirty-two-year-old man with metastatic carcinoma of his lung, which is an uncommon radiological manifestation.

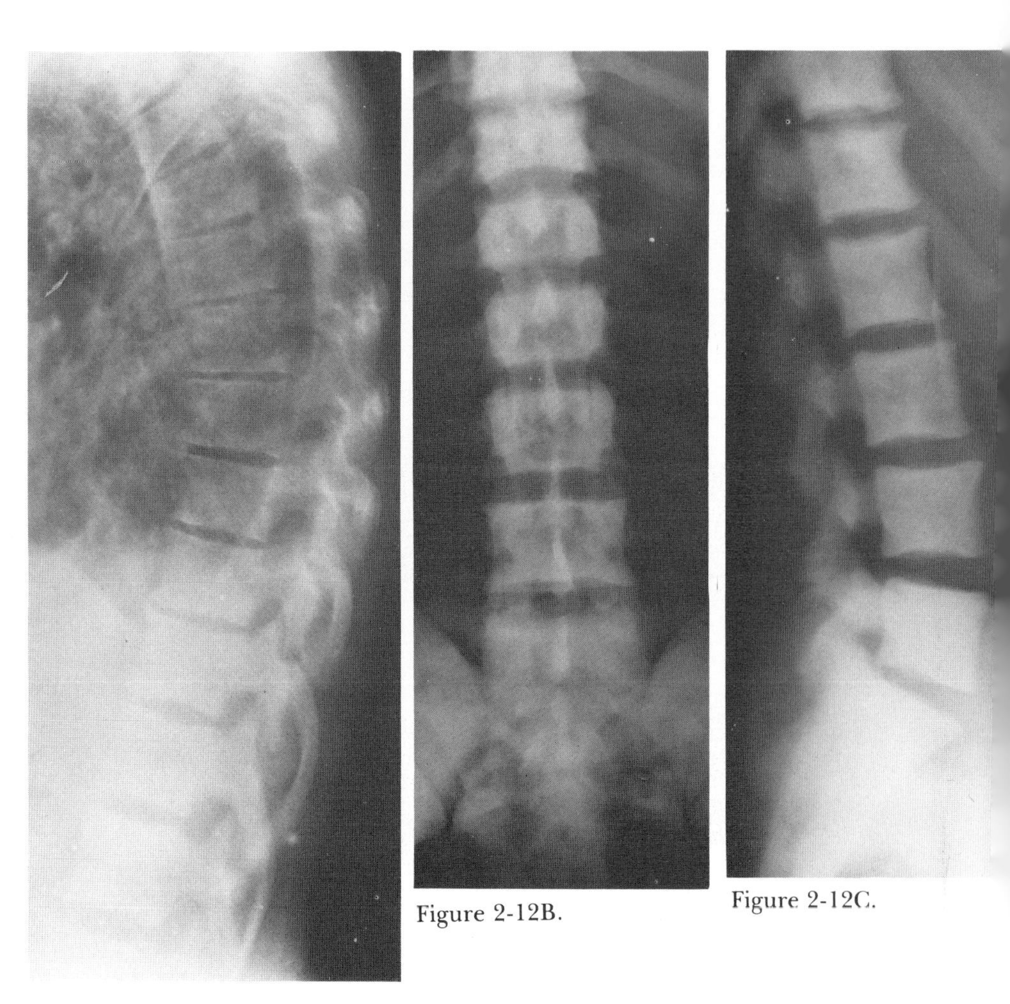

Figure 2-12B.

Figure 2-12C.

Figure 2-12A.

Figure 2-12. X-rays of the thoracic and lumbar spine of this forty-nine-year-old female with metastatic breast carcinoma show extensive osteoblastic metastasis throughout the entire thoracolumbar spine, which is an unusual roentgenographic appearance of breast carcinoma.

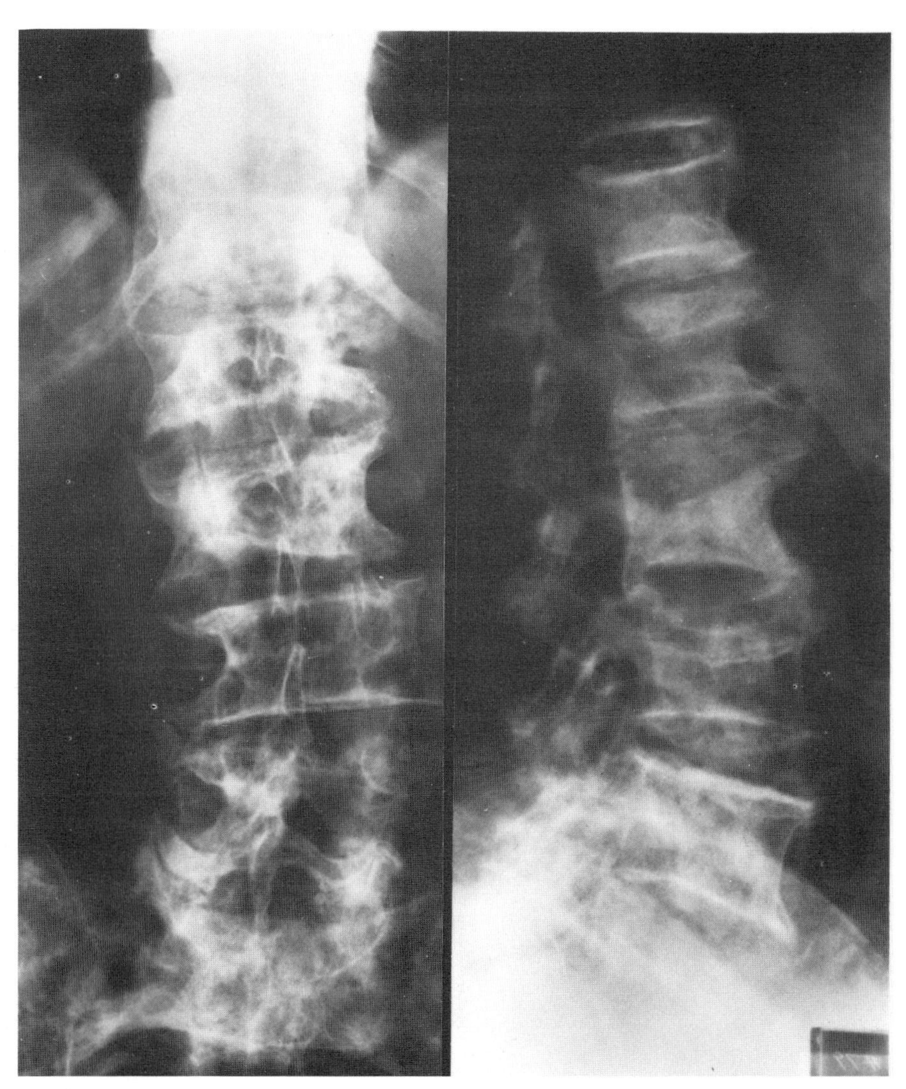

Figure 2-13. Lumbar spine x-rays showing a mixed osteolytic and osteoblastic metastasis from a prostatic carcinoma of an eighty-three-year-old man. Note the many biconcave vertebral bodies and the associated, expanded biconvex intervertebral disks.

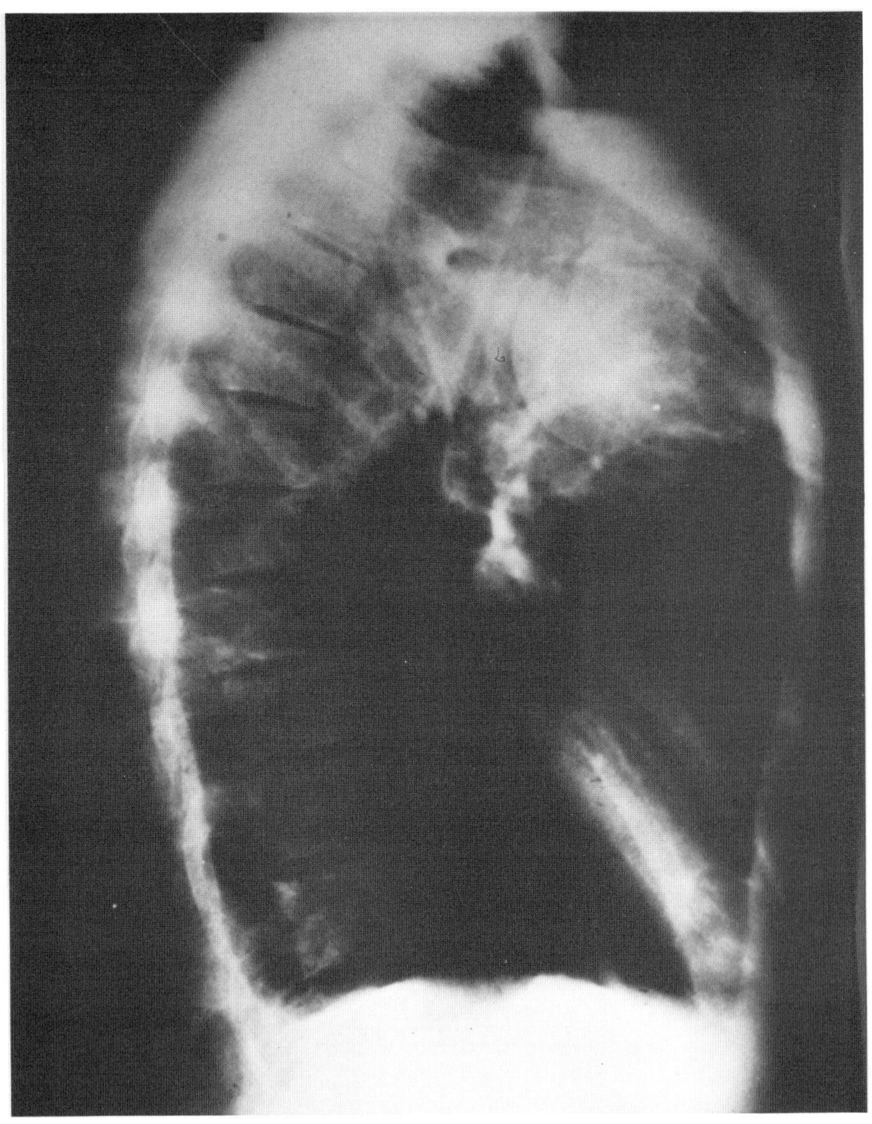

Figure 2-14. This forty-seven-year-old man had extensive mixed osteoblastic and osteolyti metastasis to his thoracolumbar spine that originated in a squamous cell carcinoma of th tongue.

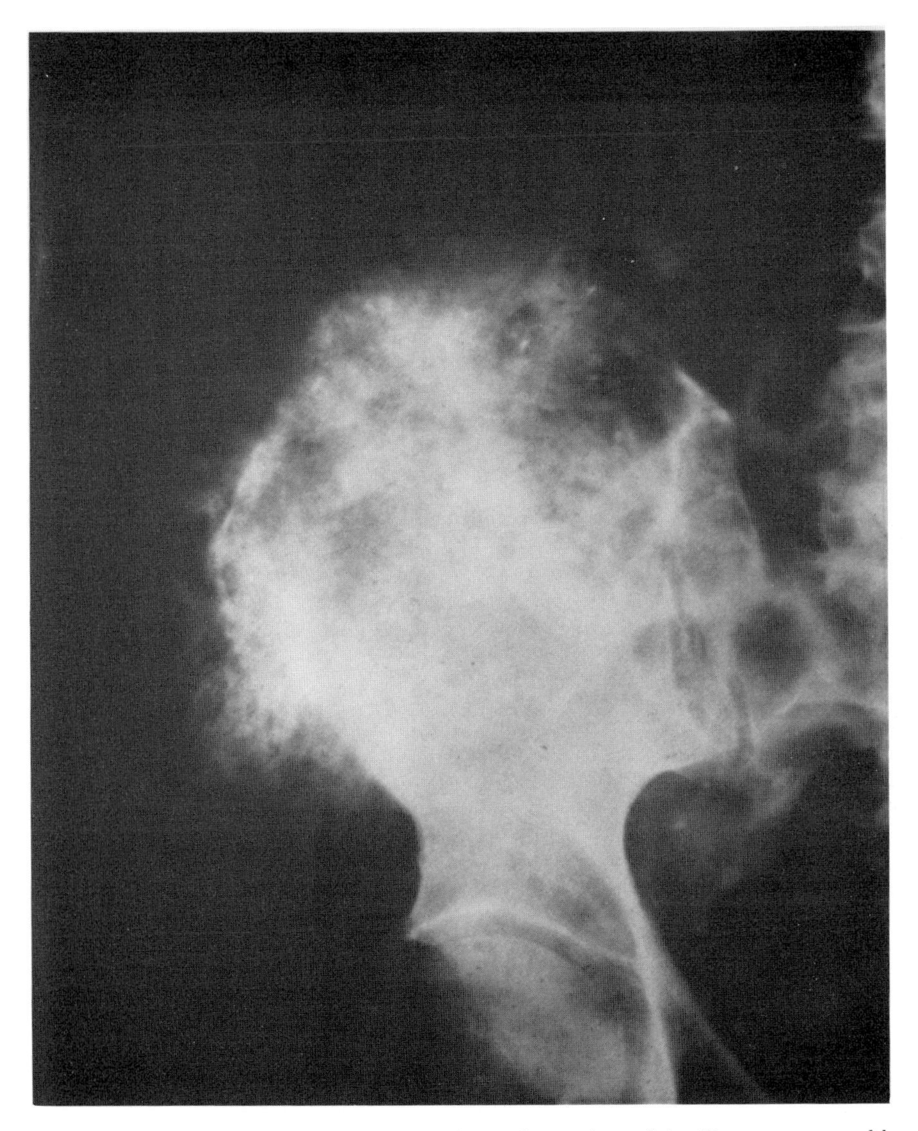

Figure 2-15. This exuberant periosteal new bone formation of the ilium was caused by a metastatic colonic adenocarcinoma of a sixty-three-year-old white male. Osteoblastic osteogenic sarcoma of the ilium can have the same radiological appearance.

spinal soft tissue mass caused by the metastatic tumor is often present, but periosteal new bone formation (Figure 2-15) is an uncommon feature of spinal metastases.

It should be pointed out that routine spinal x-rays are relatively insensitive in detecting obscure spinal metastases. For example, Figures 2-16A, 2-16B, and 2-16C show a case of widespread spinal metastases from a prostatic carcinoma that is clearly demonstrated by bone scan, but is completely invisible on routine spinal roentgenographs. Several studies had shown that osteolytic lesions less than one centimeter in diameter and vertebrae with less than 50 percent of decalcification are usually not clearly demonstrated by routine roentgenographic examination.[155-157] However, bone scans with radioactive isotopes[158-191] have greatly improved our ability to detect early metastases, which will enable us to provide cancer patients with individualized optimal courses of treatment. In addition, computer assisted tomography (CAT) scanning[192-193] and myelography are invaluable in defining the level and size of the metastatic spinal tumor and the exact location of spinal cord or nerve compression. They can also differentiate between intradural and extradural compression and may further reveal the presence of clinically asymptomatic tumor deposits in different portions of the spinal canal. The contrast material, e.g. pantopaque, is sometimes purposely left in the subarachnoid space so that the patient's postsurgical or postradiotherapeutic status of the metastatic intraspinal tumor can be followed on a regular basis by means of fluoroscopic or routine roentgenographic examination. Recently, immunocytochemical methods[194-198] employing radiolabeled antibodies to tumor cell components and their secreted products have been successfully used in detecting inconspicuous micrometastases which are uniformly invisible to various forms of radiological examination.

It should be mentioned that primary and secondary pulmonary malignancies, e.g. bronchogenic carcinomas and metastatic carcinomas and sarcomas, can sometimes produce an unusual disease called pulmonary hypertrophic osteoarthropathy[199-213] (or ossifying periostitis of Bamberger-Marie[214-215]). It is characterized by the presence of symmetrical clubbing of the fingers and toes, arthritis, and chronic periostitis of the long and short tubular bones of the upper and lower extremities (Figures 2-17A to 2-17C and 2-18A to 2-18C). Stintz (1978)[216] found the frequency of occurrence of pulmonary hypertrophic osteoarthropathy in patients who died of bronchial carcinoma to be 7 percent. Pulmonary hypertrophic osteoarthropathy is also associated with pleural methotheliomas;[217-218] lung abscess, tuberculosis, and bronchiectasis;[219] Hodgkin's disease;[220] and cystic fibrosis.[221-222] Nathanson and Riddlesberger (1980)[223] reported a 5 percent incidence of pulmonary hypertrophic osteoarthropathy in

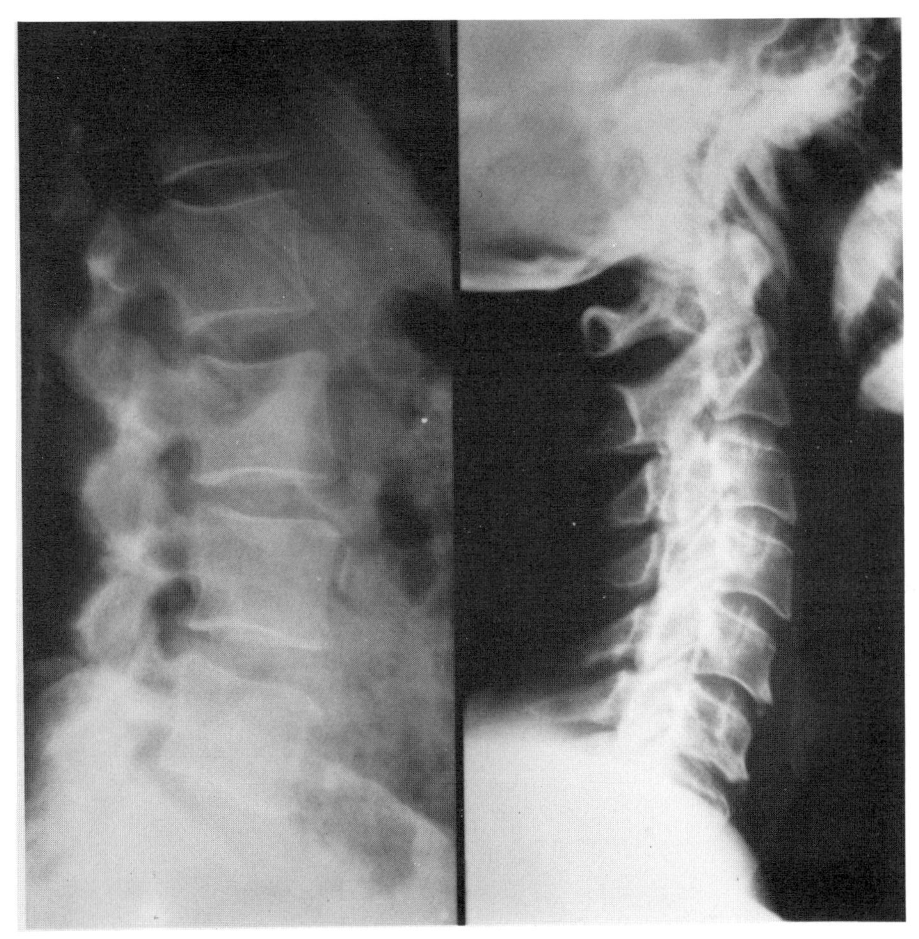

Figure 2-16A.

cystic fibrosis. Clinical experience has shown that the osteoarthropathy usually regresses after surgical removal of the primary or metastatic intrathoracic tumor or after effective chemotherapy and radiotherapy. Furthermore, symptomatic relief of the distressful osteoarthropathy has been achieved by administration of indomethacin, adrenergic blockade with propranolol and Dibenzyline®,[224] laparotomy,[225] and surgical and medical vagotomy,[226-227] which eliminates the reflexogenic afferent stimulus mediated by the vagus nerve.

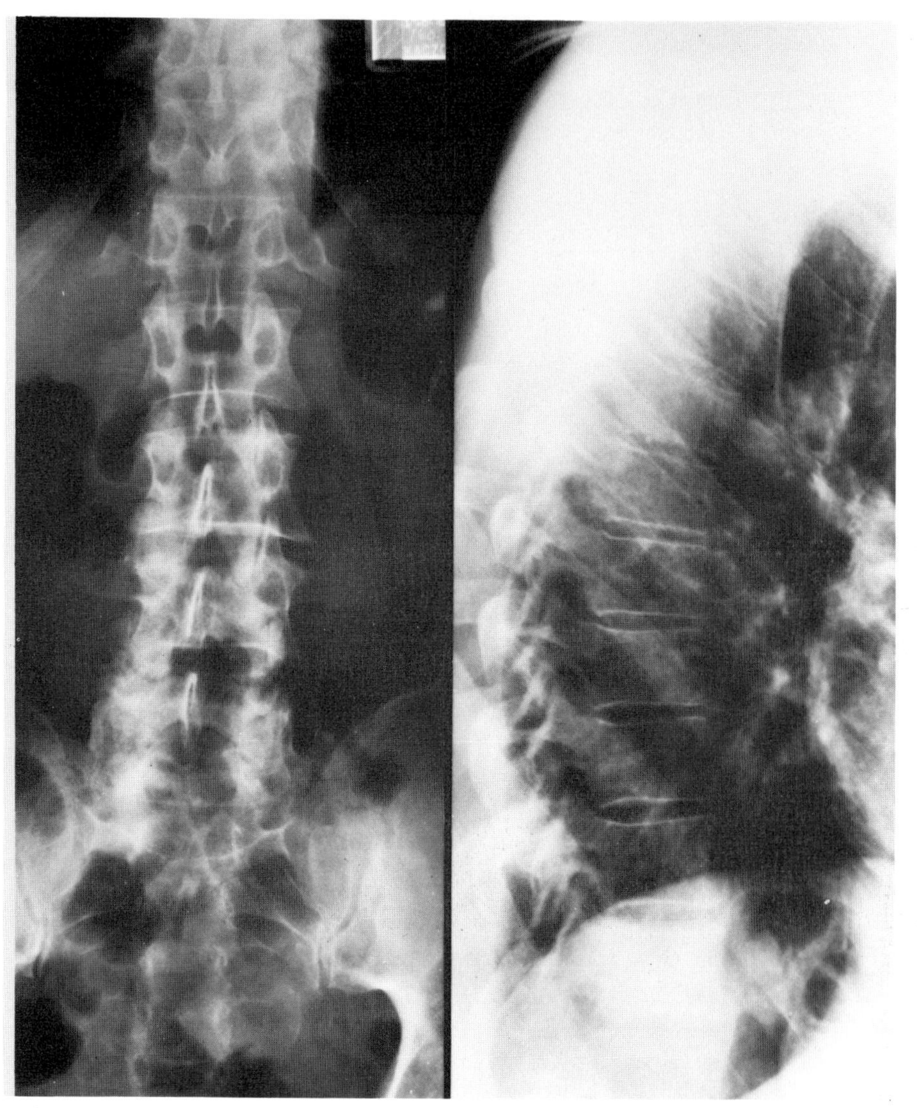

Figure 2-16B.

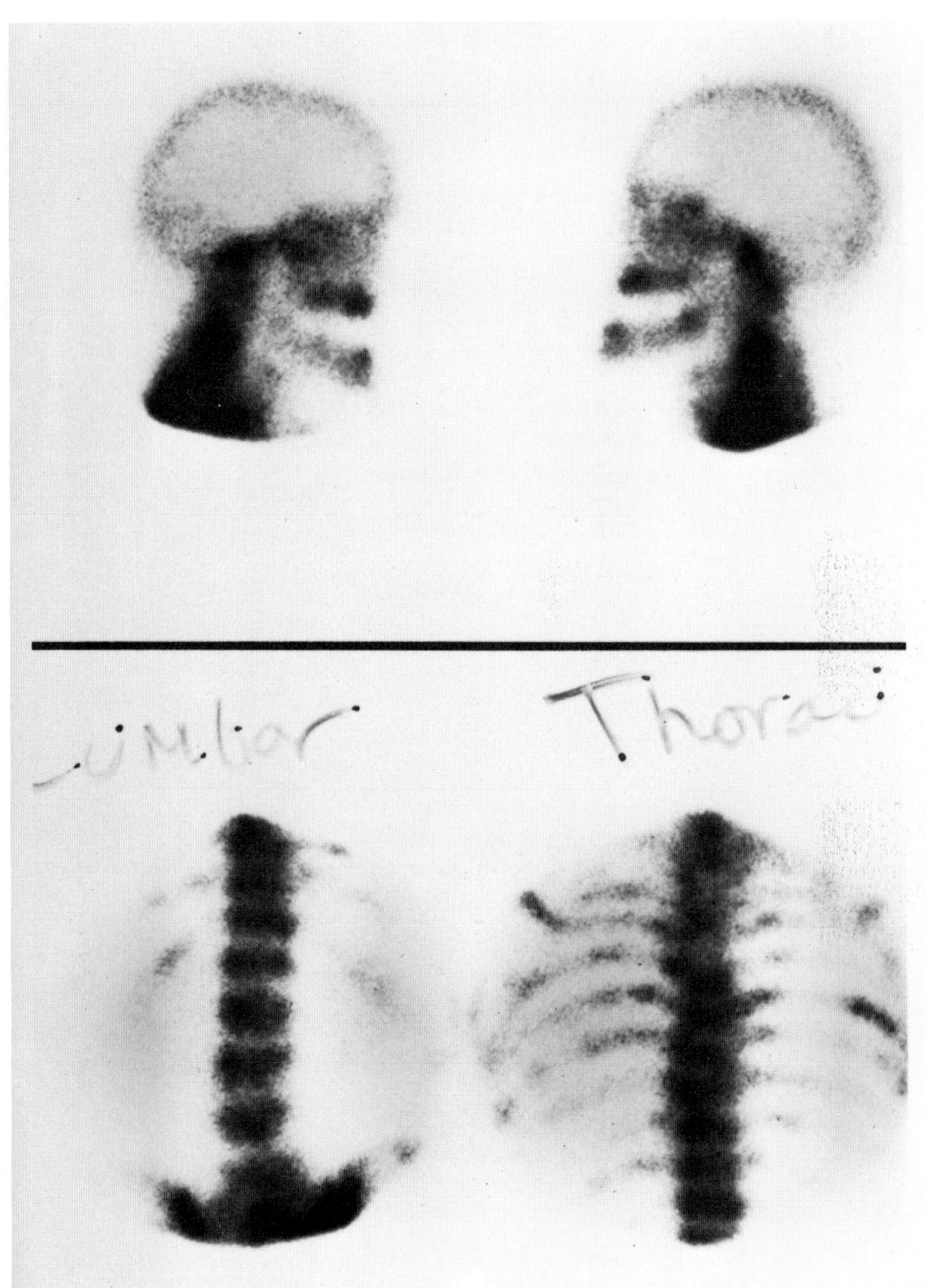

Figure 2-16C.

Figure 2-16. Routine cervical, thoracic, and lumbar spine x-rays of this sixty-two-year-old man show complete absence of any osteolytic or osteoblastic lesions. However, bone scan clearly shows multiple hot spots throughout the entire spine, suggesting of widespread spinal metastases. Further investigations revealed that the patient indeed had metastatic prostatic carcinoma that later became roentgenographically visible when the lesions got big enough.

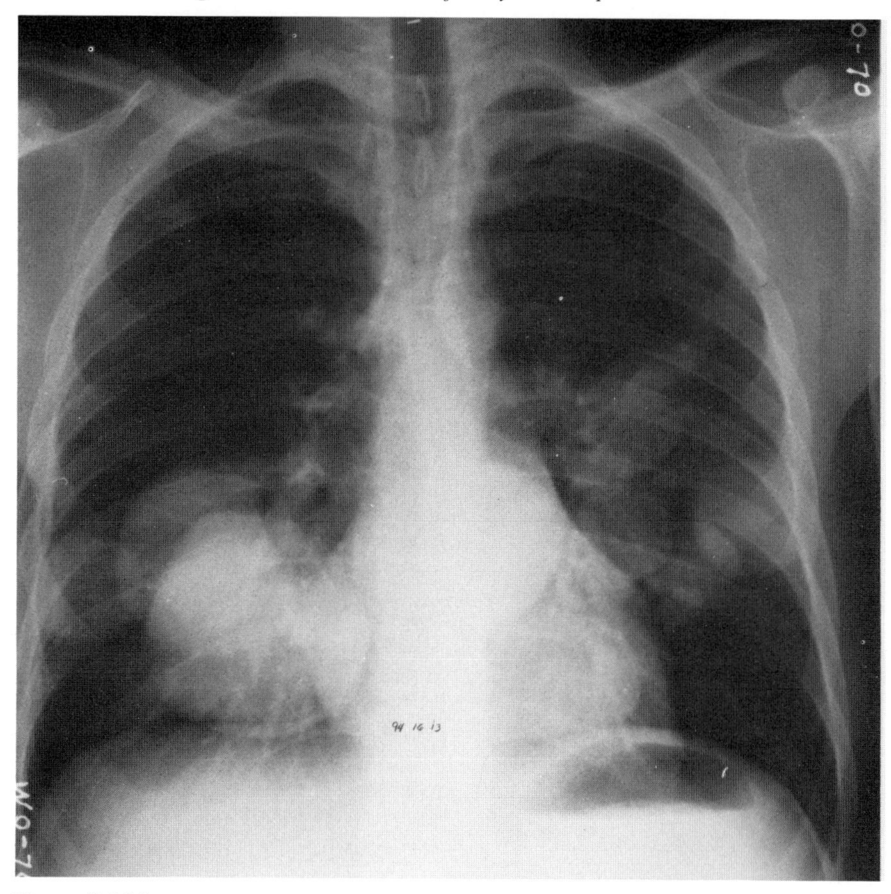

Figure 2-17A.

Figure 2-17A. This thirty-five-year-old white male with cannon-ball shaped metastases in both lungs caused by a metastasizing poorly differentiated liposarcoma of his thigh also had pulmonary hypertrophic osteoarthropathy.

Figure 2-17B. X-rays of the elbows of the same patient shown in Figure 2-17A show periosteal elevation of the distal humeri.

Figure 2-17C. X-rays of the ankle and wrist belonging to the same patient shown in Figure 2-17A show periosteal new bone formation of the distal fibula, tibia, radius and ulna, and the diaphyseal portion of the first metacarpal.

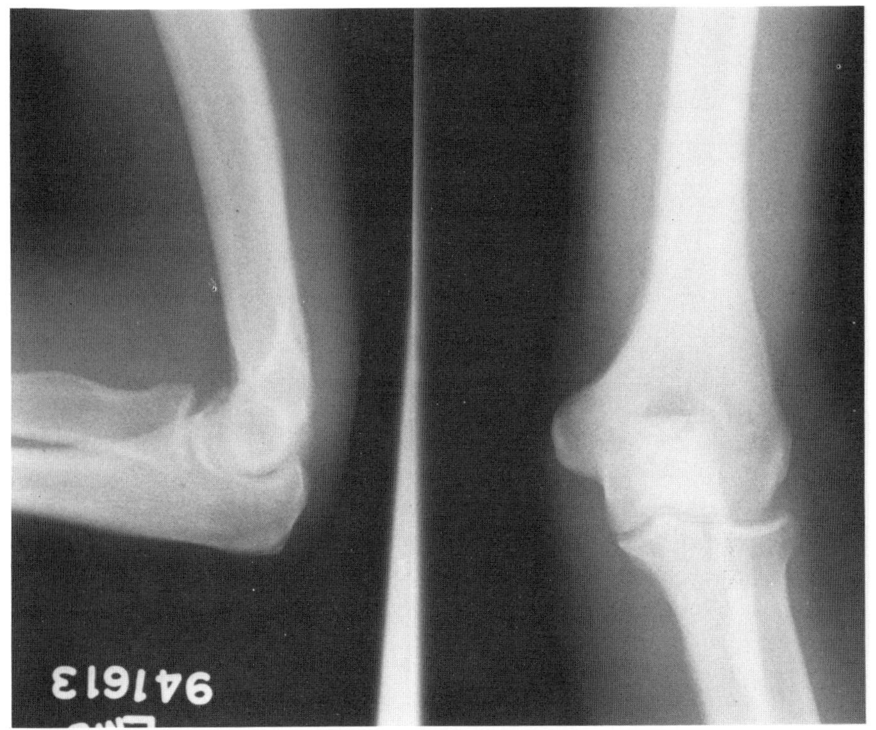

Figure 2-17B.

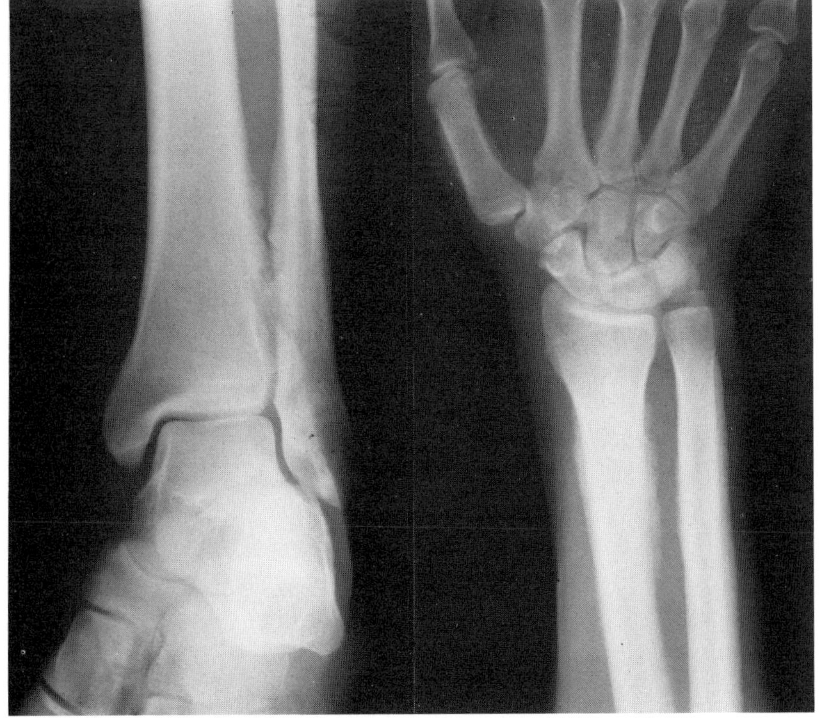

Figure 2-17C.

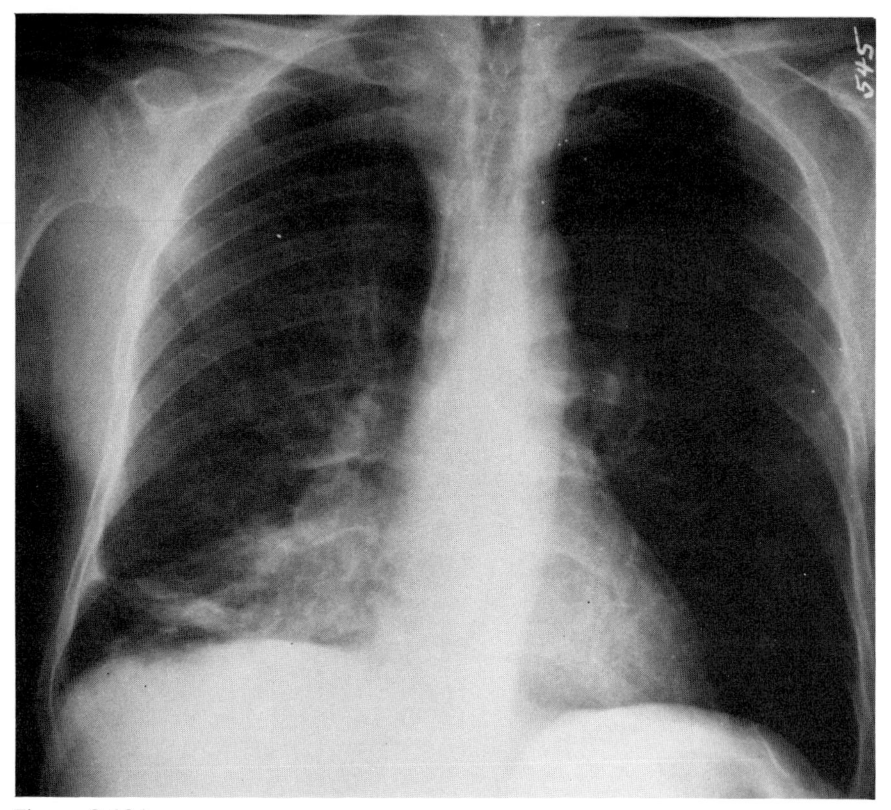

Figure 2-18A.

Figure 2-18A. This fifty-nine-year-old man with bronchogenic carcinoma of lung and pulmonary hypertrophic osteoarthropathy manifested clinically in pain and swelling of both upper and lower extremities. Note the radiopaque tumor in the lower right lung field.

Figure 2-18B. X-rays of both femora belonging to the patient shown in Figure 2-18A show extensive periosteal new bone formation throughout the femoral shafts.

Figure 2-18C. X-rays of the forearms belonging to the patient in Figure 2-18A show periosteal new bone formation in both radii and ulnae.

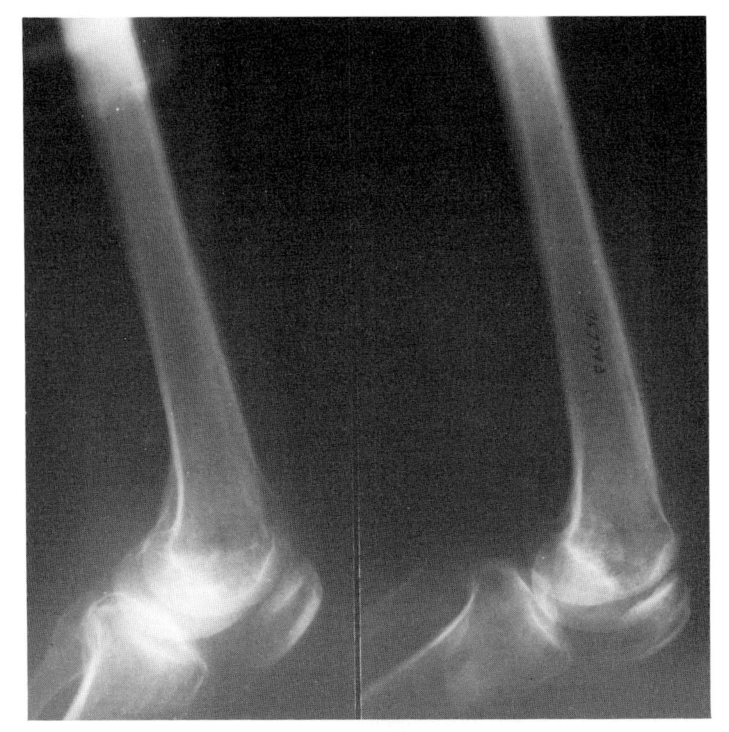

Figure 2-18B.

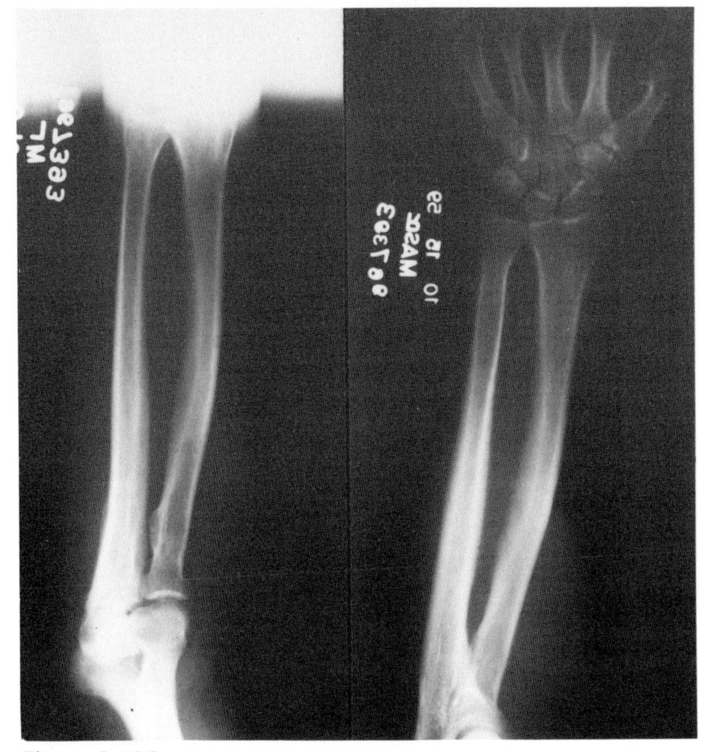

Figure 2-18C.

PATHOLOGIC FEATURES

Gross Pathology

Since many different carcinomas and sarcomas metastasize to the spine, their gross appearance shows a wide spectrum of variations. The osteolytic lesions are usually occupied by relatively soft, yellowish-white, grayish-white, or reddish tumor tissues in which foci of necrosis, hemorrhage, and cystic degeneration are frequently present (Figures 2-19 to 2-23). Metastatic spinal tumors with high collagen contents such as scirrhous carcinoma of the breast and well differentiated fibrosarcoma are firm and tough and may have a whitish or grayish-white appearance.

In contrast, densely osteoblastic lesions tend to be hard, white, or yellowish-white, and the trabecular space may be filled by new bone formed in

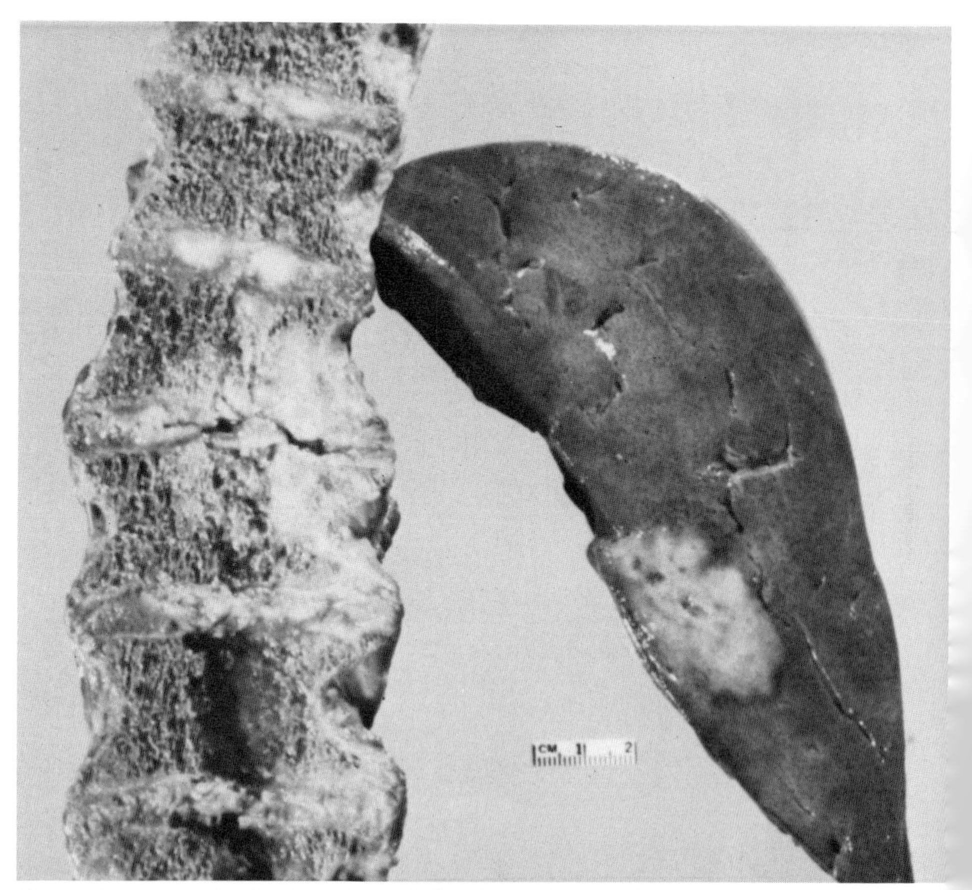

Figure 2-19. Longitudinal section of the thoracolumbar junction showing patches of yellowish-white tumor tissue that has replaced the vertebral bony trabeculae. The metastatic tumor tissue originated in the liver, which was purposely placed next to the spine to show the similarity in tumor appearance between the primary and metastatic tumor sites.

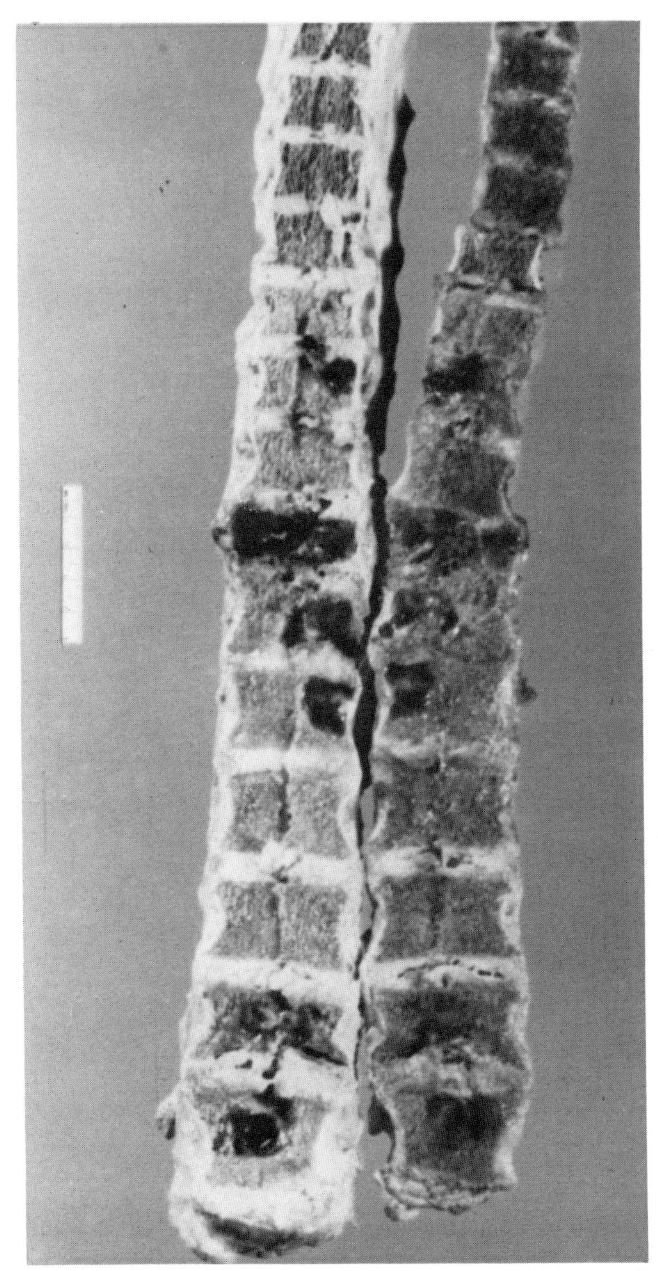

Figure 2-20. A longitudinal section through the spine of a patient who died of metastatic carcinoma of stomach showing many deformed vertebrae in which hemorrhage and cystic changes caused by the metastatic gastric carcinoma can be found.

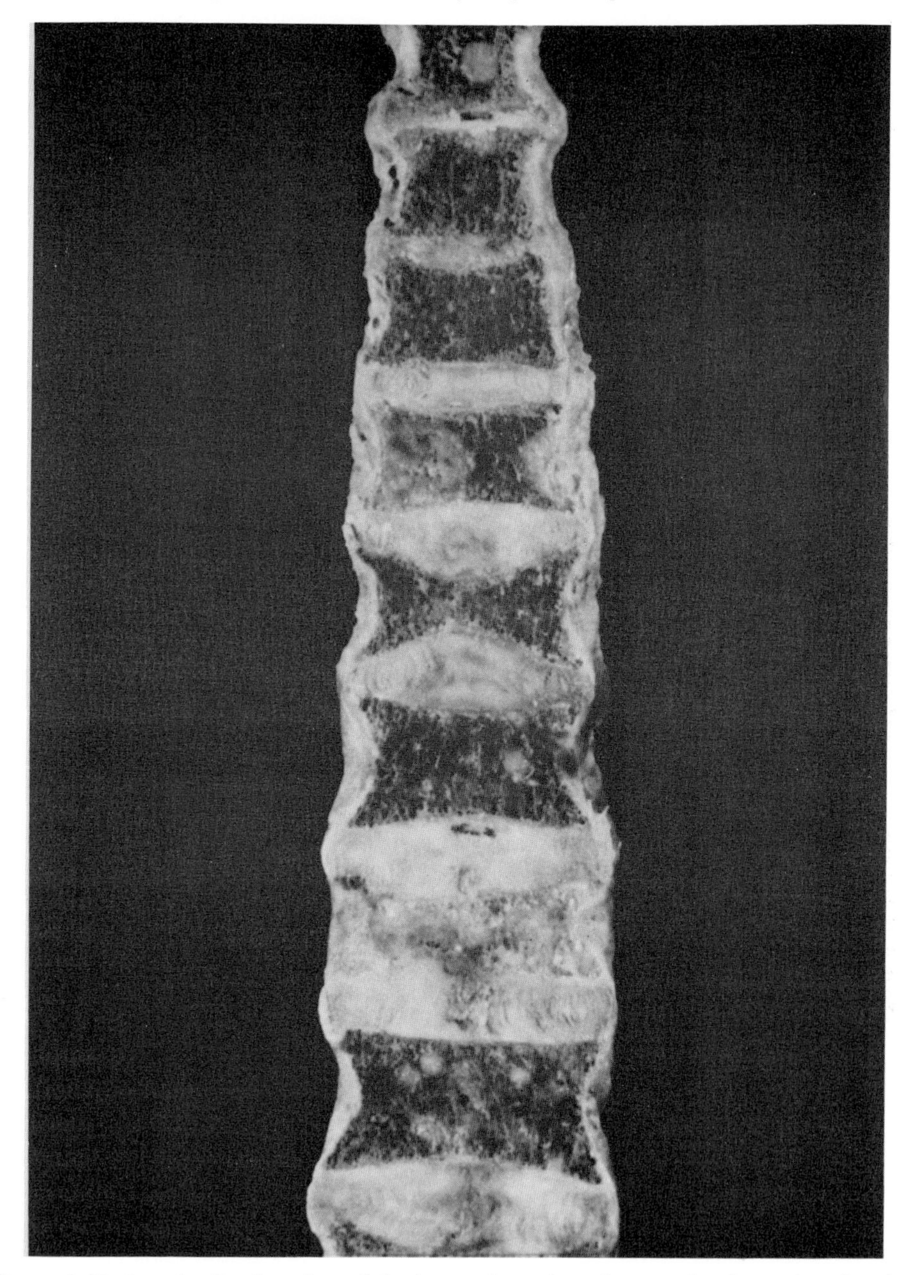

Figure 2-21. Longitudinal section of the lower thoracic and upper lumbar spine showing many roundish foci of metastatic breast carcinoma associated with deformed vertebral bodies and expanded intervertebral disks.

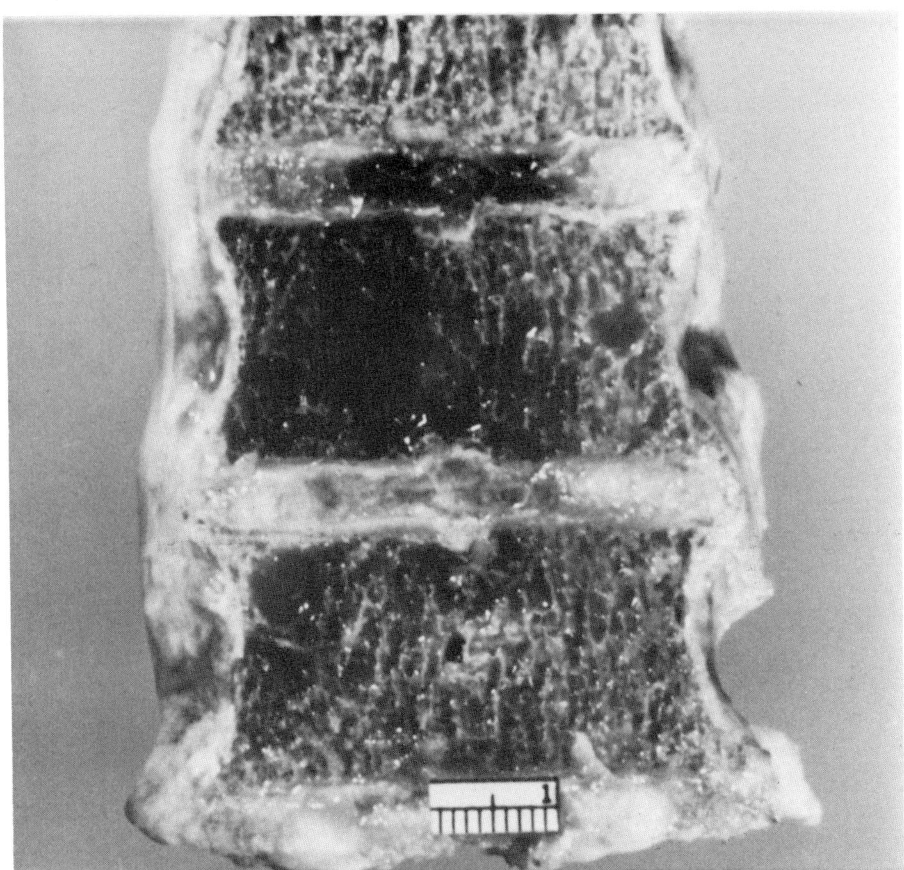

Figure 2-22. Longitudinal section of lower thoracic spine from a patient who died of metastatic carcinoma of the lung showing replacement of vertebral bony trabeculae by tumor tissue that has a hemorrhagic appearance. Note the same tumor has also invaded one of the intervertebral disks.

response to the presence of the cancer. When the spinal metastasis is caused by a chondrosarcoma, the typical appearance of a cartilaginous tumor such as its lobulated configuration, bluish-white color, foci of calcification, and firm consistency can sometimes be seen. In addition, destruction of the vertebral bodies and their posterior arches, compression vertebral fractures, tumor infiltration of the paraspinal soft tissues, compression of the spinal cord or nerves by the collapsed vertebrae or by epidural spinal metastases, etc., can be easily seen at autopsies.

Microscopic Pathology

In the presence of a monostotic spinal tumor, accurate histologic diagnosis is of vital importance because the treatment of metastatic spinal

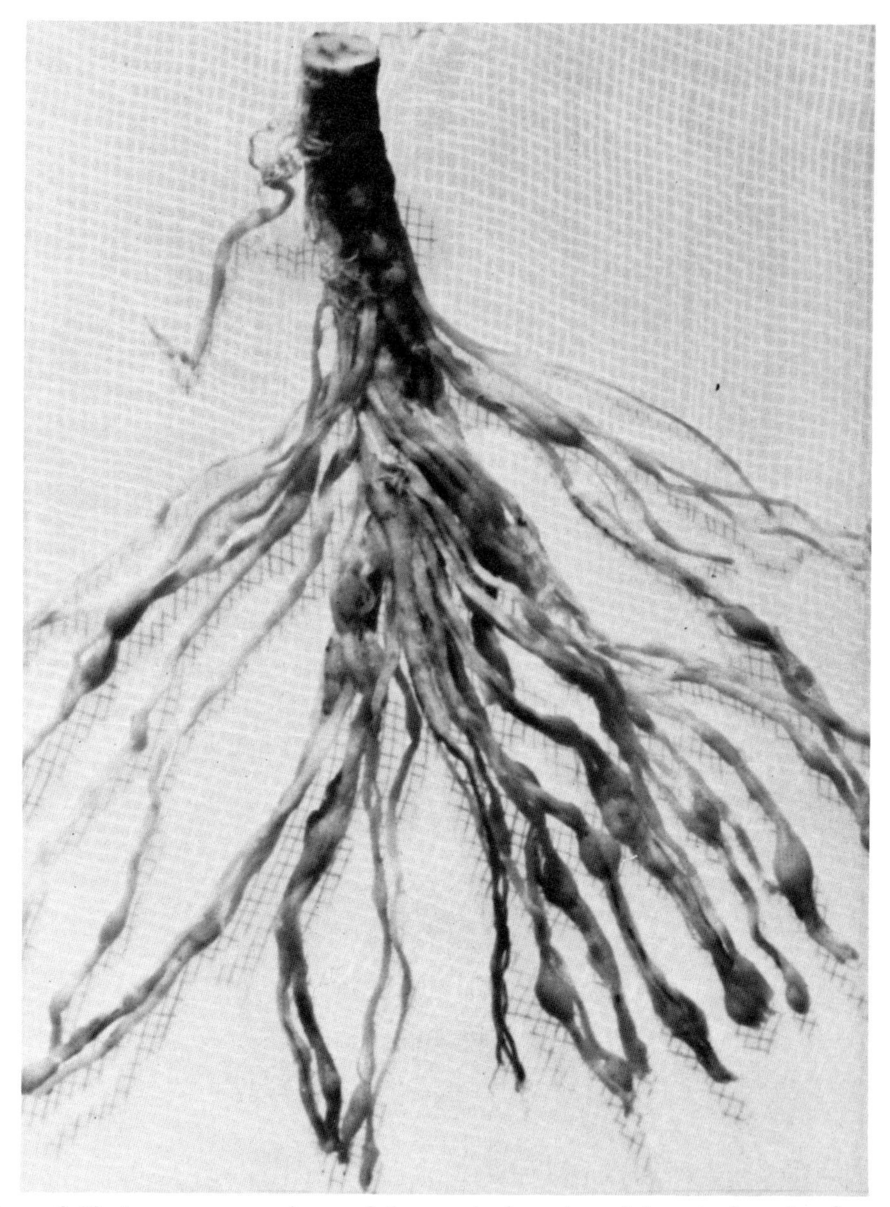

Figure 2-23. An autopsy specimen of the terminal portion of the spinal cord and cauda equina showing many knobby enlargements caused by proliferation of a metastatic breast carcinoma in the neural elements.

tumors is basically palliative in nature whereas radical eradicative surgery is usually the treatment of choice in dealing with localized primary malignant spinal tumors. Normally, the differentiation of metastatic spinal carcinomas from primary spinal sarcomas is fairly easy because carcinoma cells tend to be large with abundant cytoplasm and well defined cytoplasmic borders (Figures 2-24 and 2-25) and can form cuboidal or columnar glandular structures bound by a distinct basement membrane.

Some metastatic spinal tumors have such a typical histologic appearance that their origins can be ascertained at a glance. For example, metastatic thyroid carcinoma may show follicular structures formed by cuboidal or columnar epithelial cells and containing eosinophilic colloidal substance (Figure 2-26). Metastatic hypernephroma (renal cell carcinoma or clear cell carcinoma of the kidney) contains large cells with abundant pale foamy cytoplasm and hyperchromatic and pyknotic nuclei (Figure 2-27).

Metastatic spinal tumors consisting of glandular cuboidal or columnar epithelium can originate in bronchus, salivary glands, stomach, small intestine, large intestine, gallbladder, pancreas, uterus, breast, etc. (Figure 2-28 to 2-31). Metastatic squamous cell carcinoma of the spine consisting of sheets or cords of epidermal cells in which keratinous nests or "epithelial pearls" are frequently present. Metastatic malignant melanoma of the spine with typical intracytoplasmic melanin pigment can both come from skin, oronasopharynx, larynx, lung, esophagus, genitalia, cervix, anorectal region, etc. (Figure 2-32 to 2-35).

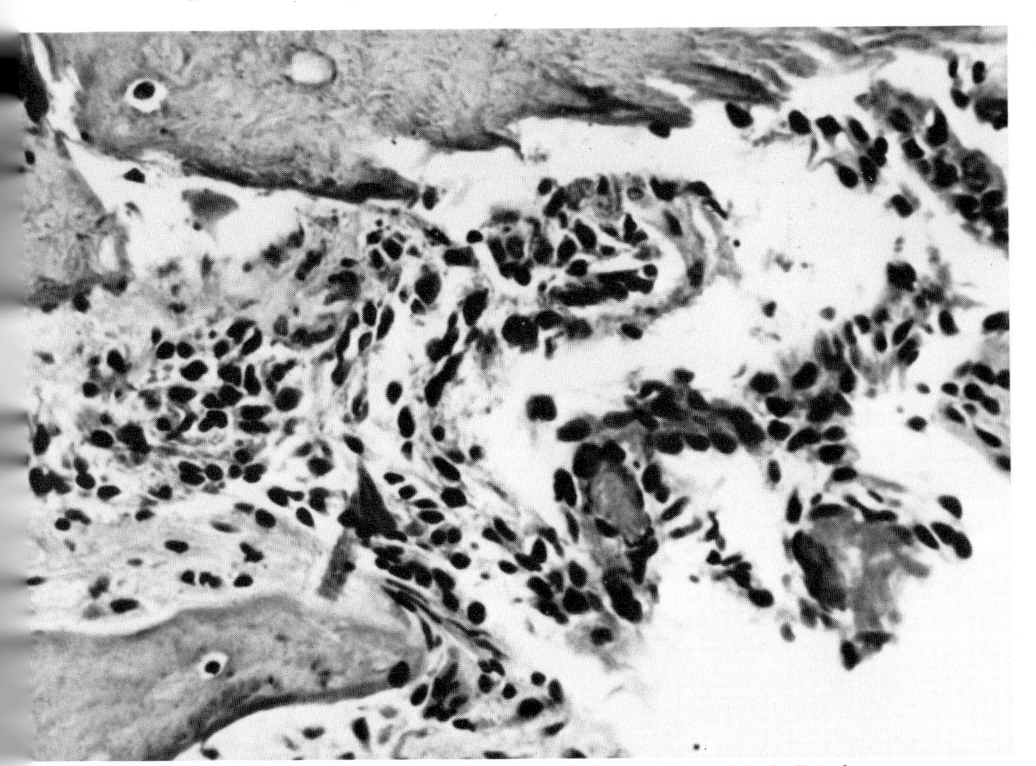

Figure 2-24. This photomicrograph (reduced 15% from 300×, H. & E.) shows many hyperchromatic breast carcinoma cells with a relatively distinct cytoplasmic border.

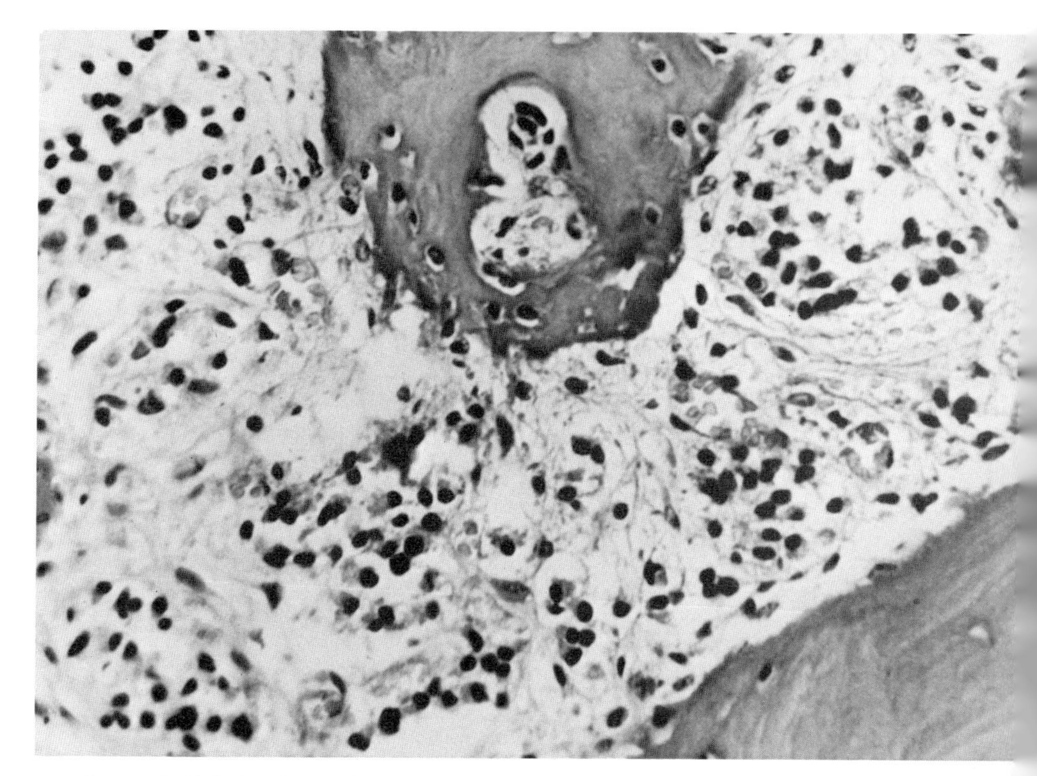

Figure 2-25. This photomicrograph (reduced 15% from 300×, H. & E.) shows invasion of bone by many hyperchromatic prostatic carcinoma cells with fairly well-defined cytoplasmic borders.

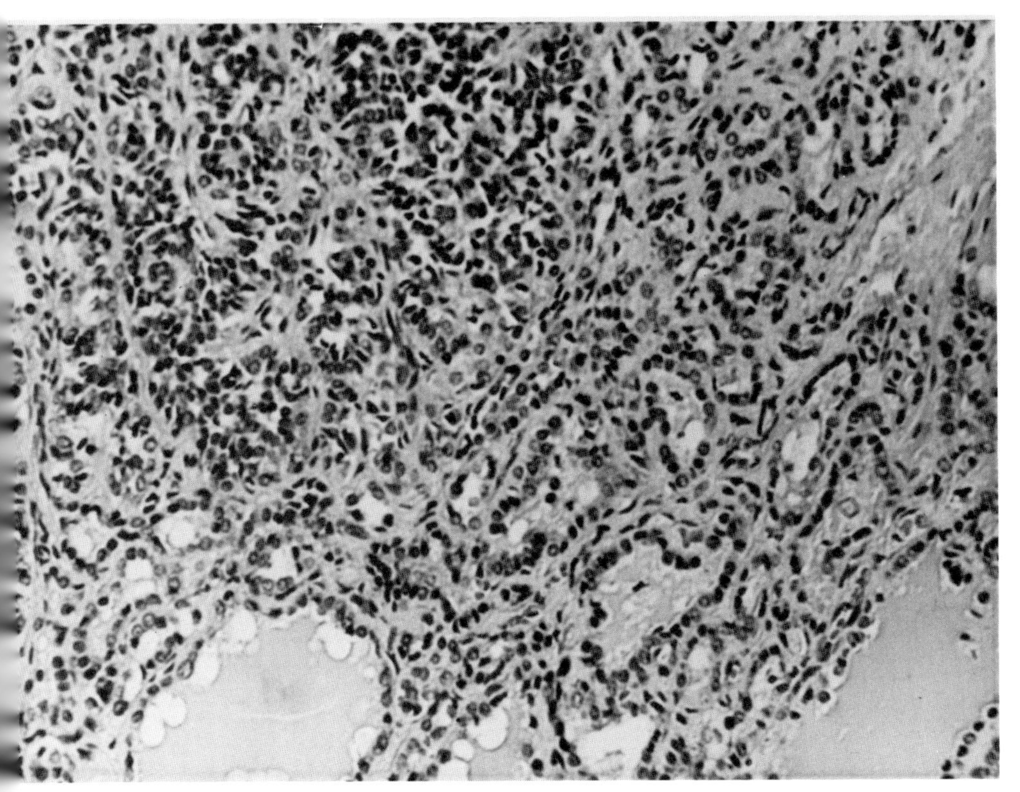

Figure 2-26. This photomicrograph (reduced 13% from 250×, H. & E.) shows the typical thyroid follicles lined by cuboidal epithelium and filled with an eosinophilic colloidal substance, the precursor of thyroid hormones.

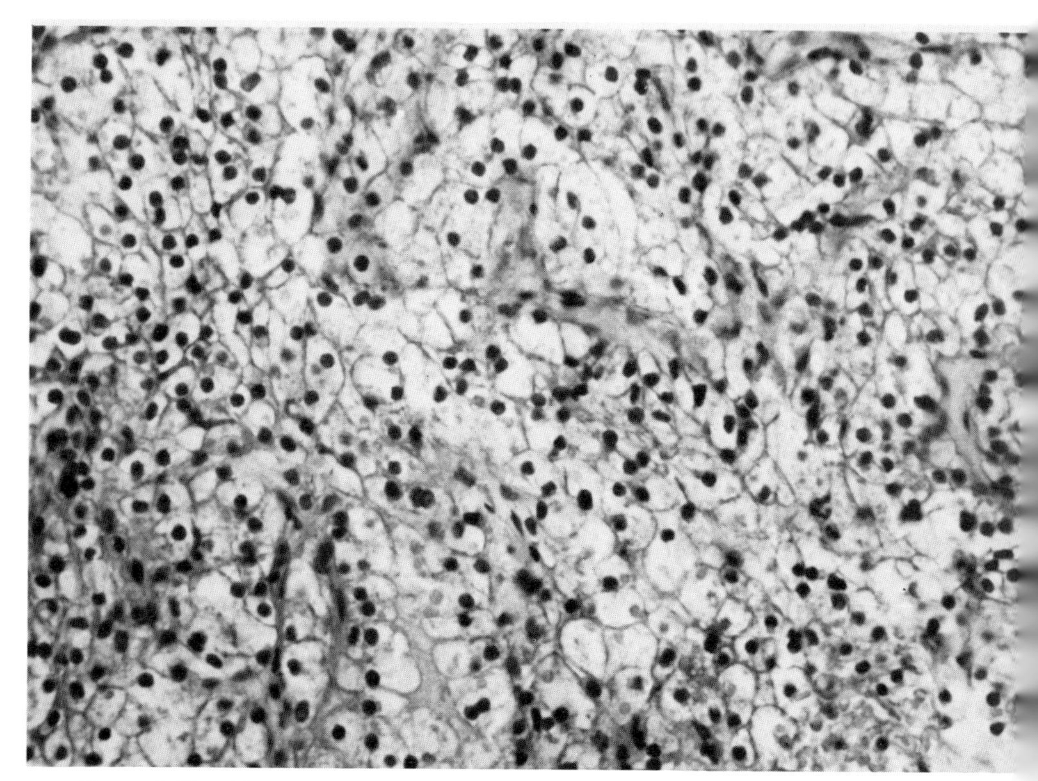

Figure 2-27. This photomicrograph (reduced 15% from 450×, H. & E.) shows the typical large hypernephroma (renal cell carcinoma) cells with round and eccentric nuclei and abundant pale foamy cytoplasm.

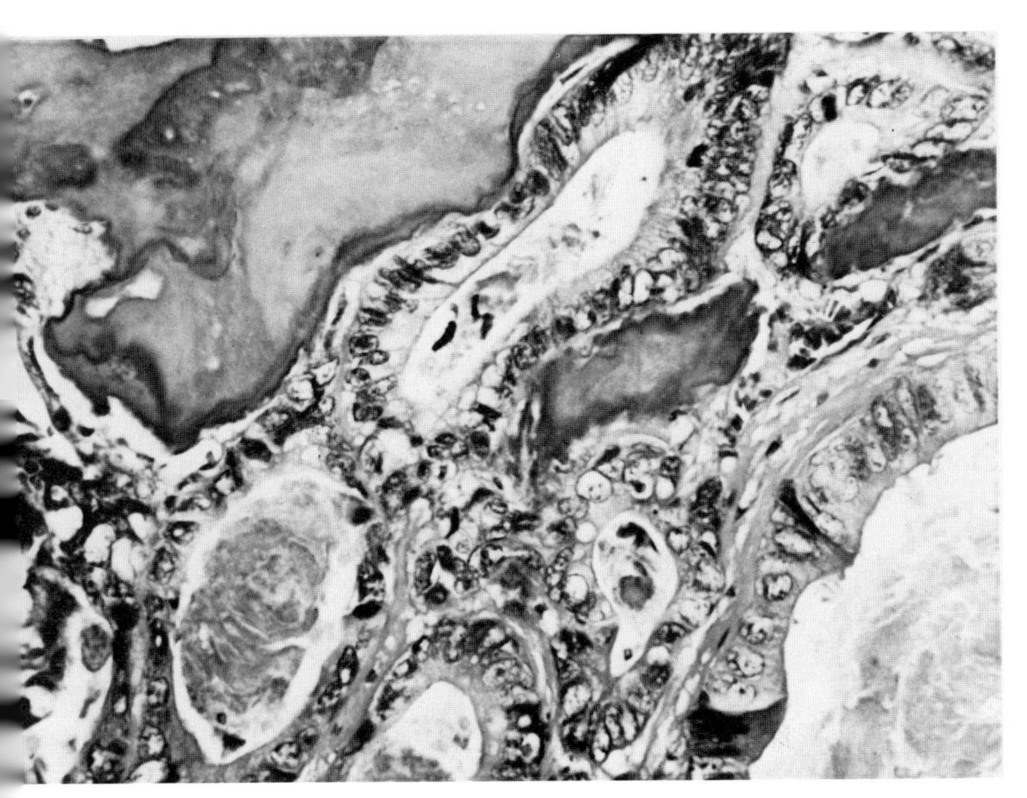

Figure 2-28. This photomicrograph (reduced 15% from 250×, H. & E.) shows intraosseous invasion of glandular structures from a colonic carcinoma, formed by columnar epithelial cells and delineated by a basement membrane.

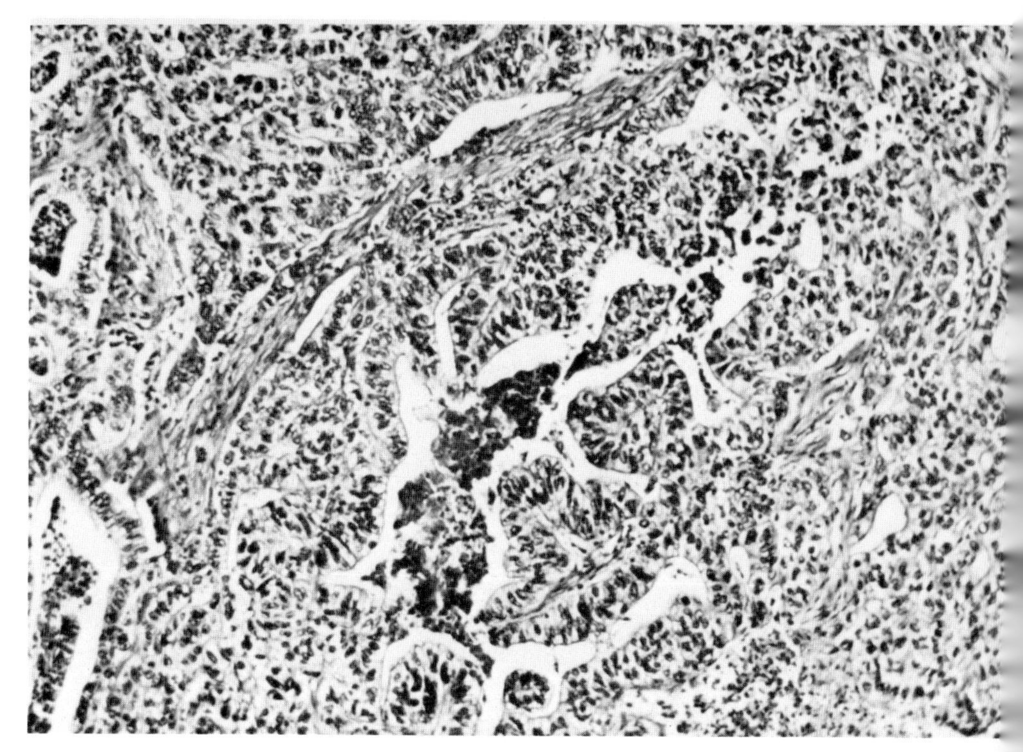

Figure 2-29. This photomicrograph (reduced 17% from 100×, H. & E.) shows sheets of tightly packed columnar epithelial cells that have formed many glandular structures in which desquamated epithelial cells can be found. These cells have their origin in a gastric carcinoma.

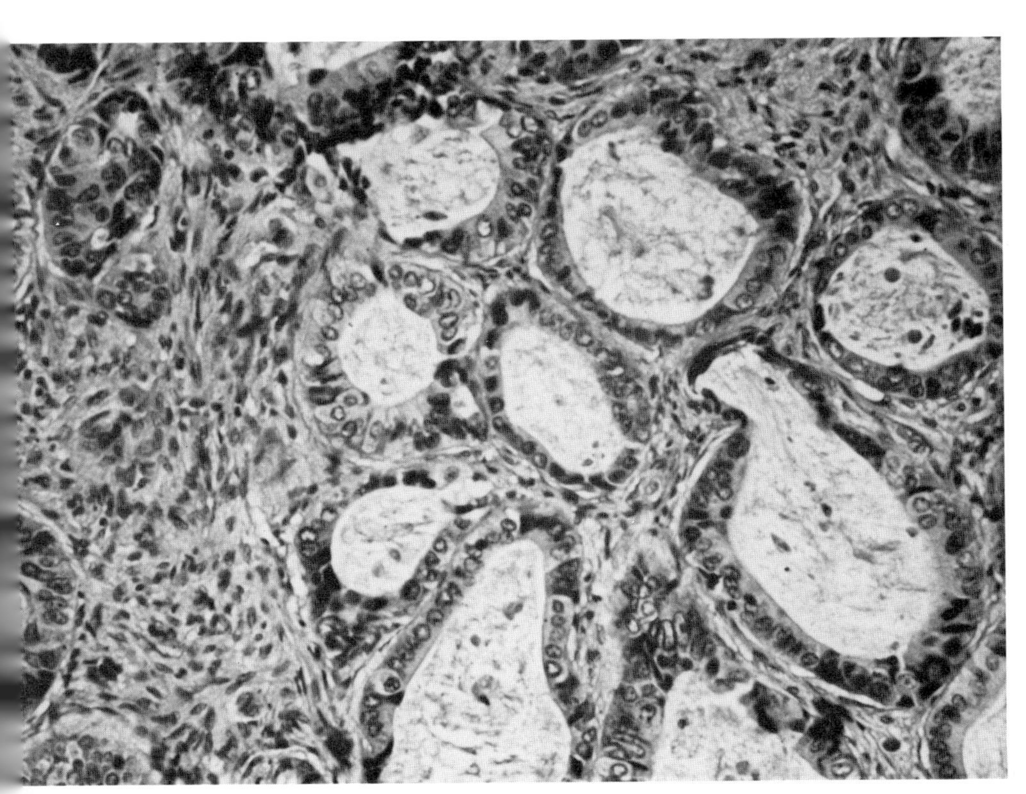

Figure 2-30. This photomicrograph (reduced 15% from 160×, H. & E.) shows glandular structures formed by metastatic adenocarcinoma cells of the lung.

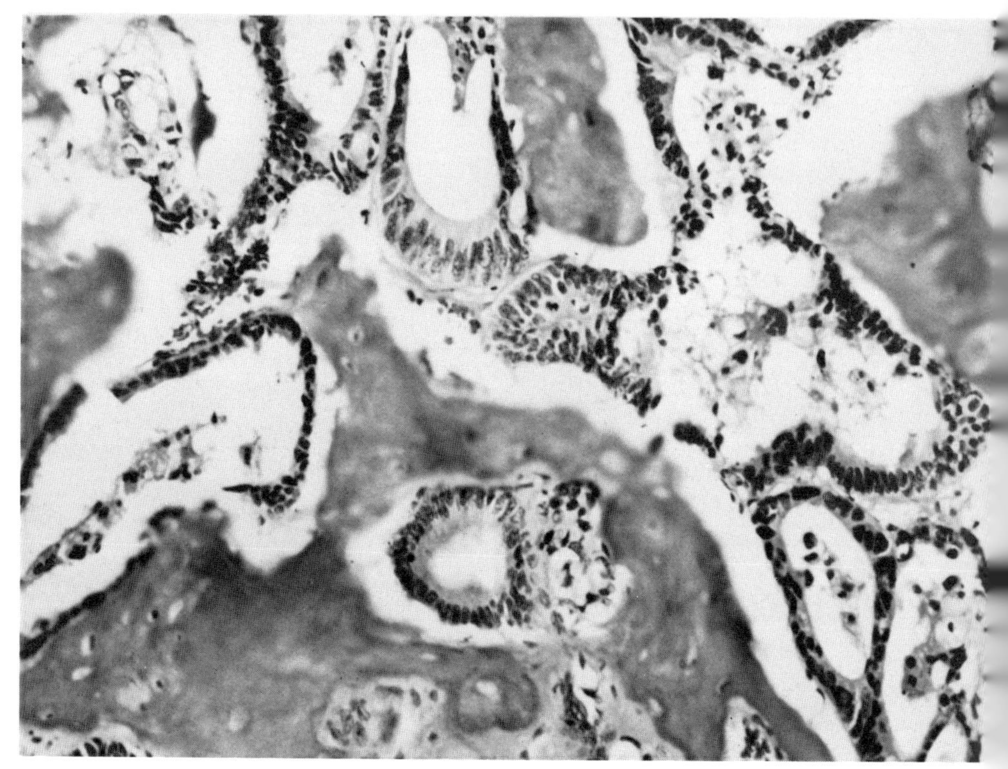

Figure 2-31. This photomicrograph (reduced 15% from 160×, H. & E.) shows many glandular structures formed by columnar epithelial cells that show extensive bone infiltration. These adenocarcinoma cells had their origin in the rectum.

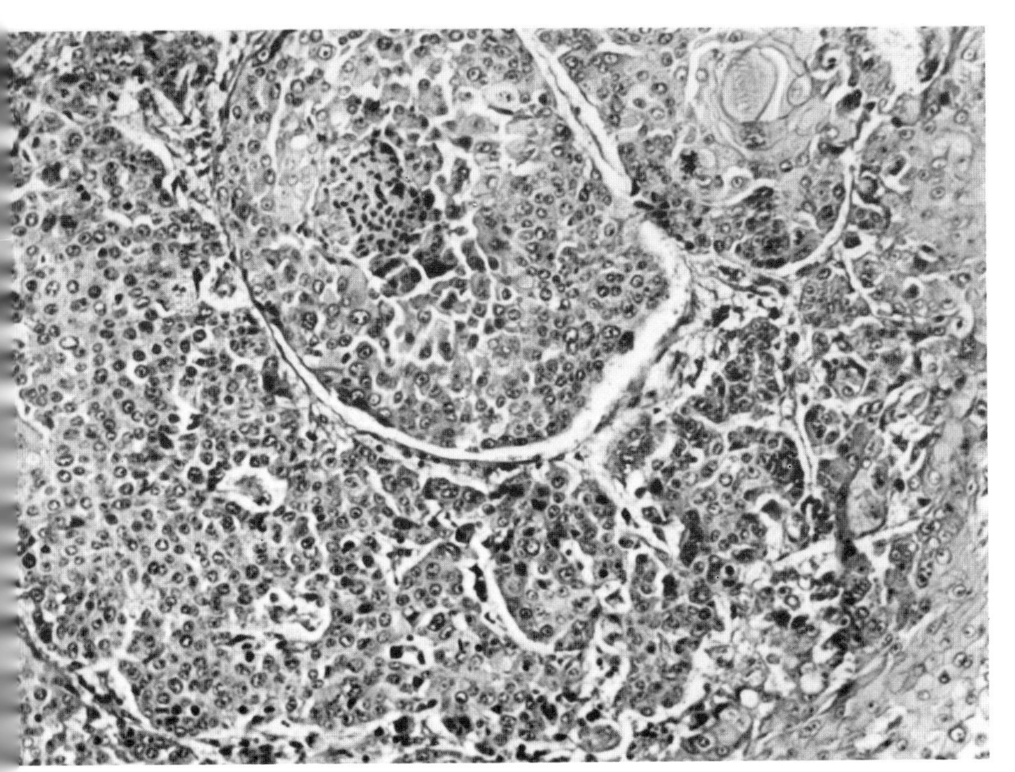

Figure 2-32. This photomicrograph (reduced 15% from 115×, H. & E.) shows a tightly packed sheet of metastatic epidermoid carcinoma cells from the lung that contains some desquamated cells and a so-called epithelial pearl in the upper right corner of the picture.

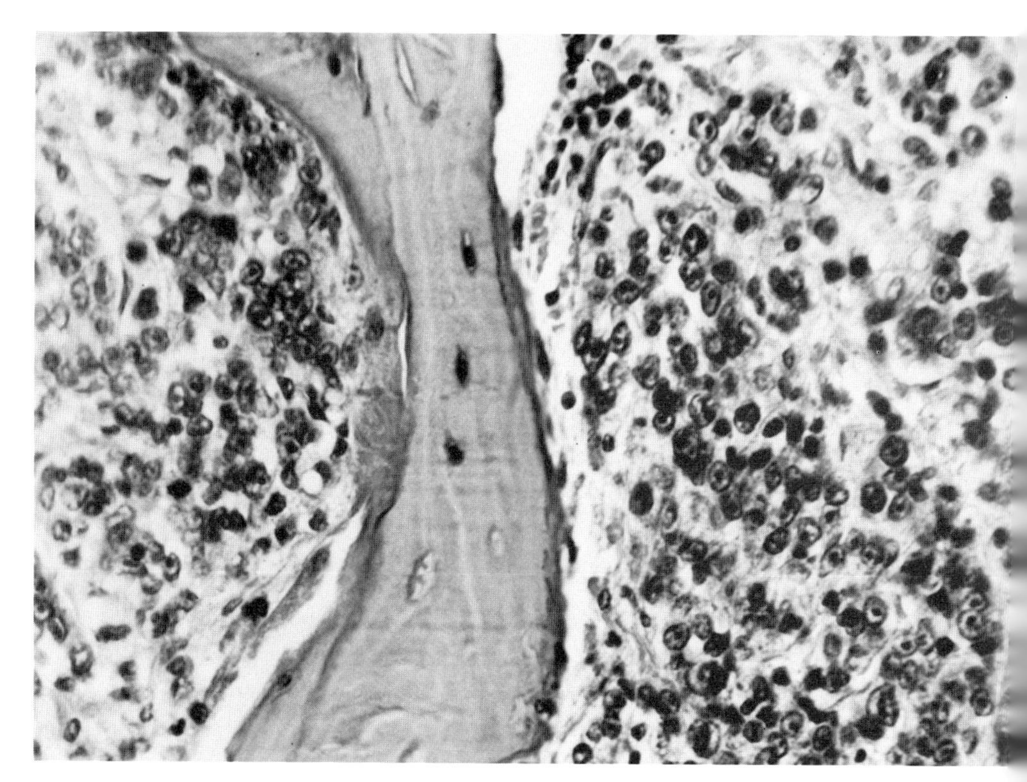

Figure 2-33. This photomicrograph (reduced 15% from 300 ×, H. & E.) shows destruction of vertebral bone by loosely arranged metastatic epidermoid carcinoma cells that came from the nasopharynx.

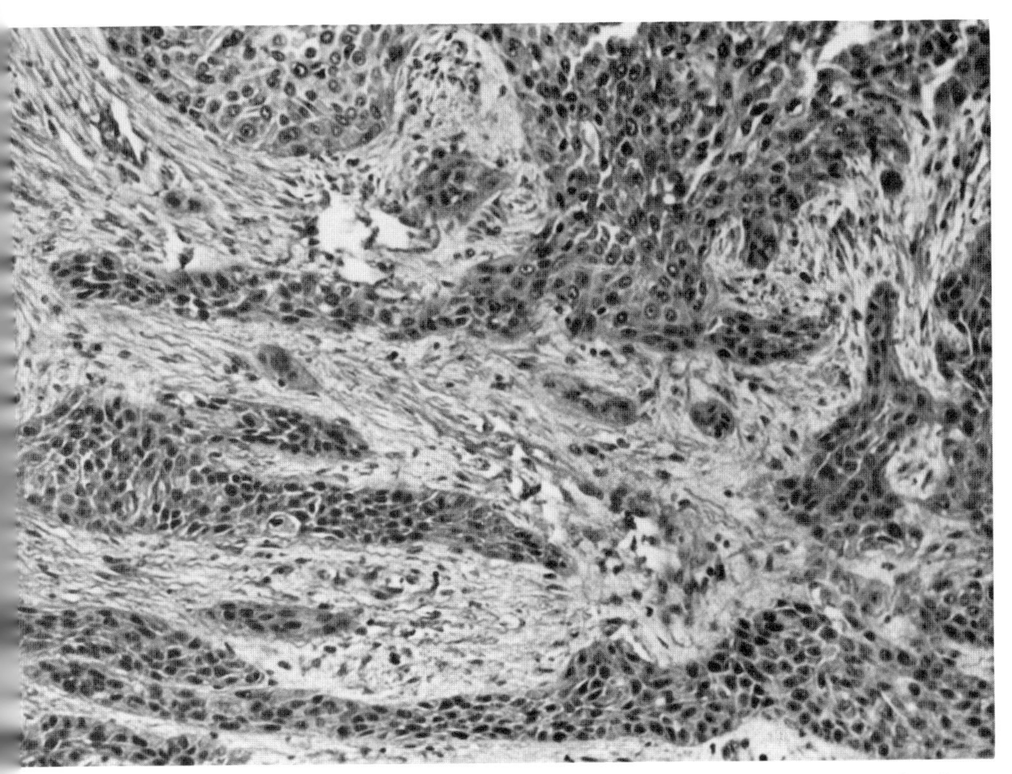

Figure 2-34. This photomicrograph (reduced 15% from 115×, H. & E.) shows cords of metastatic squamous cell carcinoma that originated in the cutaneous tissue of the arm.

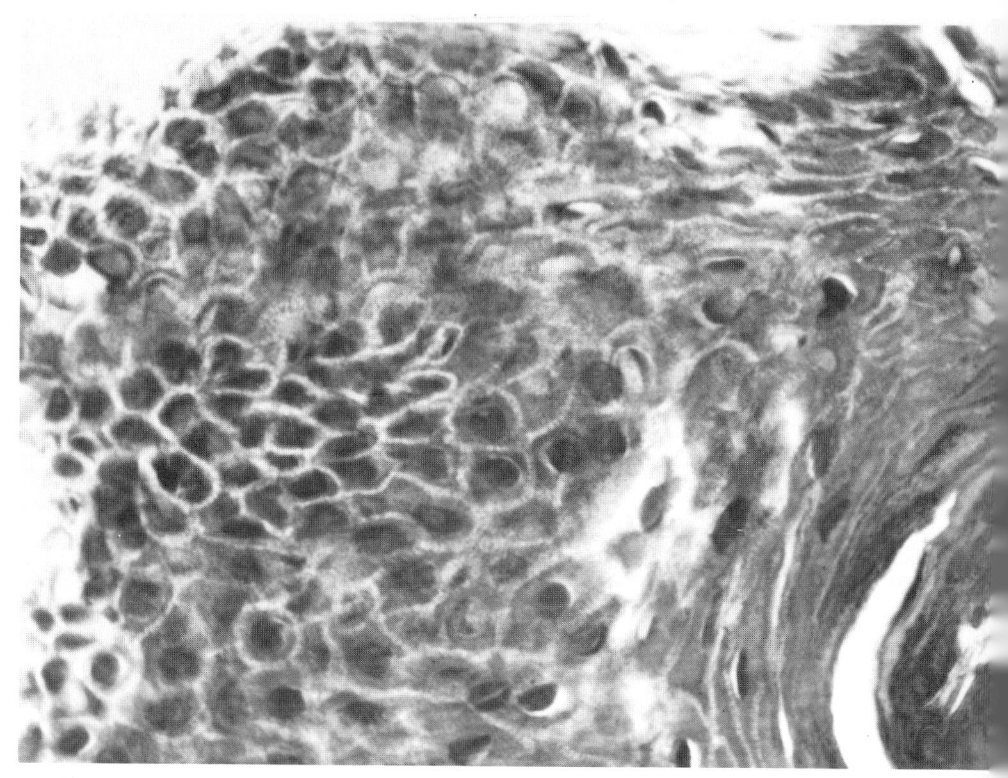

Figure 2-35. This photomicrograph (reduced 15% from 900×, H. & E.) shows many malignant melanoma cells with a clear zone around each individual cell, which clearly delineates the cytoplasmic border. Note the presence of intracytoplasmic melanin pigment.

The diagnostic problem arises when the biopsy of a spinal tumor reveals only immature and poorly differentiated cells which can be of either metastatic origin or primary sarcoma of the spine. Under this circumstance, extensive laboratory, radiological and other diagnostic studies should be employed to look for the primary site of the spinal tumor. It should be emphasized that the presence of polyostotic involvement of a spinal tumor favors the diagnosis of metastasis in spite of the fact that all diagnostic studies fail to reveal a primary site for the spinal tumor.

TREATMENT

Since patients with spinal metastases very likely have other metastases as well, chemotherapy, hormonal therapy, immunotherapy, and total body hyperthermia, which were discussed in Chapter 1, can be individually or collectively employed in treating the systemic metastases. In addition radiotherapy[228-248] and surgery[249-262] can play a very important regional role in providing pain relief and preserving and restoring neurological functions, e.g. ambulation and bladder and bowel control.

Radiotherapy is quite effective in shrinking radiosensitive tumors such as malignant lymphomas, multiple myeloma, seminoma, neuroblastoma, Ewing's sarcoma, etc., and carries a much lower mortality and morbidity rate. Therefore, it should be the primary method of treatment for all treatable spinal metastases. Furthermore, if the neurological deficit is mild and its progression is slow, radiotherapy can still be used as the primary modality of treatment for even radioresistant spinal tumors that may show favorable response to radiotherapy.

On the other hand, the indications for surgical treatment of spinal metastases include the following: spinal instability caused by destruction of spinal structural elements, e.g. pedicles, articular facets, vertebral bodies, etc., by the metastatic tumor; compression of spinal cord or nerves by bony elements caused by pathological vertebral fracture; failure of radioresistant tumor to respond to radiotherapy; previous radiation exposure of the spinal cord which may make further radiotherapy exceed the spinal cord tolerance for radiation; spinal tumor whose origin cannot be found and biopsy is necessary to rule out the possible presence of a malignant primary spinal tumor; and repeat surgical decompression for recurrent tumor for which radiotherapy for one reason or another cannot be used. Needless to say, prior to any surgical intervention, myelography and CAT scan are indispensable in determining the level and size of the tumor mass that has caused spinal cord and nerve compression and in distinguishing between intradural and extradural compression.

When the compression is in the ventral compartment of the spinal canal, a transthoracic or costotransversectomy approach should be used to provide decompression whereas a posterior laminectomy approach can be used to relieve pressure on neural elements in the posterior and lateral compartments of the spinal canal. When significant spinal instability is present, immediate stability can be achieved by repairing the spinal structural defects with methylmethacrylate which can be reinforced with metal pins or rods to gain maximal stability to last for the remainder of the cancer victim's life. Harrington rods and spinal plates can also be used to provide additional spinal support. Cervical and back braces, lumbosacral and thoracolumbar corsets, plaster and plastic casts, halo apparatus, etc., can also furnish external support and, therefore, provide palliative symptomatic relief for patients with distressful spinal metastases, especially in those situations where surgery and radiotherapy are both contraindicated. It should be stressed that hypercalcemia produced by extensive bone metastases, especially by the osteolytic metastatic tumors, should be vigorously treated with proper hydration, corticosteroids and calcitonin[263-266] in order to prevent a potentially fatal outcome and other possible long-term morbidities such as uremia secondary to hypercalcemia-induced nephrocalcinosis.

PROGNOSIS

With the exception of metastasis to the upper portion of the cervical spine where severe spinal compression can interfere with respiration and cause rapid demise, spinal metastasis in itself is generally not fatal. The following is a list of the more common causes of death in patients with metastatic carcinomas and sarcomas.[267-274]

ORGAN FAILURES.

- Lung — Pulmonary edema, infarct, embolus and fibrosis; pleural effusion; and pneumothorax.
- Heart — Pericardial effusion, myocardial infarct due to tumor emboli in coronary blood vessels, congestive heart failure, arteriosclerotic heart disease, etc.
- Central nervous system — Metastases to brain, meninges, and upper cervical spine; brain infarct caused by tumor emboli; and radiation necrosis of the brain.
- Liver — Liver failure commonly accompanied by ascites due to extensive hepatic metastasis or primary hepatic malignancies.
- Kidney — Renal failure due to renal metastasis, primary renal malignancies and hypercalcemia-induced nephrocalcinosis.

HEMORRHAGE. Tumor-induced or drug-induced thrombocytopenia, hemorrhage of organs caused by tumor invasion and hemorrhage secondary to disseminated intravascular coagulation and palliative surgical procedures.

INFECTIONS. Pneumonia, urinary tract infection, peritonitis, mediastinitis, cholecystitis, septicemia, meningitis, etc., of bacterial, fungal, viral, or protozoan etiology caused by leukopenia and weakened body defense mechanisms.

HYPERCALCEMIA. Through its adverse effects on the central nervou[s] system, heart and kidneys.

The duration of the cancer patients' survival time after the appearance of their spinal metastases will depend on the nature of the metastatic tumor; its response to various modalities of cancer therapy; the presence or absence of other serious diseases; and the patients' age, general health nutritional status, electrolyte and acid-base balance, metabolic state psychological status, etc.

REFERENCES

1. Anderson, C., and Rorabeck, C. H.: Skeletal metastases of an intracranial malignant hemangiopericytoma. *J Bone & Joint Surg, 62-A*:145-148, 1980.
2. Arseni, C. N., Simionescu, A. M., and Horwath, L.: Tumors of the spine. A follow-up study of 350 patients with neurological consideration. *Acta Psychiat et Neurologica Scandinav, 34*:398-410, 1960.

3. Auerbach, O., and Trubowitz, S.: Primary carcinoma of liver with extensive skeletal metastases and panmyelophthesis. *Cancer, 3:*837, 1950.
4. Bertin, E. J.: Metastasis to bone as the first symptom of cancer of the gastrointestinal tract. *Am J Roentgenol, 51:*614, 1944.
5. Black, P.: Spinal metastasis: Current status and recommended guidelines for management. *Neurosurgery, 5:*726-746, 1979.
6. Cantu, R. C.: Corticosteroids for spinal metastases. *Lancet, 2:*912, 1968.
7. Chade, H. O.: Metastatic tumours of the spine and spinal cord. In Vinken, P. J., and Bruyn, G. W. (Eds.): *Hand Book of Clinical Neurology.* Amsterdam, North-Holland Publishing Co., 1976, Vol. 20, pp. 415-433.
8. Cohen, D. M., Dahlin, D. C., and MacCarty, C. S.: Apparently solitary tumors of the vertebral column. *Pro Staff Meet Mayo Clin, 39:*509, 1964.
9. Copeland, M.: Bone metastases: Study of 334 cases. *Radiology, 16:*198, 1931.
10. Corrin, B., and Meadows, J. C.: Skeletal metastases from cerebellar medulloblastoma. *Br Med J, 2:*485-486, 1967.
11. Ehrlich, J. C., and Kaneko, M.: Metastasizing "adenoma" of the thyroid gland. A brief reconsideration with report of two cases. *J Mt Sinai Hosp, 24:*804, 1957.
12. Geist, R. M., and Portmann, U. V.: Primary malignant tumors of the nasopharynx. *Am J Roentgenol, 68:*262, 1952.
13. Ferreira, A. M., and Mendes, J. R.: Regression of bone metastases from renal cell carcinoma achieved by combined therapy. *Eur Urol, 2:*100-101, 1976.
14. Goldman, R. L., Winterling, A. N., and Winterling, C. C.: Maturation of tumors of the sympathetic nervous system. Report of long-term survival in two patients, one with disseminated osseous metastases, and review of cases from the literature. *Cancer, 18:*1510-1516, 1965.
15. Guri, J. P.: Tumors of the vertebral column. *Surg Gynec & Obstet, 87:*583-598, 1948.
16. Gyepes, M. T., and D'Angio, G. J.: Extracranial metastases from central nervous system tumors in children and adolescents. *Radiology, 87:*55, 1966.
17. Harris, J. H., Jr., and Libshitz, H.: Basal cell carcinoma of skin metastasizing to bone. *J Canadian Assn Radiol, 23:*217, 1972.
18. Henderson, D. W., Raven, J. L., Pollard, J. A., and Walters, M. N.: Bone marrow metastases in disseminated alveolar rhabdomyosarcoma: Case report with ultrastructural study and review. *Pathology, 8:*329-341, 1976.
19. Hoke, H. F., Jr., and Harrelson, A. B.: Granular cell ameloblastoma with metastasis to the cervical vertebrae. Observations on the origin of the granular cells. *Cancer, 20:*991-999, 1967.
20. Jackson, R.: Metastasizing basal cell carcinoma: A case report. *Canadian J Surg, 9:*411-414, 1966.
21. Kirkpatrick, D. B., Dawson, E., Haskell, C. M., and Batzdorf, U.: Metastatic carcinoid presenting as a spinal tumor. *Surg Neurol, 4:*283-287, 1975.
22. Lafferty, J. O., and Pendergrass, E. P.: Carcinoma of testes with metastasis to bone. *Am J Roentgenol, 63:*95, 1950.
23. Outerbridge, R. E.: Malignant adenoma of thyroid with secondary metastases to bone with discussion of so-called "benign metastasizing goiter." *Ann Surg, 125:*282, 1947.
24. Patchefsky, A. S., Keller, I. B., and Mansfield, C. M.: Solitary vertebral column metastasis from occult sclerosing carcinoma of the thyroid gland: Report of a case. *Am J Clin Pathol, 53:*596-601, 1970.
25. Pearson, B. W., Unni, K. K., Sizemore, G. W., and Norman, S. G.: Case report: Cellular medullary carcinoma as cervical metastases of undetermined origin. *Otolaryngol, Head, Neck Surg, 87:*640-644, 1979.

26. Pendergrass, E. P., and Selman, J.: Dysgerminoma of ovary with widespread metastases. *Radiology, 46:*377, 1946.
27. Russo, P. E.: Malignant melanoma in infancy. *Radiology, 48:*15, 1947.
28. Scott, M., Kellet, G., and Peale, A.: Angioblastic meningioma (hemangiopericytoma) of the cerebellar fossa with metastases to temporal bone and the lumbar spine *Surg Neurol, 2:*35-38, 1974.
29. Shiraishi, S., Ohkubo, Y., and Saito, T.: Regression of multiple osseous metastatic renal cell carcinoma. *Clin Orthop, 138:*246-249, 1979.
30. Sugimura, M., Yamauchi, T., Yashikawa, K., Takeda, N., Sakita, M., and Miyazaki T.: Malignant ameloblastoma with metastasis to the lumbar vertebra: Report of case. *J Oral Surg, 27:*350-357, 1969.
31. Tyler, A. F.: Epithelioma of lip metastatic to the vertebra. *Am J Roentgenol, 48:*76 1942.
32. Whitehouse, G. H., and Griffiths, G. J.: Roentgenologic aspects of spinal involvement by primary and metastatic Ewing's tumor. *J Can Assoc Radiol, 27:*290-297, 1976
33. Wolf, E., and Vickery, A. L.: Primary fibrosarcoma of heart with vertebral metastasis *Arch Path, 43:*244, 1947.
34. Abrams, H. L.: Skeletal metastases in carcinoma. *Radiology, 55:*534-538, 1950.
35. Abrams, H. L., Spiro, R., and Goldstein, N.: Metastases in carcinoma. *Cancer, 3:*74 1950.
36. Antoni, N. R. E.: Tumoren der Virbelsaule einschliesslicm des Epiduralen Spinal raumes. In Bumke, O. and Foerster, O.: *Handbuch der Neurologie.* Berlin, Springer, 1936, Vol. X, pp. 51-109.
37. Geschickter, C. F., and Copeland, M. M.: *Tumors of Bone,* ed 3. Philadelphia, J. B Lippincott, 1949.
38. Stein, R. J.: "Silent" skeletal metastases in cancer. *Am J Clin Path, 13:*34-41, 1943
39. Toumey, J. W.: Metastatic malignancy of the spine. *J Bone & Joint Surg, 25:*292-30 1943.
40. Young, J. M., and Funk, F. J., Jr.: Incidence of tumor metastases to the lumbar spine A comparative study of roentgenographic changes and gross lesions. *J Bone & Joint Surg, 35-A:*55-64, 1953.
41. Batson, O. V.: The function of the vertebral veins and their role in the spread of metastases. *Ann Surg, 112:*138, 1940.
42. Batson, O. V.: The vertebral vein system as a mechanism for the spread of metastases *Am J Roentgenol, 48:*715, 1942.
43. Codman, D. R., and DeLong, R. P.: The role of the vertebral venous system in the metastasis of cancer to the spinal column. Experiments with tumor-cell suspensions in rats and rabbits. *Cancer, 4:*610, 1951.
44. Wu, K. K., and Guise, E. R.: Metastatic tumors of the hand: A report of six cases. *Hand Surg, 3:*271-276, 1978.
45. Wu, K. K., and Guise, E. R.: Metastatic tumors of the foot. *South Med J, 71:*807-80 1978.
46. Wu, K. K., Winkelman, N. Z., and Guise, E. R.: Metastatic bronchogenic carcinoma the finger simulating acute osteomyelitis. *Orthopedics, 3:*23-28, 1980.
47. Scott, M. G.: Carcinoma of the pancreas with direct involvement of spine, stoma and colon. *Br J Radiol, 25:*671, 1952.
48. Jarvis, L. J.: Involvement of the sacrum by recurrent carcinoma of the rectum. *Am Roentgenol, 84:*339, 1960.
49. Auld, A. W., and Buerman, A.: Metastatic spinal epidural tumors: An analysis of cases. *Arch Neurol, 15:*100 108, 1966.

50. Barron, K. O., Hirano, A., Araki, S., and Terry, R. D.: Experiences with metastatic neoplasms involving the spinal cord. *Neurology, 9:*91, 1959.
51. Chang, Y. C., and Chen, R. C.: Craniospinal and cerebral metastasis of primary hepatomas: A report of 7 cases. *Taiwan I. Hsueh Hui Tsa Chih, 78:*594-604, 1979.
52. Feiring, E. H., and Hubbard, J. H., Jr.: Spinal cord compression resulting from intradural carcinoma. Report of two cases. *J Neurosurg, 23:*635-638, 1965.
53. Fisher, M. S.: Lumbar spine metastasis in cervical carcinoma: A characteristic pattern. *Radiology, 134:*631-634, 1980.
54. Gilbert, H., Apuzzo, M., Marshall, L., Kagan, A. R., Crue, B., Wagner, J., Fuchs, K., Rush, J., Rao, A., Nussbaum, H., and Chan, P.: Neoplastic epidural spinal cord compression. A current perspective. *JAMA, 240:*2771-2773, 1978.
55. Gilbert, R. W., Kim, J. H., and Posner, J. B.: Epidural spinal cord compression from metastatic tumor: Diagnosis and treatment. *Ann Neurol, 3:*40-51, 1978.
56. Halnan, K. E., and Roberts, P. H.: Paraplegia caused by spinal metastasis from thyroid cancer. *Br Med J, 3:*534-536, 1967.
57. Kennady, J. C., and Stern, W. E.: Metastatic neoplasms of the vertebral column producing compression of the spinal cord. *Am J Surg, 104:*155-168, 1962.
58. Kleinman, W. B., Kierman, H. A., and Michelsen, W. J.: Metastatic cancer of the spinal column. *Clin Orthop, 136:*166-172, 1978.
59. Mones, R. J., Dozier, D., and Berrett, A.: Analysis of medical treatment of malignant extradural spinal cord tumors. *Cancer, 19:*1842-1853, 1966.
60. Mullan, J., and Evans, J. P.: Neoplastic disease of the spinal extradural space: A review of fifty cases. *Arch Surg, 74:*900-907, 1957.
61. Olson, M. E., Chernik, N. L., and Posner, J. B.: Infiltration of the leptomeninges by systemic cancer. A clinical and pathologic study. *Arch Neurol, 30:*122, 1974.
62. Posner, J. B.: Spinal cord compression: A neurological emergency. *Clin Bull, 1:*65-71, 1971.
63. Posner, J. B.: Management of central nervous system metastases. *Semin Oncol, 4:*81-91, 1977.
64. Posner, J. B., Howieson, J., and Cvitkovic, E.: "Disappearing" spinal cord compression: Oncolytic effect of glucocorticoids (and other chemotherapeutic agents) on epidural metastases. *Ann Neurol, 2:*409-413, 1977.
65. Rogers, L.: Malignant spinal tumours and the epidural space. *Br J Surg, 45:*416-422, 1958.
66. Torma, T.: Malignant tumors of the spine and the spinal extradural space: A study based on 250 histologically verified cases. *Acta Chir Scand* (Suppl.), *225:*1-176, 1957.
67. Venkataramana, B. S., and Jakoby, R. K.: Spinal cord compression secondary to metastatic mammary carcinoma. *J Am Med Wom Assoc, 20:*953-955, 1965.
68. Wild, W. O., and Porter, R. W.: Metastatic epidural tumor of the spine: A study of 45 cases. *Arch Surg, 87:*825-830, 1963.
69. Besarab, A., and Caro, J. F.: Mechanisms of hypercalcemia in malignancy. *Cancer, 41:*2276-2285, 1978.
70. Burt, M. E., and Brennan, M. F.: Hypercalcemia and malignant melanoma. *Am J Surg, 137:*790-794, 1979.
71. Jaffe, H. L., and Bodansky, A.: Serum calcium: Clinical and biochemical considerations. *J Mt Sinai Hosp, 9:*901, 1953.
72. Kennedy, B. J., Tibbetts, D. M., Nathanson, I. T., and Aub, J. C.: Hypercalcemia, a complication of hormone therapy of advanced breast cancer. *Cancer Research, 13:*445, 1953.

73. Lacey, C. G., Morrow, C. P.: Hypercalcemia in patients with squamous cell carcinoma of the cervix. *Gynecol Oncol, 7:*215-222, 1979.
74. Liston, S. L.: Hypercalcemia and head and neck cancer. Bony metastases from tongue cancer. *Arch Otolaryngol, 104:*597-600, 1978.
75. Mandell, J., Magee, M. C., and Fried, F. H.: Hypercalcemia associated with uroepithelial neoplasms. *J Urol, 119:*844-845, 1978.
76. Myers, W. P. L.: Hypercalcemia in neoplastic disease. *Cancer, 9:*1135, 1956.
77. Myer, W. P. L.: Hypercalcemia in neoplastic disease. *Arch Surg, 80:*308, 1960.
78. Olsson, A. M., and Jonsson, G.: Advanced cancer of the prostate combined with hypercalcaemia. *Scand J Urol Nephrol, 11:*293-296, 1977.
79. Plimpton, C. H., and Gellhorn, A.: Hypercalcemia in malignant disease without evidence of bone destruction. *Am J Med, 21:*750, 1956.
80. Tashima, C. K., Samaan, N. A., Blumenschein, G. R., and Hickey, R. C.: Etiologic factors of hypercalcemia in breast cancer. *Tex Med, 74:*52-55, 1978.
81. Woodard, H. Q.: Changes in blood chemistry associated with carcinoma metastatic to bone. *Cancer, 6:*1219, 1953.
82. Bonadonna, G., Merlino, J. J., Myers, W. P. L., and Sonenberg, M.: Urinary hydroxyproline and calcium metabolism in patients with cancer. *N Engl J Med, 275:*298-305, 1966.
83. Bishop, M. C., and Fellows, G. J.: Urine hydroxyproline excretion — a marker of bone metastases in prostatic carcinoma. *Br J Urol, 49:*711-716, 1977.
84. Cuschieri, A., Jarvie, R., Taylor, W. H., Cant, E., Furnival, C. M., and Blumgart, L. H.: Three-center study on urinary hydroxyproline excretion in cancer of the breast. *Br J Cancer, 37:*1002-1005, 1978.
85. Gasser, A. B., Depierre, D., and Cour Voisier, B.: Total urinary and free serum hydroxyproline in metastatic bone disease. *Br J Cancer, 39:*280-283, 1979.
86. Guzzo, C. E., Pachas, W. N., Pinals, R. S., and Krant, M. J.: Urinary hydroxyproline in patients with cancer. *Cancer, 24:*382-387, 1969.
87. Heller, W., Harimann, R., Bichler, K. H., and Schmidt, K.: Urinary hydroxyproline in healthy patients and in prostate patients with and without bone metastases. *Cu Probl Clin Biochem, 9:*249-256, 1979.
88. Hosley, H. F., Taft, E. G., Olsen, K. B., Gates, S., and Beebe, R. T.: Hydroxyproline excretion in malignant neoplastic disease. *Arch Intern Med, 118:*565-571, 1966.
89. Kelleher, P. C.: Urinary excretion of hydroxyproline, hydroxylysine and hydroxylysine glycosides by patients with Paget's Disease of bone and carcinoma with metastases in bone. *Clin Chim Acta, 92:*373-379, 1979.
90. Kontturi, M. J., Sontaniemi, E. A., and Larmi, T. K. I.: Hydroxyproline in the earl diagnosis of bone metastases in prostatic cancer. *Scand J Urol Nephrol, 8:*91, 1974
91. Platt, W. D., Doolittle, L. H., and Hartshorn, J. W. S.: Urine hydroxyproline excretion in metastatic cancer of bone. *New Engl J Med, 271:*287-290, 1964.
92. Powles, T. J., Leese, C. L., and Bondy, P. K.: Hydroxyproline excretion in patient with breast cancer and response to treatment. *Br Med J, 2:*164, 1975.
93. Grieboff, S. I., Herrmann, J. B., Smelin, A., and Moss, J.: Hypercalcemia secondar to bone metastases from carcinoma of the breast. I. Relationship between serur calcium and alkaline phosphatase values. *J Clin Endocrinol, 14:*378, 1954.
94. Jaffe, H. L.: Dignostic significance of serum alkaline and acid phosphatase values i relation to bone disease. *Bull NY Acad Med, 19:*831, 1943.
95. Van Lente, F.: Alkaline and acid phosphatase determinations in bone disease. *Orth Clin North Am, 10:*437-450, 1979.
96. Wajsman, Z., Chu, T. M., Bross, D., Saroff, J., Murphy, G. P., Johnson, D. E., Scot W. W., Gibbons, R. P., Prout, G. R., and Schmidt, J. D.: Clinical significance

serum alkaline phosphatase isoenzyme levels in advanced prostatic carcinoma. *J Urol, 119:*244-246, 1978.

97. White, D. R., Maloney, J. J., III, Muss, H. B., Vance, R. P., Barnes, P., Howard, V., Rhyne, L., and Cowan, R. J.: Serum alkaline phyosphatase determination. Value in the staging of advanced breast cancer. *JAMA, 242:*1147-1149, 1979.
98. Bennington, J. L.: Cancer of the kidney — etiology, epidemiology and pathology. *Cancer, 32:*1017-1029, 1973.
99. Bennington, J. L., and Kradjian, R. M.: *Renal Carcinoma.* Philadelphia, W. B. Saunders, 1967.
100. Beer, E.: Some aspects of malignant tumours of the kidney (B. A. Thomas oration). *Surg Gynecol Obstet, 65:*433-446, 1937.
101. Flocks, R. H., and Kadesky, M. C.: Malignant neoplasms of the kidney; an analysis of 353 patients followed five years or more. *Trans Am Assoc Genitourin Surg, 49:*105-110, 1957.
102. Klapproth, H. J.: Wilm's tumor: A report of 45 cases and an analysis of 1351 cases reported in the world literature from 1940 to 1958. *J Urol, 81:*633-648, 1959.
103. Goldberg, M. F., Tashjian, A. H., Jr., Order, S. E., and Dammin, G. J.: Renal adenocarcinoma containing a parathyroid hormone-like substance and associated with marked hypercalcemia. *Am J Med, 36:*805-815, 1964.
104. O'Grady, A. S., Morse, L. J., and Lee, J. B.: Parathyroid hormone-secreting renal carcinoma associated with hypercalcemia and metabolic alkalosis. *Ann Intern Med, 63:*858-868, 1965.
105. Bell, E. T.: Carcinoma of the pancreas. I. A clinical and pathologic study of 609 necropsied cases. II. The relation of carcinoma of the pancreas to diabetes mellitus. *Am J Pathol, 33:*499-523, 1957.
06. Ellison, E. H., and Wilson, S. D.: The Zollinger-Ellison syndrome; reappraisal and evaluation of 260 registered cases. *Ann Surg, 160:*512-530, 1964.
07. Gullick, H. D.: Carcinoma of the pancreas; a review and critical study of 100 cases. *Medicine* (Baltimore), *38:*47-84, 1959.
08. Hanno, H. A., and Banks, R. W.: Islet cell carcinoma of pancreas with metastasis. *Ann Surg, 117:*437-449, 1943.
09. Leven, N. L.: Primary carcinoma of the pancreas. *Am J Cancer, 18:*852-874, 1933.
10. Levine, M., and Danovitch, S. H.: Metastatic carcinoma to the pancreas. *Am J Gastroenterol, 60:*290-294, 1973.
11. Sallick, M. A., and Garlock, J. H.: Obstructive jaundice due to carcinoma of the pancreas; the choice of operative procedure. *Ann Surg, 115:*25-31, 1942.
12. Van Der Veer, J. S., Choufoer, J. C., Zuerido, A., Van Der Heul, R. O., Hollander, C. F., and Van Rijssel, T. G.: Metastasizing islet cell tumor of the pancreas associated with hypoglycemia and carcinoid syndrome. *Lancet, 1:*1416-1419, 1964.
13. Williams, C., Jr., Bryson, G. H., and Hume, D. M.: Islet cell tumors and hypoglycemia. *Ann Surg, 169:*757-773, 1969.
14. Zollinger, R. M., and Ellison, E. H.: Primary peptic ulceration of the jejunum associated with islet cell tumors of the pancreas. *Ann Surg, 142:*709-728, 1955.
15. Aljersjo, O., Bengmark, S., Hafstrom, L., and Rosengren K.: Accuracy of diagnostic tools in malignant hepatic lesions. *Am J Surg, 127:*663-668, 1974.
16. Al-Sarraf, M., Kithier, K., and Vaitkevicius, V. K.: Primary liver cancer. *Cancer, 33:*574-582, 1974.
17. Gall, E. A.: Primary and metastatic carcinoma of the liver; relationship to hepatic cirrhosis. *Arch Pathol, 70:*226-232, 1960.

118. Imperato, P. J., and Lipton, M. S.: Hypoglycemia in primary carcinoma of liver. *NY J Med, 65:*2707-2710, 1965.
119. Nelson, R. S., DeElizalde, R., and Howe, C. D.: Clinical aspects of primary carcinoma of the liver. *Cancer, 19:*533-537, 1966.
120. Sasaki, K., Okuda, S., Takahashi, M., and Sasaki, M.: Hepatic clear cell carcinoma associated with hypoglycemia and hypercholesterolemia. *Cancer, 47:*820-822, 1981.
121. Thompson, C. M., and Hilferty, D. J.: Primary carcinoma of the liver (Cholangioma) with hypoglycemic convulsions. *Gastroenterol, 20:*158-165, 1952.
122. Cook, W. B., Fishman, W. H., and Clark, B. G.: Serum acid phosphatase of prostate origin in the diagnosis of prostatic cancer; Clinical evaluation of 2408 tests by the Fishman-Lerner method. *J Urol, 88:*281-287, 1962.
123. Fishman, W. H., Bonner, C. D., and Homberger, F.: Serum "prostatic" acid phosphatase and cancer of the prostate. *N Engl J Med, 255:*925-933, 1950.
124. Gursel, E. O., Rezvan, M., Sy, F. A., and Veenema, R. J.: Comparative evaluation of bone marrow acid phosphatase and bone scanning of staging of prostatic cancer. *J Urol, 111:*53-57, 1974.
125. Gutman, A. B.: The development of the acid phosphatase test for prostatic carcinoma. *Bull NY Acad Med, 44:*63-76, 1968.
126. Gutman, A. B., Gutman, E. B., and Robinson, J. M.: Determination of serum "acid" phosphatase activity in differentiating skeletal metastases secondary to prostatic carcinoma from Paget's Disease of bone. *Am J Cancer, 38:*103-108, 1950.
127. Woodard, H. Q.: The interpretation of phosphatase findings in carcinoma of the prostate. *NY J Med, 47:*379-381, 1947.
128. Wray, S.: The significance of the blood acid and alkaline phosphatase values in cancer of the prostate. *J Clin Pathol, 9:*341-346, 1956.
129. Crout, J. R., Sjoerdsma, A.: Turnover and metabolism of catecholamines in patients with pheochromocytoma. *J Clin Invest, 43:*94-102, 1964.
130. Cryer, P. E., and Kissane, J. M. (eds.): Clinicopathologic conference on metastatic catecholamine-secreting paraganglioma (extra-adrenal pheochromocytoma). *Am J Med, 61:*523-532, 1976.
131. Gitlow, S. E., Dziedzic, L. B., Stauss, L., Greenwood, S. M., and Dziedzic, S. W.: Biochemical and histologic determinants in the prognosis of neuroblastoma *Cancer, 32:*898-905, 1973.
132. Kaser, H.: Catecholamine-producing neural tumors other than pheochromocytoma *Pharmacol Rev, 18:*659-665, 1966.
133. Robinson, R., Smith, P., and Whittaker, S. R. F.: Secretion of catecholamines in malignant phaeochromocytoma. *Br Med J, 1:*1422-1424, 1964.
134. Sato, T. L., Sjoerdsma, A.: Urinary homovanillic acid in pheochromocytoma. *Br Med J, 2:*1472-1473, 1965.
135. Tanigawa, H., Allison, D. J., and Assaykeen, T. A.: A comparison of the effects of various catecholamines on plasma renin activity alone and in the presence of adrenergic blocking agents. In Genest, J., and Koiw, E. (Eds.): *Hypertension.* New York, Springer Verlag, 1972, pp. 37-44.
136. Von Studnitz, W.: Chemistry and pharmacology of catecholamine secreting tumors *Pharmacol Rev, 18:*645-650, 1966.
137. Williams, C. M., and Greer, M.: Homovanillic acid and vanilmandelic acid in diagnosis of neuroblastoma. *JAMA, 183:*836-840, 1963.
138. Black, S. P. W., and Keats, T. E.: Generalized osteosclerosis secondary to metastatic medulloblastoma of cerebellum. *Radiology, 82:*395, 1964.
139. Bloch, C., and Peck, H. M.: Diffuse osteoblastic metastases from carcinoma of the stomach. Case report. *J Mount Sinai Hosp NY, 29:*451, 1962.

140. Blumer, H., Aronoff, A., Chartier, J., and Shapiro, L.: Carcinoma of the stomach with myelosclerosis: Presentation of a case and review of the literature. *Canadian MAJ, 84:*1254, 1961.
141. Fried, J. R.: Skeletal and pulmonary metastases from cancer of the kidney, prostate and bladder. *Am J Roentgenol, 55:*153, 1946.
142. Jaffe, N.: Osteoblastic metastases in carcinoma of the pancreas. *Br J Radiol, 44:*226, 1971.
143. Jaffe, N., and Antonioli, D. A.: Osteoblastic bone metastases secondary to adenocarcinoma of the pancreas. *Clin Radiol, 29:*41-46, 1978.
144. Peavy, P. W., Rogers, J. V., Jr., Clements, J. L., Jr., and Borns, J. B.: Unusual osteoblastic metastases from carcinoid tumors. *Radiology, 107:*327, 1973.
145. Pederson, R. T., Haidak, D. J., Ferris, R. A., MacDonal, J. S., and Schein, P. S.: Osteoblastic bone metastases in Zollinger-Ellison syndrome. *Radiology, 118:*63-64, 1976.
146. Thomas, B. M.: Three unusual carcinoid tumors with particular reference to osteoblastic bone metastases. *Clin Radiol, 19:*221, 1968.
147. Toomey, F. B., and Felson, B.: Osteoblastic bone metastases in gastrointestinal and bronchial carcinoids. *Am J Roentgenol, 83:*709, 1960.
148. Warren, S., Harris, P. N., and Graves, R. C.: Osseous metastases of carcinoma of the prostate. *Arch Path, 22:*139, 1936.
149. Bouchard, J.: Skeletal metastases in breast cancer; study of the character, incidence and response to roentgenotherapy. *Am J Roentgenol, 54:*156-171, 1945.
150. Kaufmann, E.: Pathologische Anatomie der Malignen Neoplasmen der Prostata. *Deutsche Ztschr F Chir, 53:*381, 1902.
151. Sharpe, W. S., and McDonald, J. R.: Reaction of bone to metastases from carcinoma of breast and prostate. *Arch Path, 33:*312-318, 1942.
152. Staley, C. J.: Skeletal metastases in cancer of the breast. *Surg Gynec Obstet, 102:*683-694, 1956.
153. Sum, P. W., Roswit, B., and Unger, S. M.: Skeletal metastases from malignant testicular tumors. A report of 10 cases with osteolytic and osteoblastic changes. *Am J Roentgenol, 83:*704, 1960.
154. Walther, H. E.: *Krebsmetastasen.* Basle, Benno Schwabe, 1948.
155. Ardan, G. M.: Bone destruction not demonstratable by radiography. *Brit J Radiol, 24:*107, 1951.
156. Bachman, A. L., and Sproul, E. E.: Correlation of radiographic and autopsy findings in suspected metastases in the spine. *Bull NY Acad Med, 31:*146, 1955.
157. Borak, J.: Relationship between the clinical and roentgenological findings in bone metastases. *Surg Gynec Obstet, 75:*599, 1942.
158. Belitsky, P., Ghose, T., Path, F. R., Aquino, J., Tai, J., and Macdonald, A. S.: Radionuclide imaging of metastases from renal-cell carcinoma by 131 I-labeled antitumor antibody. *Radiology, 126:*515-517, 1978.
159. Brereton, H. D., Line, B. R., Londer, H. N., O'Connell, J. F., Kent, C. H., and Johnson, R. E.: Gallium scans for staging small cell lung cancer. *JAMA, 240:*666-667, 1978.
160. Cancroft, E. T., Montorfano, D., and Goldfarb, C. R.: Metastases to bone from malignant thymoma detected by technetium phosphate and gallium-67 scintigraphy. *Clin Nucl Med, 3:*312-314, 1978.
161. Charkes, N. D., Sklaroff, D. M., and Young, I. A.: Critical analysis of strontium bone scanning for detection of metastatic cancer. *Am J Radiol, 96:*647-656, 1966.
162. Citrin, D. L., Hougen, C., Zweibel, W., Schlise, S., Pruitt, B., Ershler, W., Davis, T. E., Harberg, J., and Cohen, A. I.: The use of serial bone scans in assessing response to bone metastases to systemic treatment. *Cancer, 47:*680-685, 1981.

163. Donato, A. T., Ammerman, E. G., and Sullesta, O.: Bone scanning in the evaluation of patients with lung cancer. *Ann Thorac Surg, 27:*300-304, 1979.
164. Fitzgerald, P. J., Foote, F. W., and Hill, R. F.: Concentration of I^{131} in thyroid cancer shown by radioautography. *Cancer, 3:*86, 1950.
165. Fitzpatrick, J. M., Constable, A. R., Sherwood, T., Stephenson, J. J., Chisholm, G. D., and O'Donoghue, E. P.: Serial bone scanning: The assessment of treatment response in carcinoma of the prostate. *Br J Urol, 50:*555-561, 1978.
166. Fogelman, I., Citrin, D. L., McKillop, J. H., Turner, J. G., Bessent, R. G., and Greig, W. R.: A clinical comparison of TC-99M HEDP and TC-99 MDP in the detection of bone metastases: Concise Communication. *J Nucl Med, 20:*98-101, 1979.
167. Front, D., Hardoff, R., and Iosilevsky, G.: Scintigraphic assessment of technetium 99M-Diphosphonate uptake, vascularity and vessel permeability in human bone tumours. *Br J Radiol, 52:*34-35, 1979.
168. Galasko, C. S. B., and Doyle, F. H.: The destruction of skeletal metastases from mammary cancer. A regional comparison between radiology and scintigraphy, *Clin Radiol, 23:*295, 1972.
169. Goldstein, H., McNeil, B. J., Zufall, E., Jaffe, N., and Treves,S.: Changing indications for bone scintigraphy in patients with osteosarcoma. *Radiology, 135:*177-180, 1980.
170. Hahn, P., Vikterlof, K. J., Kydman, H., Beckman, K. W., and Blom, O.: The value of wholebody bone scan in the preoperative assessment in carcinoma of the breast. *Eur J Nucl Med, 4:*207-210, 1979.
171. Hooper, R. G., Beechler, C. R., and Johnson, M. C.: Radioisotope scanning in the initial staging of bronchogenic carcinoma. *Am Rev Resp Dis, 118:*279-281, 1978.
172. Howman-Giles, R. B., Gilday, D. L., and Ash, J. M.: Radionuclide skeletal survey in neuroblastoma. *Radiology, 131:*497-502, 1979.
173. Kies, M. S., Baker, A. W., and Kennedy, P. S.: Radionuclide scans in staging of carcinoma of the lung. *Surg Gynecol Obstet, 147:*175-176, 1978.
174. Kim, E. E., Deland, F. H., and Maruyama, Y.: Decreased uptake in bone scans (cold lesions) in metastatic carcinoma. Two case reports. *J Bone & Joint Surg, 60-A:*844-846, 1978.
175. Legge, D. A., Tauxe, W. N., Pugh, D. G., and Utz, D. C.: Radioisotope scanning of metastatic lesions of bone. *Mayo Clin Proc, 45:*755-761, 1970.
176. McGregor, B., Tulloch, A. G., Quinlan, M. F., and Lovegrove, F.: The role of bone scanning in the assessment of prostatic carcinoma. *Br J Urol, 50:*178-181, 1978.
177. McKillop, J. H., Blumgart, L. H., Wood, C. B., Fogelman, I., Furnival, C. M., Greig, W. R., and Citrin, D. L.: The prognostic and therapeutic implications of positive radionuclide bone scan in clinically early breast cancer. *Br J Surg, 65:*649-652, 1978.
178. McNeil, B. J.: Rationale for the use of bone scans in selected metastatic and primary bone tumors. *Semin Nucl Med, 8:*336-345, 1978.
179. McNeil, B. J., and Hanley, J.: Analysis of serial radionuclide bone images in osteosarcoma and breast carcinoma. *Radiology, 135:*171-176, 1980.
180. Meckelenburg, R. L.: Bone scanning and cancer. *Del Med J, 51:*377-378, 1979.
181. Meyer, J. E., and Messer, R. J.: Extradural metastatic breast carcinoma detected on a bone scan. *Cancer, 40:*3074-3075, 1977.
182. Murray, I. P.: Bone scanning in the child and young adult. Part I. *Skeletal Radiol, 5:*1-14, 1980.
183. Pabst, H. W., and Langhammer, H.: Detection and differential diagnosis of bone lesions by scintigraphy. *Eur J Nucl Med, 2:*261-268, 1977.

184. Parthasarathy, K. L., Landsberg, R., Bakshi, S. P., Donoghue, G., and Merrin, C.: Detection of bone metastases in urogenital malignancies utilizing 99MTC-labelled phosphate compounds. *Urology, 11:*99-102, 1978.
185. Rubin, P.: The detection of occult metastatic cancer by radioactive bone scans. *JAMA, 210:*1079, 1969.
186. Seabold, J. E., Haynie, T. P., Deasis, D. N., Samaan, N. A., Glenn, H. L., and Jahns, M. F.: Detection of metastatic adrenal carcinoma using 131 I-6-Beta-Iodomethyl-19-Norcholesterol total body scans. *J Clin Endocrinol Metab, 45:*788-797, 1977.
187. Siddiqui, A. R., Wellman, H. N., Weetman, R. M., and Smith, W. L.: Bone scanning in management of metastatic osteogenic sarcoma. *Clin Nucl Med, 4:*6-11, 1979.
188. Sklaroff, D. M., and Charles, N. D.: Diagnosis of bone metastasis by photoscanning with strontium 85. *JAMA, 188:*121, 1964.
189. Valdez, V. A., Bonnine, J. M., Martin, I. T., and Herrera, N. E.: Abnormal liver and bone scans in a case of a metastatic neuroblastoma. *Clin Nucl Med, 3:*337-338, 1978.
190. Wilson, G. S., Rich, M. A., and Brennan, M. J.: Evaluation of bone scan in preoperative clinical staging of breast cancer. *Arch Surg, 115:*415-419, 1980.
191. Wolfe, J. A., Rowe, L. D., and Lowry, L. D.: Value of radionucleotide scanning in the staging of head and neck carcinoma. *Ann Otol Rhinol Laryngol, 88:*832-836, 1979.
192. DeSantos, L. A., Goldstein, H. M., Murray, J. A., and Wallace, S.: Computed tomography in the evaluation of musculoskeletal neoplasms. *Radiology, 128:*89-94, 1978.
193. Nakagawa, H., Huang, Y. P., Malis, L. K., and Wolf, B. S.: Computed tomography of intraspinal and paraspinal neoplasms. *J Comput Assist Tomogr, 1:*377-390, 1977.
194. Ballou, B., Levine, G., Hakala, T. R., and Solter, D.: Tumor location detected with radioactivity labeled monoclonal antibody and external scintigraphy. *Science, 206:*844-846, 1979.
195. Belitsky, P., Ghose, T., Aquino, J., Norvell, S. T., and Blair, H. A.: Radionuclide imaging of metastases from renal-cell carcinoma by ^{131}I-labeled antitumor antibody. *Radiology, 126:*515-517, 1978.
196. Goldenberg, D. M., Deland, F., Kim, E., Bennett, S., Primus, F. J., Van Nagell, Jr., J. R., Estes, N., Desimone, P., and Rayburn, P.: Use of radiolabeled antibodies to carcinoembryonic antigen for the detection and localization of diverse cancers by external photoscanning. *N Engl J Med, 298:*1384-1388, 1978.
197. Goldenberg, D. M., Kim, E. E., Deland, F. H., Bennett, S., and Primus, F. J.: Radioimmunodetection of cancer with radioactive antibodies to carcinoembryonic antigen. *Cancer Res, 40:*2984-2992, 1980.
198. Sloane, J. P., Ormerod, M. G., and Neville, A. M.: Potential pathological application of immunocytochemical methods to the detection of micrometastases. *Cancer Res, 40:*3079-3082, 1980.
199. Ameri, M. R., Alebouyeh, M., and Donner, M. W.: Hypertrophic osteoarthropathy in childhood malignancy. *Am J Radiol, 130:*992-993, 1978.
200. Aufses, A. H., and Aufses, B. H.: Hypertrophic osteoarthropathy in association with pulmonary metastases from extrathoracic malignancies. *Dis Chest, 38:*399-402, 1960.
201. Bangotra, A. K., Parashar, S., and Bhandary, S. V.: Pulmonary hypertrophic osteoarthropathy — a case report. *Clinican, 44:*548-551, 1980.
202. Diwan, R. V.: Hypertrophic pulmonary osteoarthropathy and its occurrence with pulmonary metastases from osteogenic sarcoma — case report and review of literature. *J Assoc Physicians India, 26:*651-655, 1978.

203. Ennis, G. C., Cameron, D. P., and Burger, H. G.: On the aetiology of hypertrophic pulmonary osteoarthropathy in bronchogenic carcinoma: Lack of relationship to elevated growth hormone levels. *Aust Nz. J Med, 3:*157-161, 1973.
204. Fam, A. G., and Gross, E. G.: Hypertrophic osteoarthropathy, phalangeal and synovial metastases associated with bronchogenic carcinoma. *J Rheumatol, 6:*680-686, 1979.
205. Gall, E. A., Bennett, G. A., and Bauer, W.: Generalized hypertrophic osteoarthropathy. *Am J Path, 27:*349, 1951.
206. Hansen, J. L.: Bronchial carcinoma presenting as arthralgia. *Acta Med Scand* (Suppl.), *266:*467, 1952.
207. Howard, C. P.,Telander, R. L., Hoffman, A. D., and Burgert, E. O.: Hypertrophic osteoarthropathy in association with pulmonary metastasis from osteogenic sarcoma. *Mayo Clin Proc, 53:*538-541, 1978.
208. Mendlowitz, M.: Clubbing and hypertrophic osteoarthropathy. *Medicine, 21:*269, 1942.
209. Rothendler, H. H.: Pulmonary hypertrophic osteoarthropathy. *Bull Hosp Joint Dis, 7:*43, 1946.
210. Schumacher, H. R.: Articular manifestations of hypertrophic pulmonary osteoarthropathy in bronchogenic carcinoma. *Arthritis Rheum, 19:*629-636, 1976.
211. Semple, T., McCluskie, R. A.: Generalized hypertrophic osteoarthropathy in association with bronchial carcinoma. *Br Med J, 1:*754-759, 1955.
212. Shapiro, S.: Ossifying periostitis of Bamberger-Marie (secondary hypertrophic pulmonary osteoarthropathy). *Bull Hosp Joint Dis, 2:*77, 1941.
213. Wilson, K. S., and Naidoo, A.: Hypertrophic osteoarthropathy. *Mayo Clin Proc 54:*208-209, 1979.
214. Bamberger, E.: Ueber Knochenveranderungen Bei Chronischen Lungen-und Herz krankheiten. *Ztschr F Klin-Med, 18:*193, 1891.
215. Marie, P.: De L'osteo-arthropathie hypertrophiante pneuminque. *Rev De Med, 10:*1 1890.
216. Stintz, S.: The frequency of the pulmonary hypertrophic osteoarthropathy in autopsies with bronchial carcinoma. *Zentralbl Allg Pathol Pathol Anat, 122:*249-255 1978.
217. Engelmann, C.: Localized primary pleural tumors (solitary mesothelioma). *Gaz Me Fr, 99:*136-145, 1974.
218. Wierman, W. H., Clagett, O. T., and MacDonald, J. R.: Articular manifestations in pulmonary diseases: An analysis of their occurrence in 1024 cases in which pulmonary resection was performed. *JAMA, 155:*1459, 1954.
219. Cavanaugh, J. J. A., Holman, G. H.: Hypertrophic osteoarthropathy in childhood. *Pediatr, 66:*27-40, 1965.
220. Kay, J. C., Rosenberg, M. A., and Burd, R.: Hypertrophic osteoarthropathy and childhood Hodgkin's Disease. *Pediatr Radiol, 112:*177-178, 1974.
221. Athreya, B. H., Borns, P., Rosenlund, M. L.: Cystic fibrosis and hypertrophic osteoarthropathy in children. Report of three cases. *Am J Dis Child, 129:*634-637, 1975.
222. Grossman, H., Denning, C. R., and Baker, D. H.: Hypertrophic osteoarthropathy in cystic fibrosis. *Am J Dis Child, 107:*1-6, 1964.
223. Nathanson, I., Riddlesberger, M. M., Jr.: Pulmonary hypertrophic osteoarthropathy in cystic fibrosis. *Radiology, 135:*649-651, 1980.
224. Reardon, G., Collins, A. J., and Bacon, P. A.: The effect of adrenergic blockade in hypertrophic pulmonary osteoarthropathy. *Postgrad Med J, 52:*170-173, 1976.

225. Greco, F. A., and Kushner, I.: Loss of symptoms of pulmonary hypertrophic osteoarthropathy after laparotomy. *Ann Intern Med, 81:*555-556, 1974.
226. Flavell, G.: Reversal of pulmonary osteoarthropathy by vagotomy. *Lancet, 1:*260, 1956.
227. Lopez-Enriquez, E., Morales, A. R., and Robert, F.: Effect of atropine sulfate in pulmonary hypertrophic osteoarthropathy. *Arthritis Rheum, 23:*822-824, 1980.
228. Charbord, P., L'Heritier, C., Cukersztein, W., Lumbroso, J., and Tubiana, M.: Radioiodine treatment in differentiated thryoid carcinomas. Treatment of first local recurrences and of bone and lung metastases. *Ann Radiol* (Paris), *20:*783-786, 1977.
229. Correns, H. J., Mebel, M., Buchali, K., Schnorr, D., Seidel, C., and Mitterlechner, E.: 89 strontium therapy of bone metastases of carcinoma of the prostatic gland. *Eur J Nucl Med, 4:*33-35, 1979.
230. Garmatis, C. J., and Chu, F. C.: The effectiveness of radiation therapy in the treatment of bone metastases from breast cancer. *Radiology, 126:*235-237, 1978.
231. Gilbert, H. A., Kagan, A. R., Nussbaum, H., Rao, A. R., Satiman, J., Chan, P., Allen, B., and Forsythe, A.: Evaluation of radiation therapy for bone metastases: Pain relief and quality of life. *Am J Radiol, 129:*1095-1096, 1977.
232. Jenkins, R. D.: Radiation treatment of Ewing's sarcoma and osteogenic sarcoma. *Can J Surg, 20:*530-536, 1977.
233. Khan, F. R., Glicksman, A. S., Shu, F. C. H., and Nickerson, J. J.: Treatment by radiotherapy of spinal cord compression due to extradural metastases. *Radiology, 89:*495-500, 1967.
234. Kumar, P. P.: Role of radiotherapy in the management of breast cancer. *J Natl Med Assoc, 69:*787-792, 1977.
235. Kumar, P. P., Bahrassa, F., and Espinoza, M. C.: The role of radiotherapy in management of metastatic bone disease. *J Natl Med Assoc, 70:*909-911, 1978.
236. O'Mara, R. E.: New 32P compounds in therapy for bone lesions. In Spencer, R. P. (Ed.): *Therapy in Nuclear Medicine.* New York, Grune & Stratton, 1978, pp. 257-260.
237. Pistenma, D. A., Bagshaw, N. A., and Freiha, F. S.: Extended-field radiation therapy for prostatic adenocarcinoma: Status report of a limited prospective trial. In *Clinical Conference on Cancer.* 23rd M. D. Anderson Hospital and Tumor Institute, Houston, 1978. Cancer of the Genitourinary Tract. New York, Raven Press, 1979, pp. 229-247.
238. Qasim, M. M.: Techniques and results of half body irradiation (HBI) in metastatic carcinomas and myelomas. *Clin Oncol, 5:*65-68, 1979.
239. Rengachary, S. S., Lee, S. H., and Watanabe, I.: Spinal epidural radiation necrosis simulating metastatic neoplasm. *Surg Neurol, 10:*101-103, 1978.
240. Roberts, D. J., Jr.: 32P-sodium phosphate treatment of metastatic malignant disease. *Clin Nucl Med, 4:*92-93, 1979.
241. Seidlin, S. M., Marinelli, L. D., and Oshry, E.: Radioactive iodine therapy; effect on functioning metastases of adenocarcinoma of the thyroid. *JAMA, 132:*838, 1946.
242. Seydel, H. G., Creech, R. H., Mietlowski, W., and Perez, C.: Radiation therapy in small cell lung cancer. *Semin Oncol, 5:*288-298, 1978.
243. Slawson, R. G.: Radiation therapy for germinal tumors of the testes. *Cancer, 42:*2216-2223, 1978.
244. Solisio, E. O., Akbiyik, K., and Alexander, L. L.: Spinal cord compression from metastatic breast carcinoma: Treatment by radiation therapy alone. *J Natl Med Assoc, 71:*229-230, 1979.

245. Vikram, B., and Chu, F. C.: Radiation therapy for metastases to the base of the skull. *Radiology, 130:*465-568, 1979.
246. Wara, W. M., Phillips, T. L., Sheline, G. E., and Schwade, J. G.: Radiation tolerance of the spinal cord. *Cancer, 35:*1558-1562, 1975.
247. Winston, M. A.: Radioisotope therapy in bone and joint disease. *Semin Nucl Med, 9:*114-120, 1979.
248. Wolfson, S. A., Reznick, S., and Gunther, L.: Early diagnosis of malignant metastases to the spine: A clinical syndrome. *JAMA, 116:*1044-1048, 1941.
249. Apuzzo, M. L., Weibs, M. H., Minassian, H. V.: Epidural spinal metastases: Factors related to selection of cases for decompressive laminectomy. *Bull L A Neurol Soc, 42:*63-70, 1977.
250. Brice, J., and McKissock, W.: Surgical treatment of malignant extradural spinal tumours. *Br Med J 1:*1341, 1965.
251. Cross, G. O., White, H. L., and White, L. P.: Acrylic prosthesis of the fifth cervical vertebra in multiple myeloma. Technical note. *J Neurosurg, 35:*112-114, 1971.
252. Dunn, E. J.: The roll of methyl methacrylate in the stabilization and replacement of tumors of the cervical spine. A project of the cervical spine research society. *Spine, 2:*15-24, 1977.
253. Eftekhar, N. S., and Thurston, C. W.: Effect of irradiation on acrylic cement with special reference to fixation of pathological fractures. *J Biomech, 8:*53-56, 1975.
254. Hall, A. J., and McKay, N. N. S.: The results of laminectomy for compression of the cord and cauda equina by extradural malignant tumor. *J Bone & Joint Surg, 55-B:*497-505, 1973.
255. Harrington, K. D.: The use of methylmethacrylate for vertebral-body replacement and anterior stabilization of pathological fracture-dislocations of the spine due to metastatic malignant disease. *J Bone & Joint Surg, 63-A:*36-46, 1981.
256. Livingston, K. E., and Perrin, R. G.: The neurosurgical management of spinal metastases causing cord and cauda equina compression. *J Neurosurg, 49:*839-843, 1978.
257. Panjabi, M. M., Hopper, W., White, A. A., III, and Keggi, K. J.: Posterior spine stabilization with methylmethacrylate. Biomechanical testing of a surgical specimen. *Spine, 2:*241-247, 1977.
258. Raycroft, J. F., Hockman, R. P., and Southwick, W. O.: Metastatic tumors involving the cervical vertebrae: Surgical palliation. *J Bone & Joint Surg, 60-A:*763-768 1978.
259. Scoville, W. B., Palmer, A. H., Samra, K., and Chong, G.: The use of acrylic plastic for vertebral replacement or fixation in metastatic disease of the spine. A technical note. *J Neurosurg, 27:*274-279, 1967.
260. Smith, R.: An evaluation of surgical treatment for spinal cord compression due to metastatic carcinoma. *J Neurol Neurosurg Psychiatry, 28:*152-158, 1965.
261. White, W. A., Patterson, R. H., Jr., and Bergland, R. M.: Role of surgery in the treatment of spinal cord compression by metastatic neoplasm. *Cancer, 27:*558 561, 1971.
262. Wright, R. L.: Malignant tumor in the spinal extradural space. Results of surgical treatment. *Ann Surg, 159:*227-231, 1963.
263. Baker, W. H.: Abnormalities in calcium metabolism in malignancy, effects of hormonal therapy. *Am J Med, 21:*714, 1956.
264. Koelmeyer, T. D., and Stephens, E. J.: Synthetic human calcitonin in the treatment of hypercalcaemia of metastatic breast cancer: Preliminry report. *NZ Med J, 87:*434 435, 1978.

265. Myers, W. P. L.: Cortisone in the treatment of hypercalcemia in neoplastic disease. *Cancer, 11:*83, 1958.
266. Vaughan, C. B., and Vaitkevicius, V. K.: The effects of calcitonin in hypercalcaemia in patients with malignancy. *Cancer, 34:*1268-1271, 1974.
267. Hagemeister, F. B., Jr., Buzdar, A. U., Luna, M. A., and Blumenschein, G. R.: Causes of death in breast cancer. *Cancer, 46:*162-167, 1980.
268. Hakulineu, T., and Teppo, L.: Causes of death among female patients with cancer of the breast and intestines. *Ann Clin Res, 9:*15-24, 1977.
269. Inagake, J., Rodriguez, V., and Bodey, G. P.: Causes of death in cancer patients. *Cancer, 33:*568-573, 1974.
270. Klastersky, J., Daneau, D., and Verhest, A.: Causes of death in patients with cancer. *Eur J Cancer, 8:*149-154, 1972.
271. Levin, D. L., Connelly, R. R., and Devesa, S. S.: Demographic characteristics of cancer of the pancreas: Mortality, incidence, and survival, *Cancer. 47:*1456-1468, 1981.
272. Miller, A. B., Hoogstraten, B., Staquet, M., and Winkler, A.: Reporting results of cancer treatment. *Cancer, 47:*207-214, 1981.
273. Mueller, C. B., Ames, F., and Anderson, G. C.: Breast cancer in 3558 women: Age as a significant determinant in the rate of dying and causes of death. *Sug, 83:*123-132, 1978.
274. PeJovic, M. H., Wolff, J. P., Kramar, A., and Goldfarb, E.: Cure rate estimation and long-term prognosis of uterine cervix carcinoma. *Cancer, 47:*203-206, 1981.

Chapter 3

Malignant Lymphomas

CLASSIFICATION

MALIGNANT LYMPHOMAS are a group of closely related lymphorecticular neoplasms that arise in lymphocytic cells. They are located primarily in lymphnodes, thymus, spleen, liver, bone marrow, and submucosal region of respiratory and gastrointestinal tracts. Lymphocytes and histiocytes in different stages of differentiation and maturation are the basic cell types. The old classification divides lymphomas into four groups: Hodgkin's disease, reticulum cell sarcoma, lymphosarcoma, and giant follicular lymphoma. The new classification takes the different predominant cell types into consideration and pays particular attention to the cell patterns and the stages of differentiation. Table 3-I shows the contrast between the old and the new classification of lymphomas.

In passing, it should be mentioned that mycosis fungoides[1-9] is a cutaneous form of malignant lymphoma, characterized by severe pruritis, and may eventually involve lymphnodes, bone marrow, liver, spleen, lung, and other tissues.

INCIDENCE

Since Hodgkin's disease and non-Hodgkin's lymphomas are closely related diseases, they share several common clinical features: their predilection for lymphnodes and to a lesser extent for spleen, liver and bone; preferential affection for male patients with a male to female ratio of 1.5 or 2 to 1; affinity for the same bones such as vertebral column, sternum, ribs, scapula and long tubular bones; and common routes of dissemination that

TABLE 3-I
CLASSIFICATION OF LYMPHOMAS

New Classification			*Old Classification*
(I) Hodgkin's Disease	(1) Lymphocytic predominance		
	(2) Nodular sclerosis		Hodgkin's Disease
	(3) Mixed cellularity		
	(4) Lymphocytic depletion		
	Cell Pattern	*Cell Type*	
(II) Non-Hodgkin's Lymphoma	(A) Nodular (follicular)	(1) Lymphocytic, well differentiated	
			Reticulum cell sarcoma
	(B) Diffuse	(2) Lymphocytic, intermediately differentiated	
	(C) Mixed nodular and diffuse		Lymphosarcoma
		(3) Lymphocytic, poorly differentiated	
			Giant follicular lymphoma
		(4) Lymphoblastic	
		(5) Mixed cell type	
		(6) Large cell type (histiocytic)	
		(7) Burkitt's lymphoma	
(III) Mycosis Fungoides			

consist of direct extension to spine from adjacent diseased lymphnodes and metastatic spread through the lymphatic channels, systemic circulation, and the vertebral venous system (Batson's plexus). However, Hodgkin's disease does differ from non-Hodgkin's lymphomas in several important aspects.

Hodgkin's disease principally affects patients between twenty to forty years of age, whereas non-Hodgkin's lymphomas mainly victimize children under ten years of age (Burkitt's lymphoma) and adults between forty to sixty-five years of age. In addition, Hodgkin's disease shows a strong tendency to involve the lymphnodes, but the non-Hodgkin's lymphomas tend to have more extranodal involvements than Hodgkin's disease. Although clinically detectable bone involvement in lymphomas is between 10 to 20 percent of the cases,[10-15] the actual incidence of bone involvement according to several autopsy series varied from 34 percent to 78 percent.[16-17] The vertebral column, particularly the lower thoracic and upper lumbar spine, is commonly involved, although many of these vertebral lesions are not clinically apparent. Among the subtypes of Hodgkin's disease, mixed cellularity is the commonest, nodular sclerosis less common, and lymphocyte predominance and lymphocyte depletion least common. In non-Hodgkin's lymphomas, diffuse lymphocytic lymphoma (lymphosarcoma) is more common than histiocytic lymphoma (reticulum cell sarcoma), and nodular lymphocytic lymphoma (giant follicular lymphoma) is the least common.

It should be emphasized that malignant lymphoma is a dynamic disease in the sense that one histologic subtype can transform into another subtype over time and different histologic subtypes can also coexist in the same patient. Consequently, wide tissue samplings are sometimes required in order to obtain a precise diagnosis. Occasionally, malignant lymphomas can originate in certain bones such as the long tubular bones (femur, tibia, humerus, etc.), ilium, scapula, ribs, and vertebral column without any apparent lymphnode or visceral involvements. These tumors are called primary reticulum cell sarcoma of bone (reticulosarcoma)[18-43] and primary Hodgkin's disease of bone.[44-50]

CLINICAL SYMPTOMS AND SIGNS

Owing to the fact that malignant lymphomas can involve almost every system in the body, a wide spectrum of clinical symptoms and signs can be present. Constitutional symptoms such as weight loss, generalized weakness, malaise, fever, night sweats, anorexia, ease of fatigue, etc., are likely to be associated with disseminated form of malignant lymphomas. Lymphadenopathy can involve all the major lymphnode groups such as the cervical mediastinal, abdominal, pelvic, axillary, femoral and popliteal nodes. Coughs, dyspnea, and cyanosis can be caused by lymphoma-induced upper airway obstruction, marked mediastinal lymphadenopathy, pleural effusion, parenchymal involvement of the lung, and pericardial effusion. Lymphomatous involvements of the abdominal viscerae can produce abdominal pain, dysphagia, hepatosplenomegaly, palpable abdominal masses, obstipation, bowel obstruction, black stools, etc. Involvement of the urinary tract by lymphomas can bring about flank pain, hematuria, obstructive uropathy, and even renal failure. Lymphomatous involvements of the brain, meninges, cranial nerves, spinal cord, spinal nerves, dorsal root ganglia, and cauda equina can cause headaches; pain in neck, back, and upper and lower extremities; disorientation; lethargy; behavior changes; visual disturbances; facial nerve palsy; weakness, paralysis, hypesthesia, and paresthesia of upper and lower extremities; changes in deep tendon reflexes and the presence of pathologic reflexes, etc. Skeletal involvement can cause bone pain, tenderness, swelling, joint effusion, and pathologic fractures. Involvement of the skeletal portion of the vertebral column cannot only cause neck and back pain but can also produce compression of the spinal cord and nerves from compression fractures.

Subtly different clinical symptoms and signs do exist between Hodgkin's disease and non-Hodgkin's lymphomas. Patients with Hodgkin's disease tend to have good general health, frequent pruritis, fever in early stages of the disease, unilateral lower cervical and jugular lymphnode involvement with polylobulated lymphnode, and rare involvement of upper air passage and gastrointestinal tract. In contrast, patients with non-Hodgkin's lymphomas often do not have good general health, pruritis, or fever in early stages of the disease, but do have frequent upper air passage and gastrointestinal involvements, and bilateral upper cervical, jugular and epitrochlear lymphnode involvement with large ovoid lymphnodes.

It is of interest to note that Burkitt's lymphoma,[51-58] a malignant lymphoma of childhood consisting of poorly differentiated lymphocytic cells with an intense basophilic cytoplasm, has a peculiar predilection for the jaw bone of Nigerian children and can produce destruction of vertebral column, epidural deposits, paraplegia, paravertebral soft tissue mass, visceral involvements, and leukemia.[59-68] Osteonecrosis of major joints caused by cytotoxic chemotherapy, radiotherapy, and systemic corticosteroid administration is sometimes encountered in treating malignant lymphomas.[69-72] Very rarely, hypertrophic pulmonary osteoarthropathy characterized by clubbing of the digits, periostitis, and arthritis can be produced by malignant lymphomas.[73-75]

LABORATORY STUDIES

Abnormal laboratory findings[76-84] in lymphomas are reflections of the extent of the systemic lymphomatous involvements. Lymphoma-related bleedings and bone marrow involvement can produce anemia and thrombocytopenia. Bone and soft tissue destruction can cause elevated erythrocyte sedimentation rate and serum alkaline phosphatase, hypercalcemia, and increased urinary excretion of hydroxyproline. Hepatic involvement by lymphomas can bring about hyperbilirubinemia and elevated serum liver enzymes. Extensive renal involvement can produce elevated serum BUN and creatinine, hematuria, and abnormal urinalysis. When leukemia develops from a malignant lymphoma, considerable number of malignant lymphoma cells will be visible on peripheral blood and bone marrow smears. In addition, when the central nervous system is invaded by the lymphoma.[85-101] In addition to increased cerebrospinal fluid pressure, analysis of the cerebrospinal fluid will reveal elevated white blood cell count, the presence of malignant lymphoma cells, increased protein content, and decreased glucose concentration.

SPECIAL DIAGNOSTIC STUDIES

Lymphomatous involvements of the various body systems can be completely asymptomatic and not detectable by routine physical and roentgenographic examination and laboratory studies. Special diagnostic procedures are often required to determine the exact extent of involvement, which is of vital importance for both therapeutic and prognostic purposes. These special diagnostic studies consist of upper GI series, barium enema, intravenous pyelogram, arteriogram, inferior venacavogram, bone marrow biopsy, myelogram, lymphangiogram,[102-107] ultrasonogram,[108-116] bone and soft tissue scanning with radioisotopes,[117-126] computed tomography,[127-135] laparoscopy, and surgical laparotomy.[136-144]

The obvious advantages of laparotomy include the opportunity to document the exact extent of abdominal involvement by the lymphoma and to obtain representative lymphnode biopsies from various abdominal lymphnode groups (para-aortic, retrocrural, splenic, celiac, pelvic, iliac, mesenteric, etc.) and the feasibility to perform a splenectomy and liver and iliac bone biopsy at the same time. The disadvantages of laparotomy naturally include the possible surgical mortality and morbidity and its lack of general application in staging non-Hodgkin's lymphomas because of their tendency to show generalized involvements.

On the basis of the extent of involvement, malignant lymphomas can be grouped into four stages[145-148] on which the various modalities of therapy and long-term prognosis are dependent.

STAGE I. Involvement of a single lymphnode region or of a single extralymphatic organ or site.

STAGE II. Involvement of two or more lymphnode regions on the same side of the diaphragm or localized involvement of extra lymphatic organ or site and of one or more lymphnode regions on the same side of the diaphragm.

STAGE III. Involvement of lymphnode regions on both sides of the diaphragm, which may be accompanied by localized involvement of extralymphatic organ or site.

STAGE IV. Diffuse or disseminated involvement of one or more extralymphatic organs or tissues with or without associated lymphnode enlargement.

Each of these four stages can be further divided into Substage A and Substage B. Substage B means the presence of fever, night sweats, or weight loss of greater than 10 percent of the body weight where Substage A has complete absence of these three constitutional symptoms.

ROENTGENOGRAPHIC MANIFESTATIONS

By and large, primary and secondary intraosseous lesions of Hodgkin's disease and non-Hodgkin's lymphomas[149-163] have similar appearance. They tend to involve the metaphyseal and diaphyseal portions of the bone and most of them are osteolytic in nature with only a small portion of the lesions having a purely osteosclerotic or a mixture of osteosclerotic and osteolytic appearance. These lesions usually start in the intramedullary portion of the bone and can eventually perforate the cortex and extend into the surrounding soft tissues.

Periosteal reaction sometimes accompanies these lymphomatous bone lesions.[164] However, when the bone lesion is saucer-shaped and begins from the outer cortex, it is usually a secondary lymphomatous bone lesion, most likely caused by an invading diseased lymphnode. Furthermore, primary Hodgkin's disease and non-Hodgkin's lymphomas of the bone are often solitary lesions (Figure 3-1), at least at their early stages, whereas secondary lymphomatous bone lesions tend to be polyostotic and can be easily demonstrated by radioisotope bone scans.

When the spinal column is invaded by a lymphoma-infiltrated lymph-

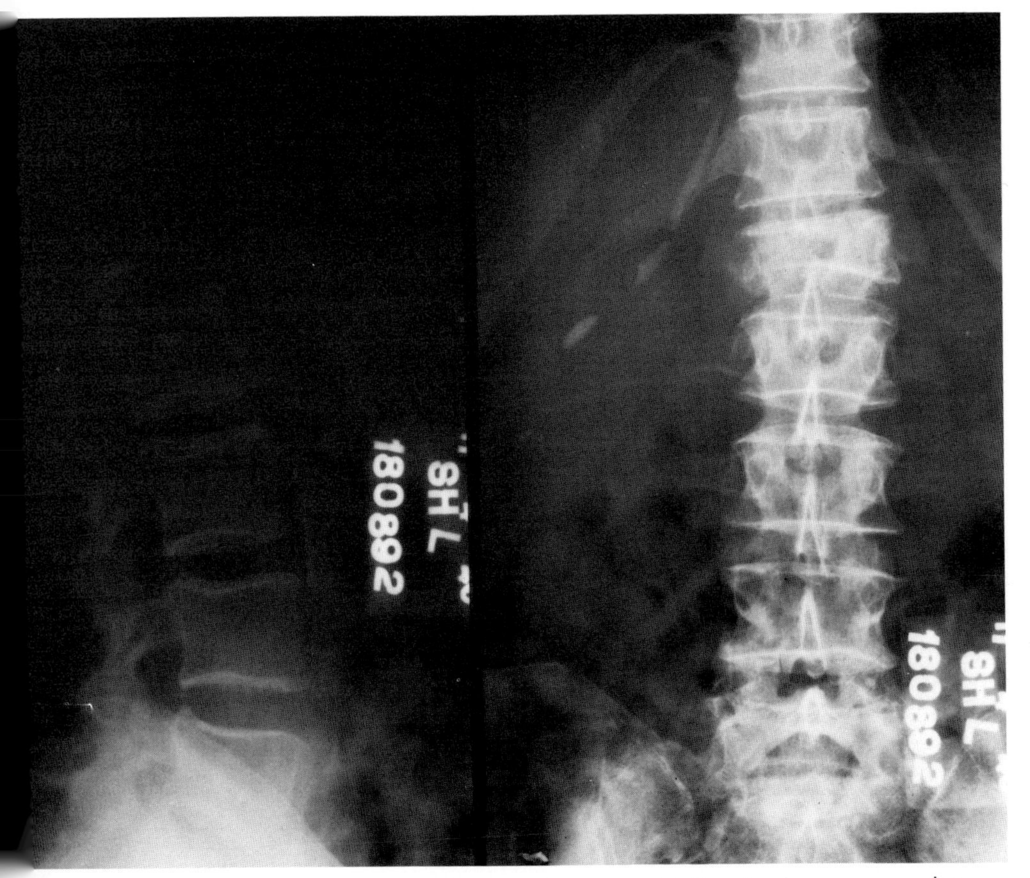

Figure 3-1. Lumbar spine x-rays of this sixty-eight-year-old female show compression fracture of the first lumbar vertebral body caused by a primary reticulum cell sarcoma (diffuse, histiocytic non-Hodgkin's lymphoma) of the spine, which was confirmed by biopsy.

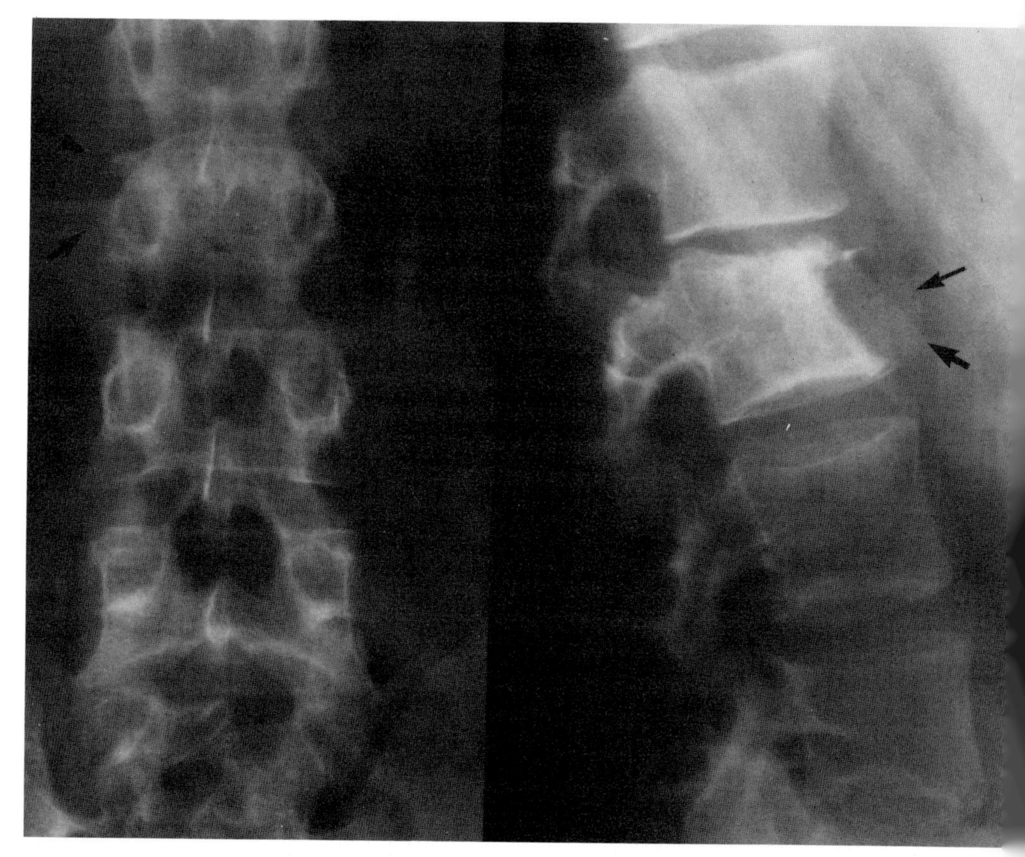

Figure 3-2. Lumbar roentgenographs of a twenty-year-old man showing a saucer-shaped erosion involving the anterior aspect of the third lumbar vertebral body caused by a large paraspinal lymphnode affected by Hodgkin's disease.

node, a saucer-shaped vertebral body destruction (Figure 3-2), enlargement of the intervertebral foramen and erosion of the pedicles can be present. Metastatic lymphomatous lesions of the spine, brought to the spinal column by the systemic circulation or the vertebral venous plexus, are predominantly osteolytic in nature and frequently involve one to several vertebral bodies (Figure 3-3) that may appear to be somewhat osteoporotic and can produce compression fracture and even extraosseous tumor extension (Figure 3-4). Although vertebral bodies are the principal sites of lymphomatous involvement, the transverse and spinous processes, pedicles, laminae and articular facets can sometimes be involved, but the intervertebral disks are usually spared.

Occasionally, Hodgkin's disease and rarely non-Hodgkin's lymphoma can induce so much osteoblastic activity in the spine that the involved vertebral body can become densely osteosclerotic, producing a so-called

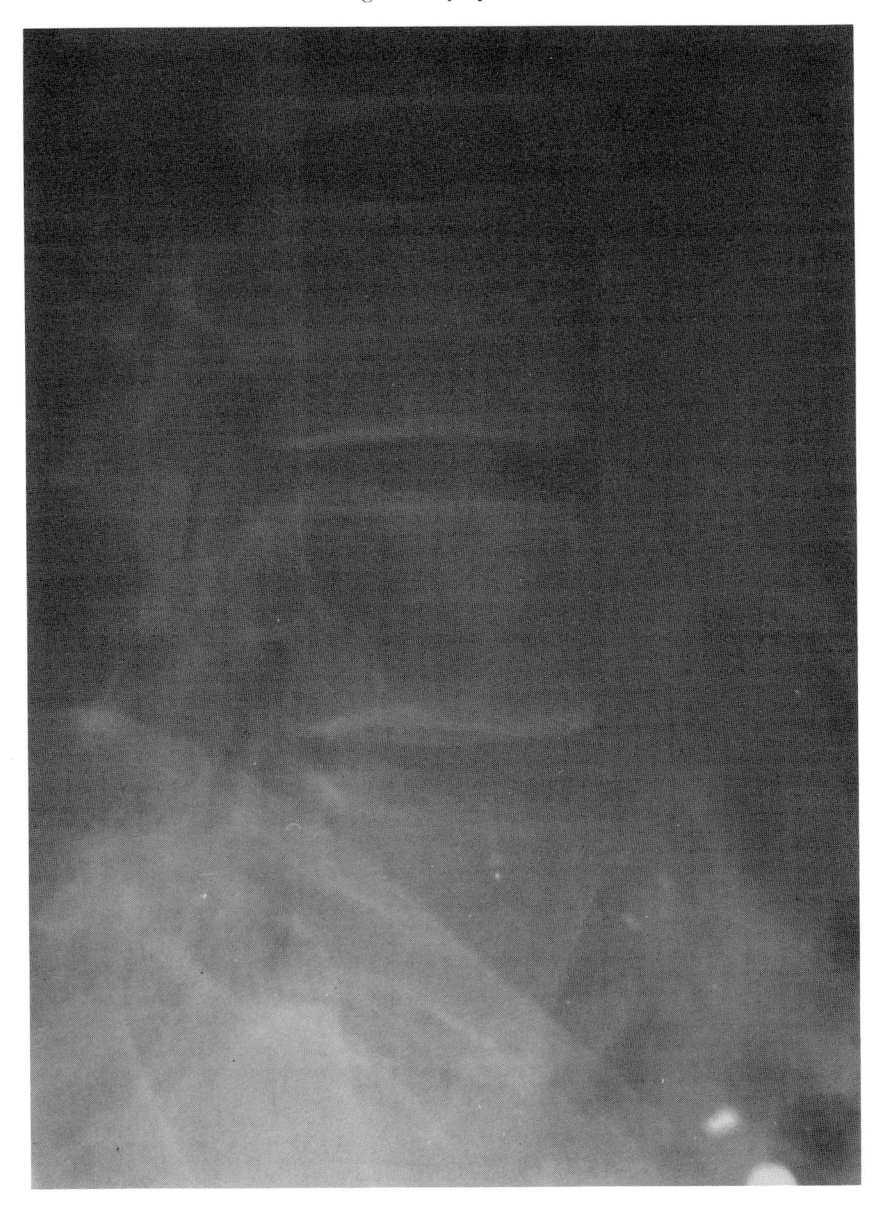

Figure 3-3. Lateral view of the lumbar spine x-ray showing radiolucency and an indistinct anterior vertebral border of the fourth lumbar vertebral body caused by proliferation of cells of Hodgkin's disease in L4.

ivory vertebra (Figure 3-5).[165-169] In addition, radiation can sometimes change an osteolytic lesion to an osteosclerotic one and progression of the disease can transform an osteosclerotic lesion to an osteolytic lesion. Mandell (1978)[170] had also observed resolution of Hodgkin's disease-induced

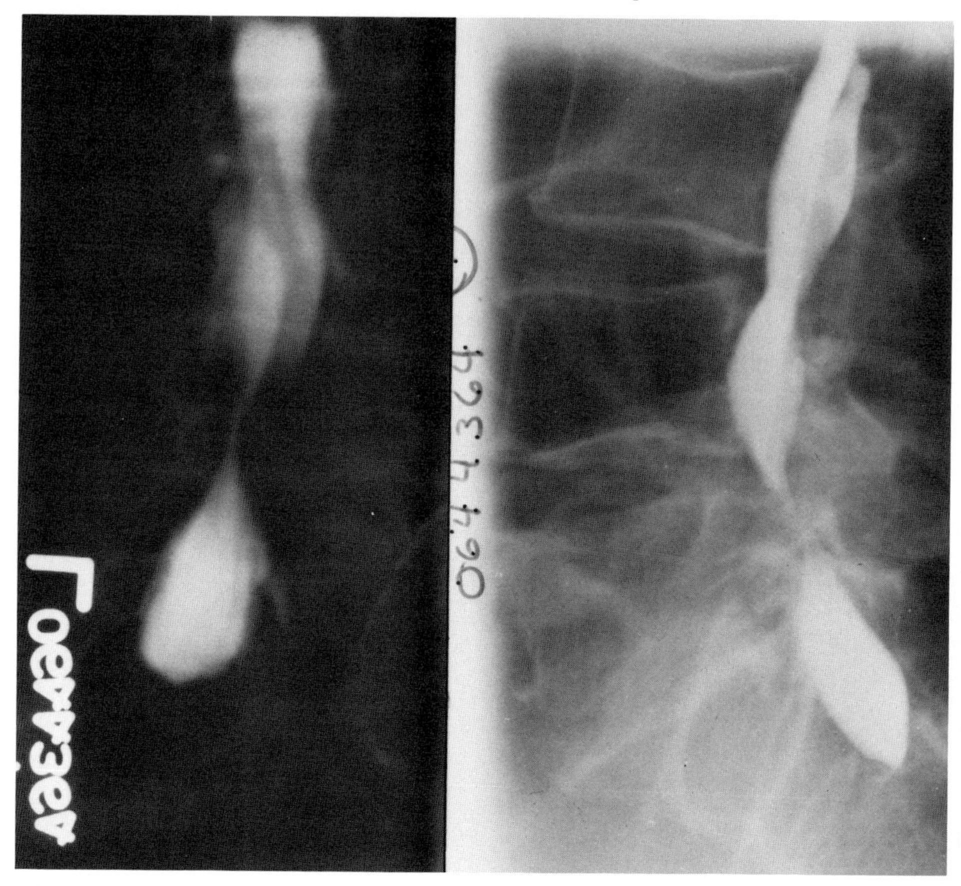

Figure 3-4. Myelogram of the lumbar spine belonging to a patient with non-Hodgkin's lymphoma (lymphosarcoma; or diffuse, lymphocytic, poorly differentiated lymphoma) shows destruction of the fifth lumbar vertebral body and extraosseous tumor extension into the spinal canal that has caused an almost complete blockage of the myelographic dye flow.

ivory vertebra to normal density with chemotherapy and radiotherapy. Calcification of the anterior spinal longitudinal vertebral ligaments in Hodgkin's disease was reported by Duncan (1973).[171]

PATHOLOGIC FEATURES

GROSS PATHOLOGY. Osteolytic lesions of malignant lymphomas usually show destruction and thinning of trabeculae by the tumor tissue, which is often soft, friable or rubbery, and grayish-red or grayish-yellow in color (Figures 3-6 through 3-10) and can be associated with cortical perforation, periosteal reaction and extraosseous tumor extension. Foci of necrosis and hemorrhage can usually be found in the large tumors. Compression fracture of the vertebrae, impingement of the spinal cord and nerves, and

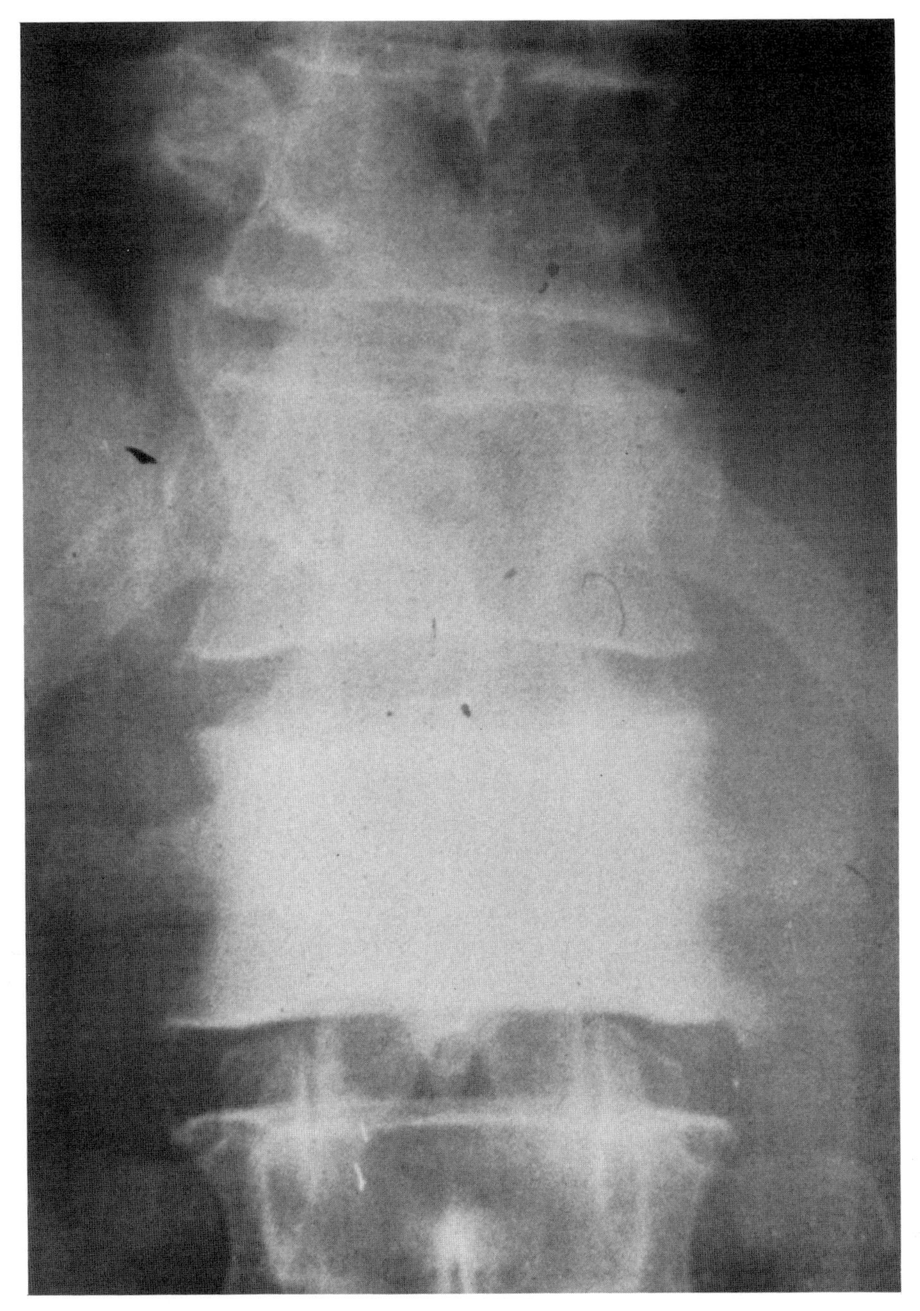

Figure 3-5. This forty-five-year-old white male with Hodgkin's disease has a densely osteosclerotic first lumbar vertebra (ivory vertebra) caused by his Hodgkin's disease.

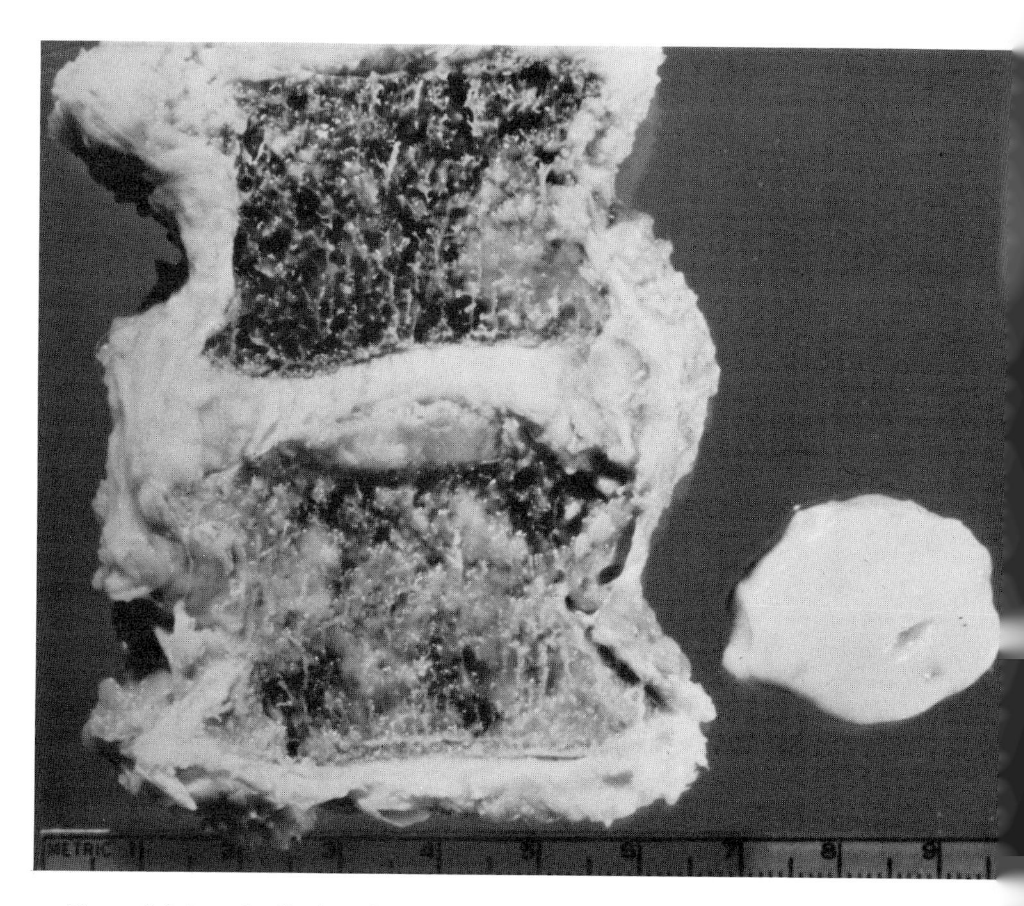

Figure 3-6. Longitudinal section of two thoracic vertebrae affected by Hodgkin's disease shows trabecular destruction and diffuse intraosseous infiltration of lymphomatous tissue. Note the homogeneous and glistening cut surface of the greatly enlarged, diseased paraspinal lymphnode placed next to the vertebrae.

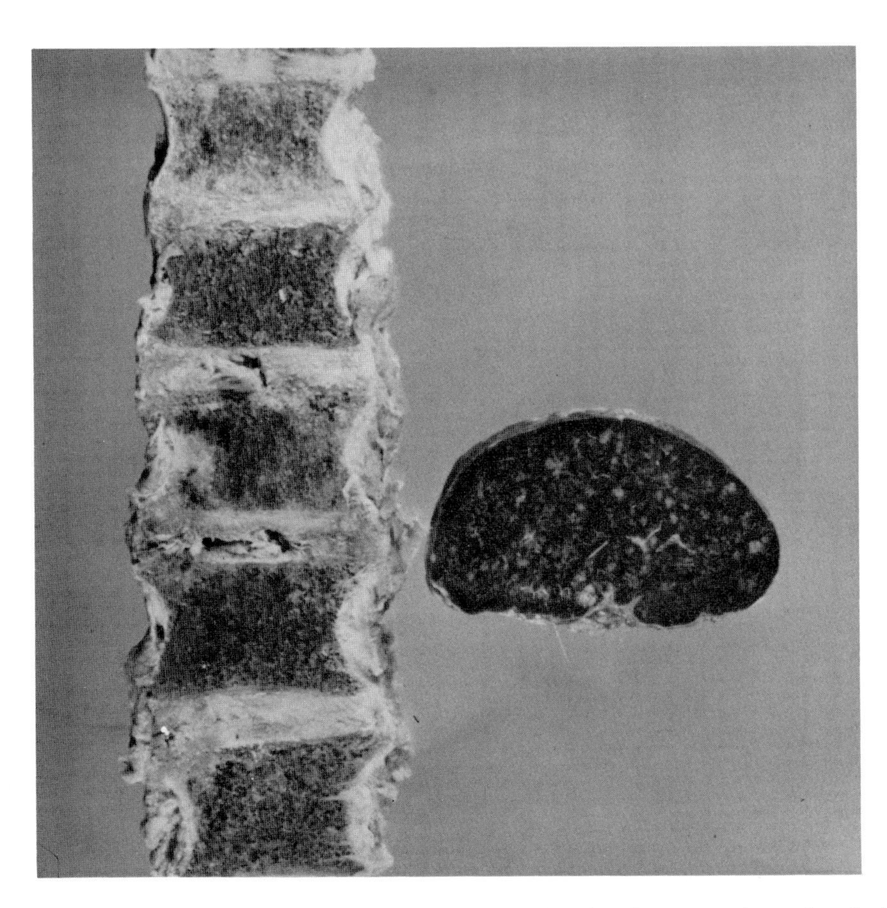

Figure 3-7. Longitudinal section of the lower thoracic spine from a patient who died of disseminated giant follicular lymphoma (nodular, lymphocytic non-Hodgkin's lymphoma) shows many yellowish-gray tumor deposits in the vertebral bodies. Note the similarity in gross tumor appearance between the intraosseous tumor foci and the intrasplenic tumor deposits.

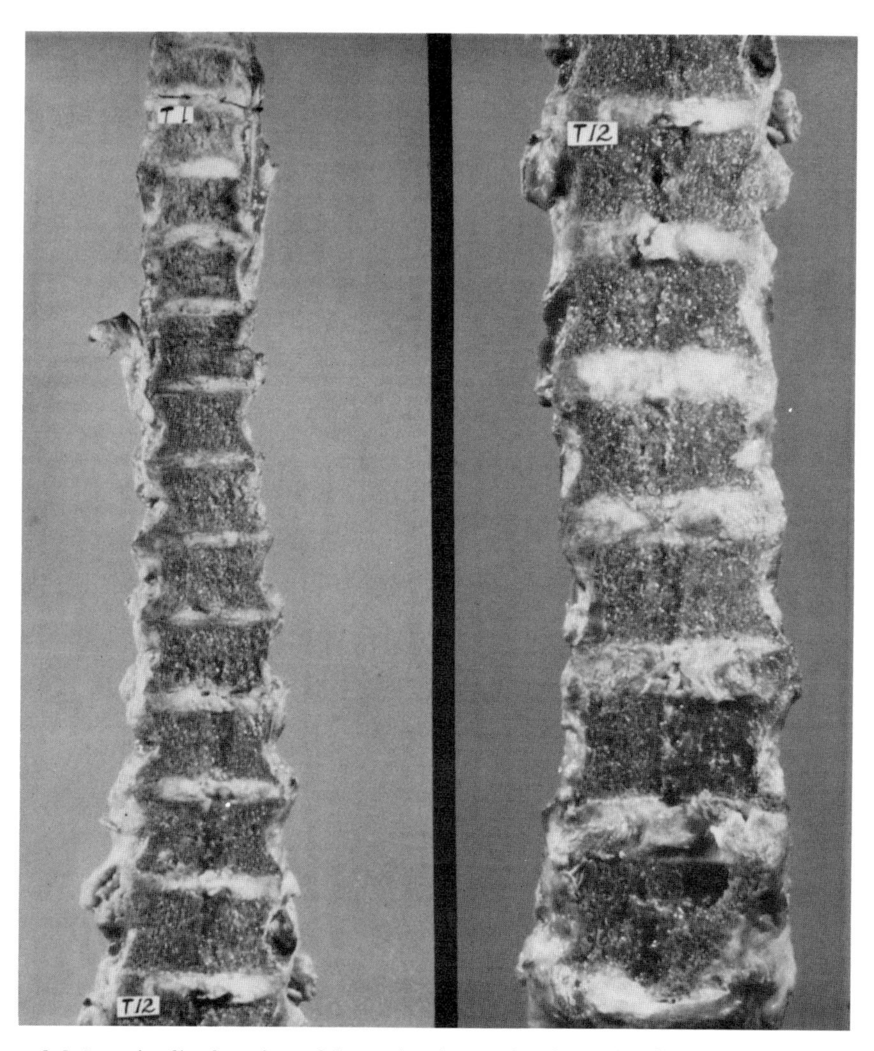

Figure 3-8. Longitudinal section of the entire thoracolumbar spine from a patient who died of non-Hodgkin's lymphoma shows diffuse intraosseous infiltration by the lymphomatous tissue. Note the cystic changes and hemorrhagic foci in the fourth and fifth vertebral bodies.

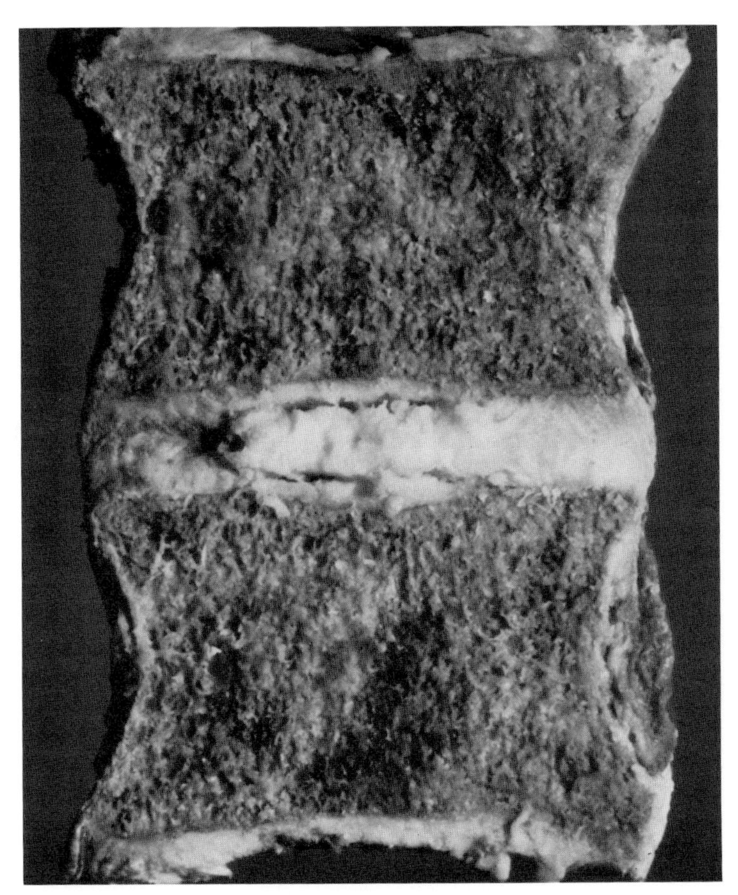

Figure 3-9. Close-up view of a longitudinal section of two thoracic vertebrae affected by disseminated non-Hodgkin's lymphoma shows extensive intraosseous infiltration of the grayish-yellow lymphomatous tissue.

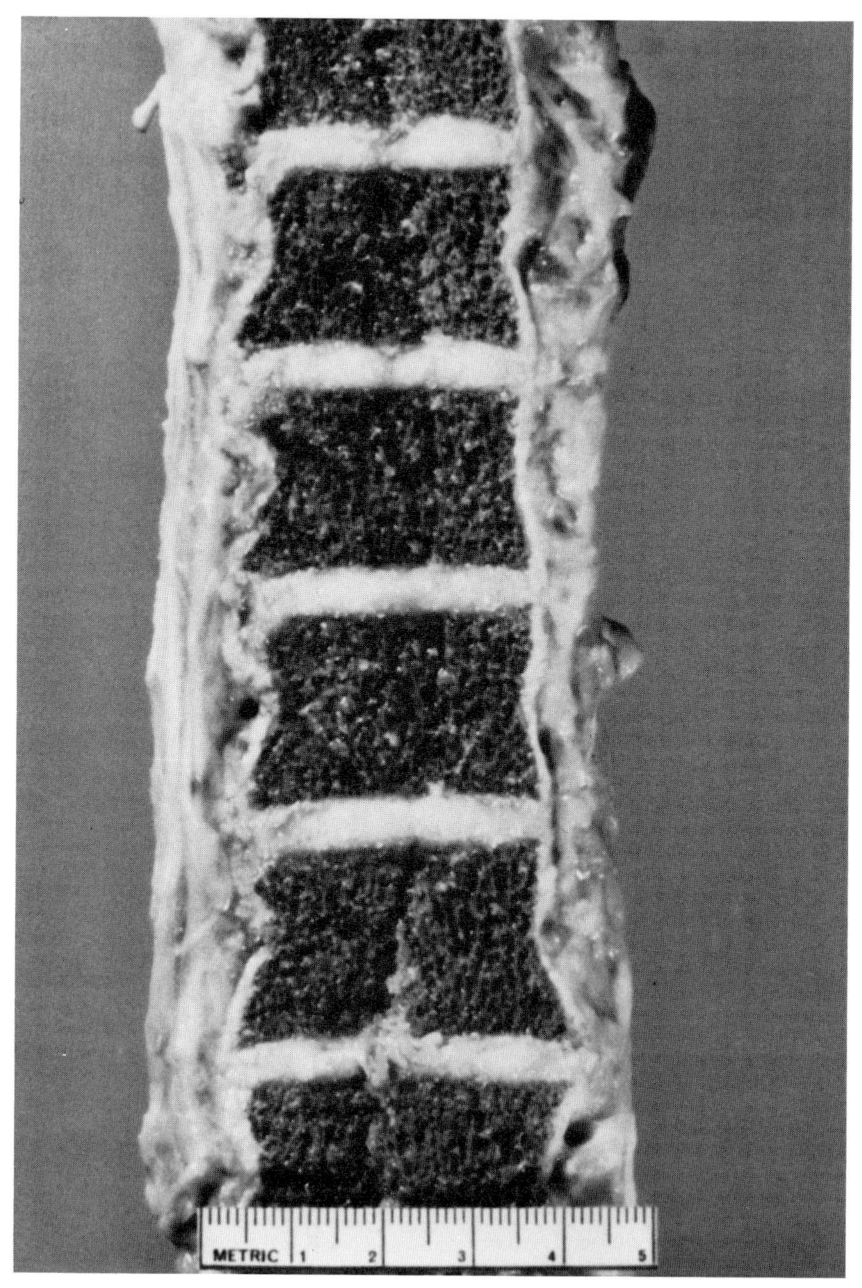

Figure 3-10. Longitudinal section of the lower thoracic and upper lumbar spine from a victim of a widely disseminated lymphosarcoma (diffuse, poorly differentiated, lymphocytic non-Hodgkin's lymphoma) shows moderate amount of osteoporosis and scattered foci of tumor tissue deposits.

direct invasion of the neural elements of the spine by the lymphomatous tissue, when present, are readily visible to the naked eyes at autopsies. In contrast, osteoblastic lesions of the spine rarely show compression fracture because the intramedullary space is frequently filled with reactive new bone formation which gives the involved vertebral body a whitish or yellowish-white and solid appearance.

MICROSCOPIC PATHOLOGY. The presence of Reed-Sternberg cell (Figure 3-11), a large cell with abundant acidophilic to basophilic cytoplasm and two or more nuclei or a lobulated nucleus with prominent acidophilic round nucleoli, in Hodgkin's disease distinguishes it from non-Hodgkin's lymphomas. The various types of Hodgkin's disease and non-Hodgkin's lymphomas can be determined by the presence of several predominant cell types, the amount of interstitial fibrous tissue, and the cellular patterns. The following is a comprehensive photomicrographic representation of the major types of Hodgkin's disease and non-Hodgkin's lymphomas:

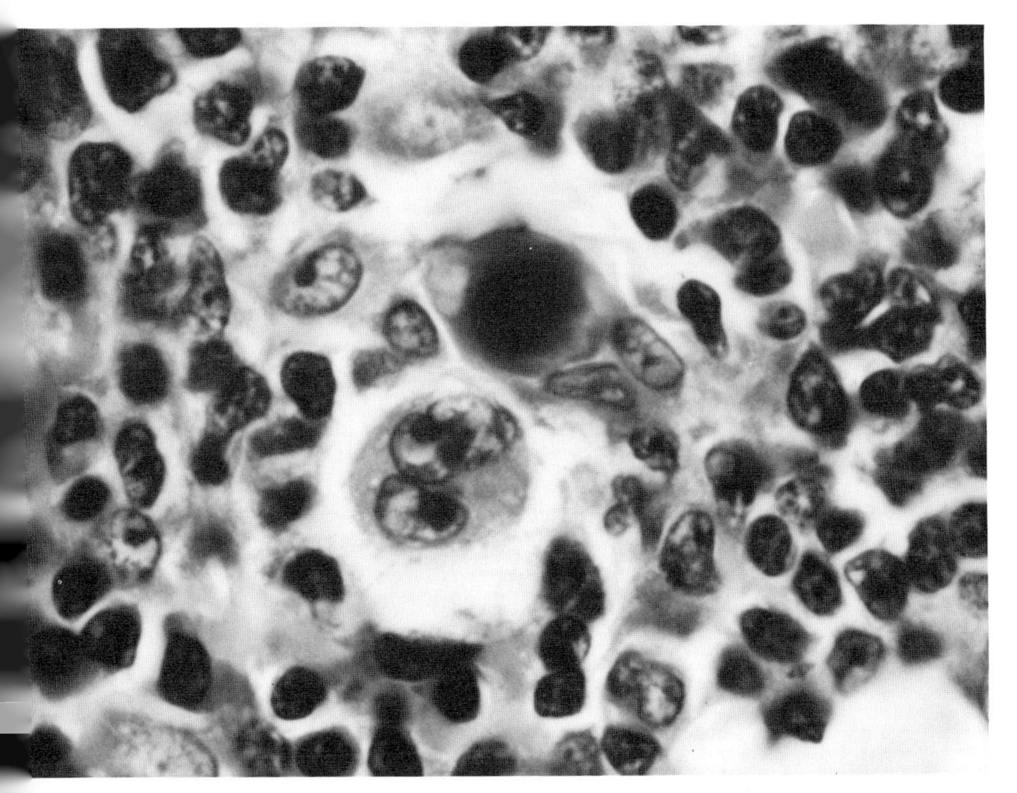

igure 3-11. This photomicrograph (reduced 15% from 1000×, H. & E.) shows a typical eed-Sternberg cell that is quite large and has a well defined cytoplasmic border, abundant ranular cytoplasm, and two reniform nuclei with prominent and hyperchromatic nucleoli nd a lacey chromatin.

Hodgkin's Disease

- Lymphocytic predominance type (Figure 3-12).
- Nodular sclerosis type (Figure 3-13).
- Mixed cellularity type (Figure 3-14).
- Lymphocytic depletion type (Figure 3-15).

Non-Hodgkin's Lymphomas

- Diffuse lymphocytic lymphoma (Figure 3-16).
- Nodular lymphocytic lymphoma (Figures 3-17A and 3-17B).
- Histiocytic lymphoma (Figure 3-18).
- Mixed cell type lymphoma (Figure 3-19).
- Burkitt's lymphoma (Figure 3-20).

TREATMENT

The treatment of choice for a particular lymphoma will naturally depend on the extent of its involvement, its histologic classification, and the presence or absence of central nervous system symptoms.[172-188] Owing to the radiosensitivity of the great majority of lymphomas, radiotherapy is

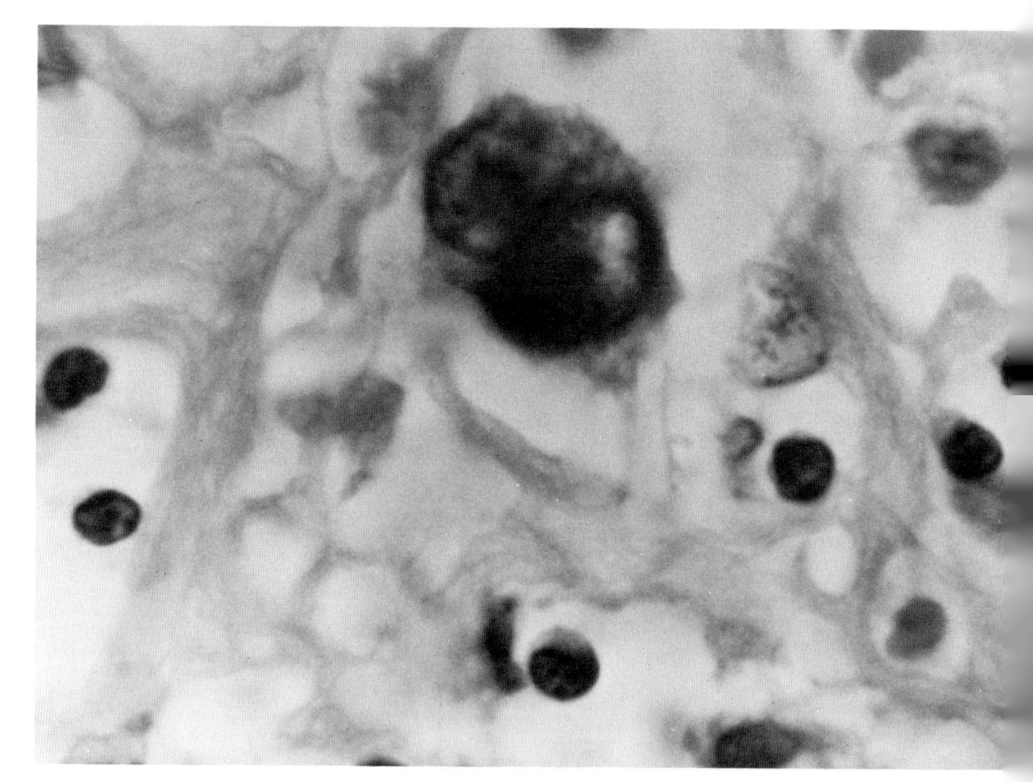

Figure 3-12. This photomicrograph (reduced 15% from 1300×, H. & E.) shows a lymphocytic predominance type of Hodgkin's disease characterized by the presence of a Reed-Sternberg cell surrounded by lymphocytic cells.

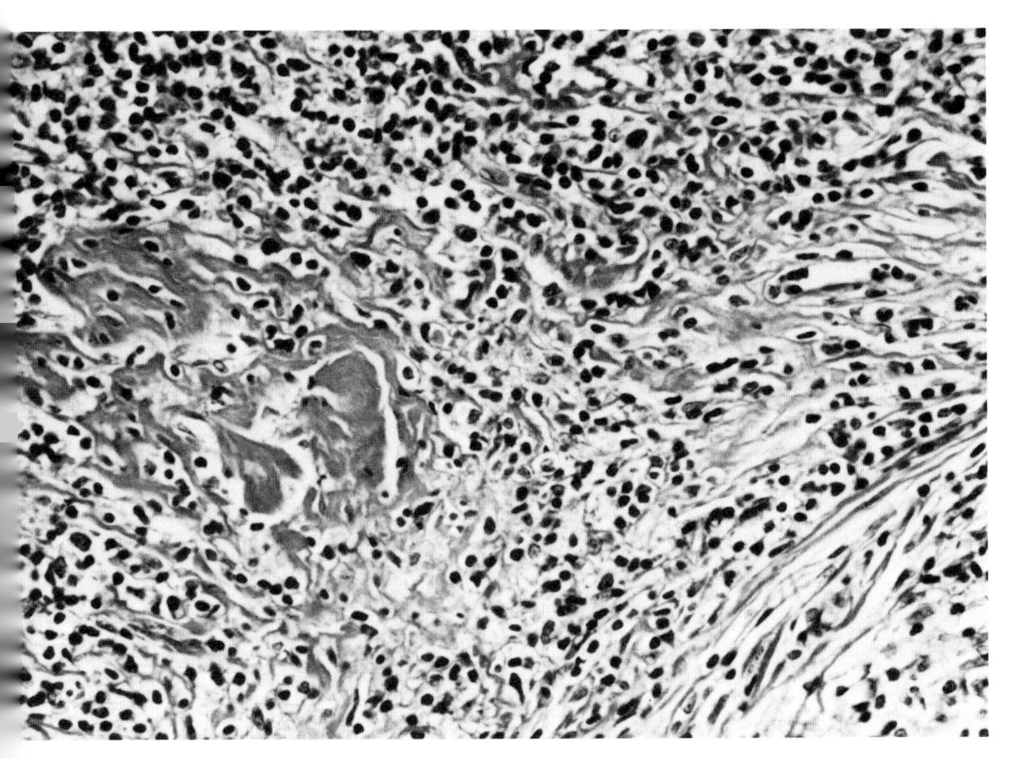

Figure 3-13. This photomicrograph (reduced 18% from 250×, H. & E.) shows the typical features of a nodular sclerosis type of Hodgkin's disease with dense strands of collagen crisscrossing the entire field. Note that the predominant cell type is lymphocytic in nature.

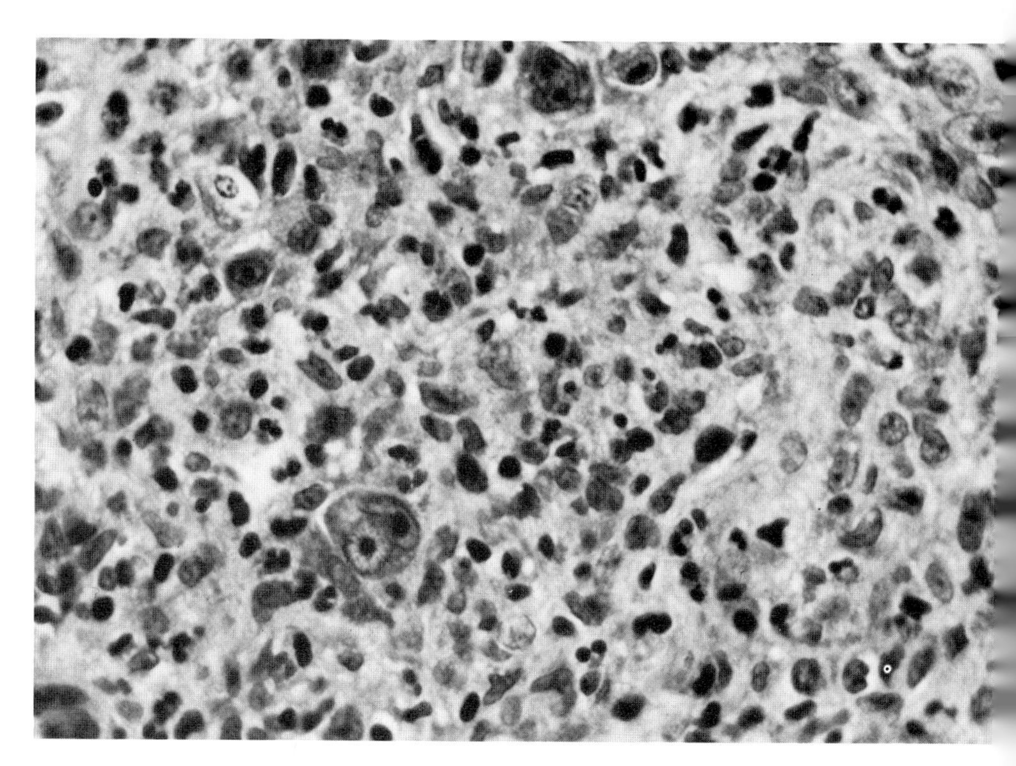

Figure 3-14. This photomicrograph (reduced 18% from 400 ×, H. & E.) illustrates a mixed cellularity type of Hodgkin's disease that contains a large, doubly-nucleated Reed-Sternberg cell and a mixture of lymphocytic and histiocytic cells.

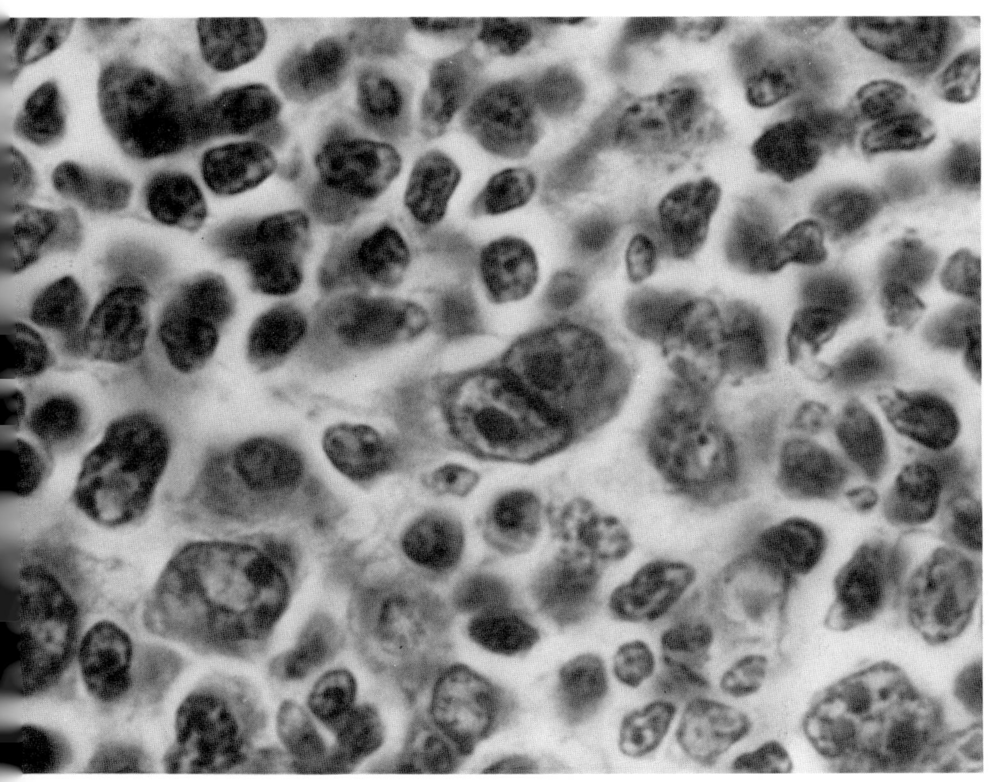

Figure 3-15. This photomicrograph (reduced 13% from 1100×, H. & E.) shows a lymphocytic depletion type of Hodgkin's disease that is characterized by the presence of a Reed-Sternberg cell in the center accompanied by purely histiocytic cells throughout the entire field.

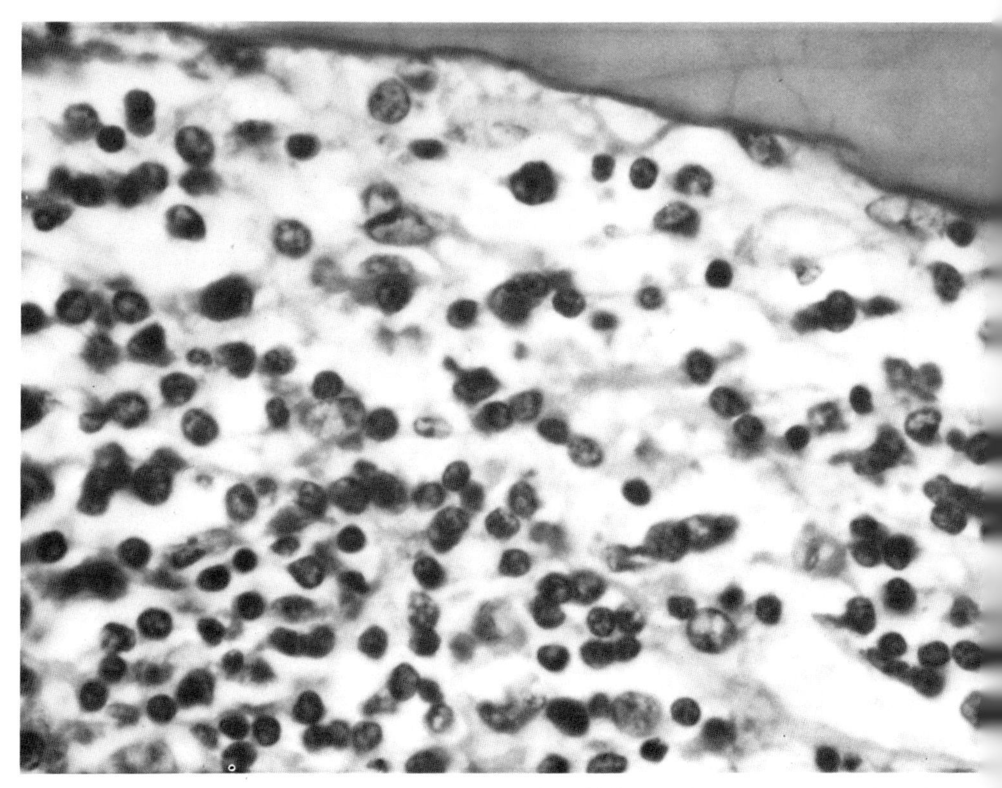

Figure 3-16. This photomicrograph (reduced 15% from 630×, H. & E.) taken from a spinal lymphosarcoma (diffuse, poorly differentiated, lymphocytic non-Hodgkin's lymphoma) shows invasion of the marrow space by many poorly differentiated lymphocytic cells that show no intention of forming any lymphoid follicles.

Figure 3-17A. This photomicrograph (reduced 15% from 16×, H. & E.) from a patient with giant follicular lymphoma (nodular lymphocytic lymphoma) shows the distinctive nodular arrangement of the tumor tissue.

Figure 3-17B. This photomicrograph (reduced 15% from 100×, H. & E.) is a close-up view of one of the follicles shown in Figure 3-17A. It shows a nodular collection of larger, paler and less mature lymphocytes surrounded by the smaller, hyperchromatic, mature lymphocytes.

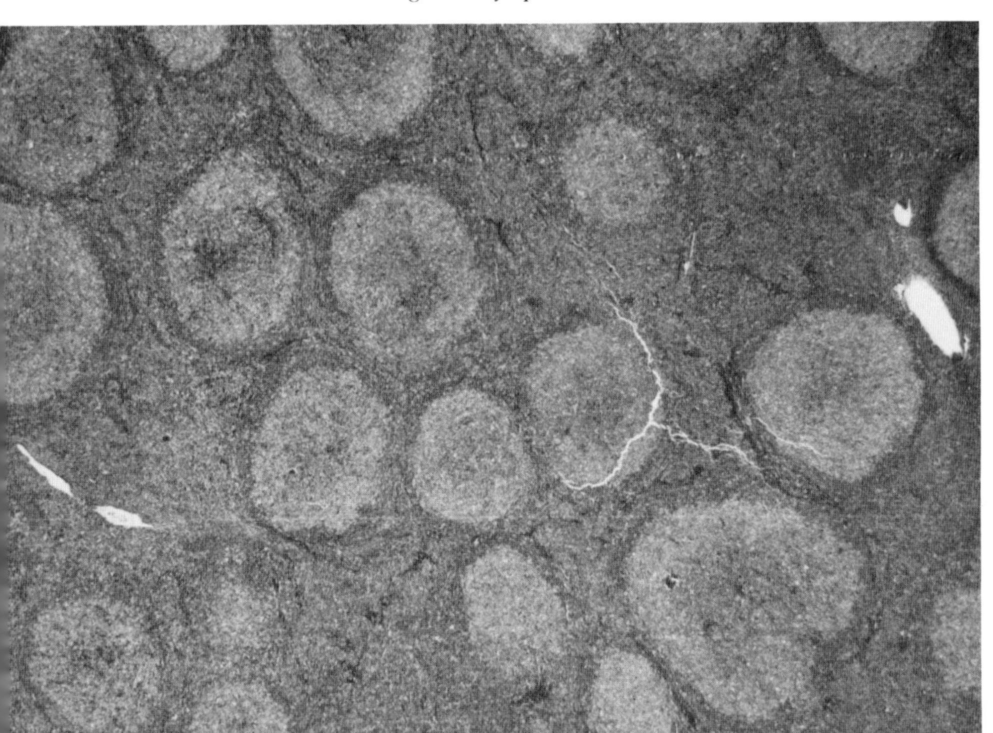

Figure 3-17A.

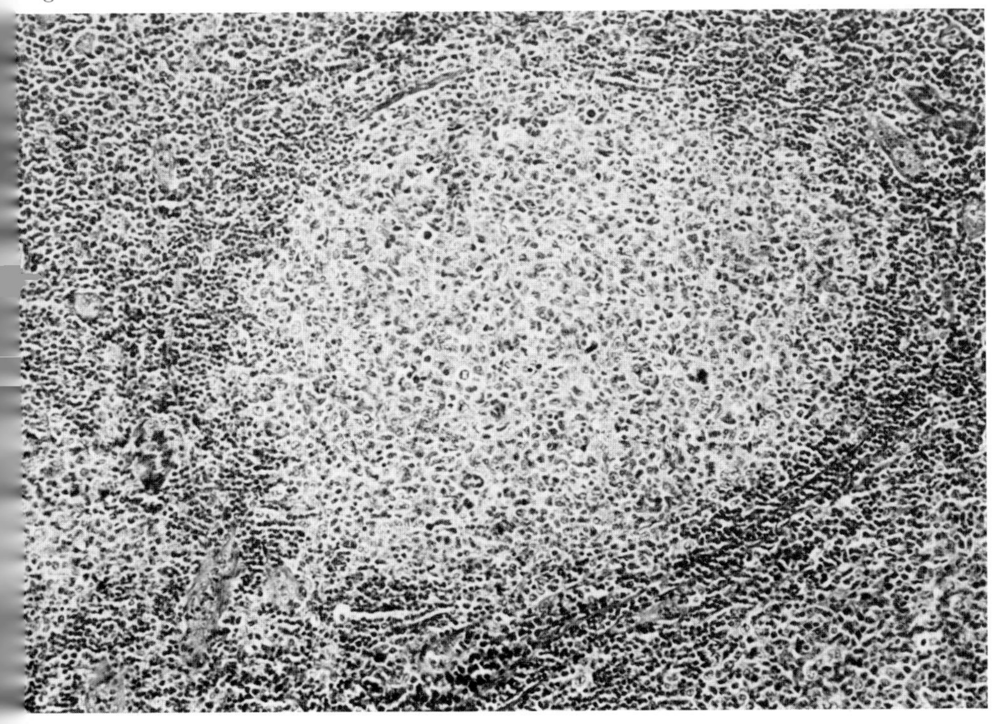

igure 3-17B.

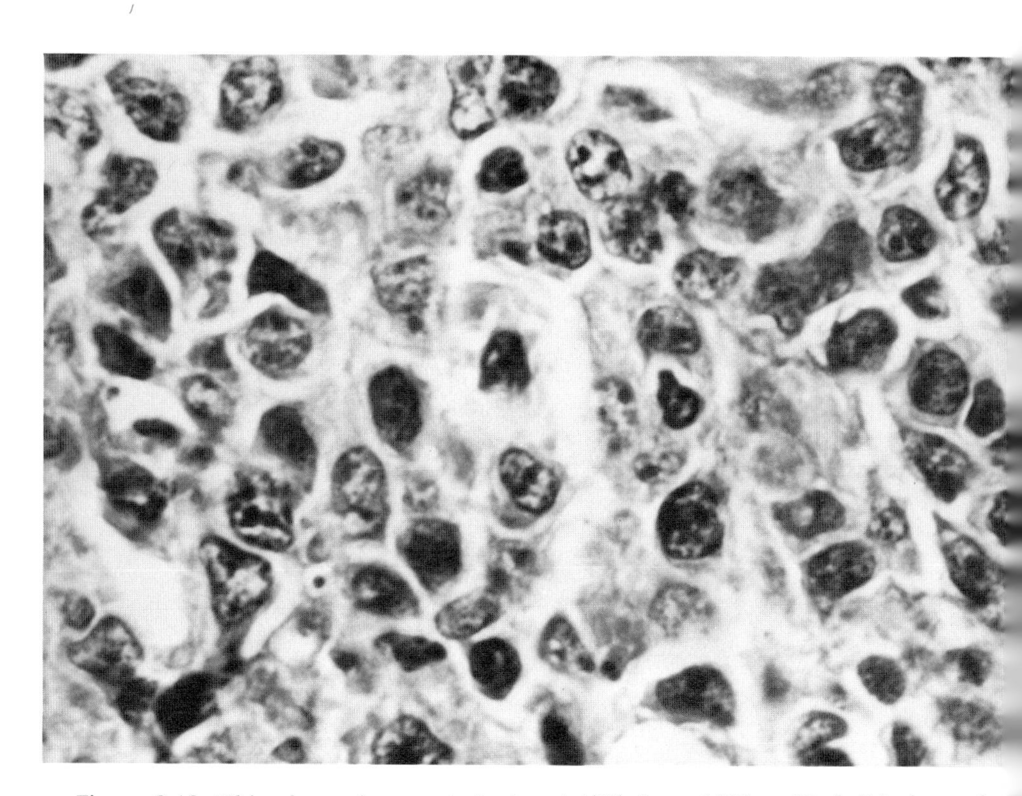

Figure 3-18. This photomicrograph (reduced 17% from 1000×, H. & E.) shows the variation in size and shape of the reticulum cell sarcoma cells (histiocytic non-Hodgkin's lymphoma) that have a pale nucleus with one or more prominent nucleoli and an indistinct cytoplasmic border.

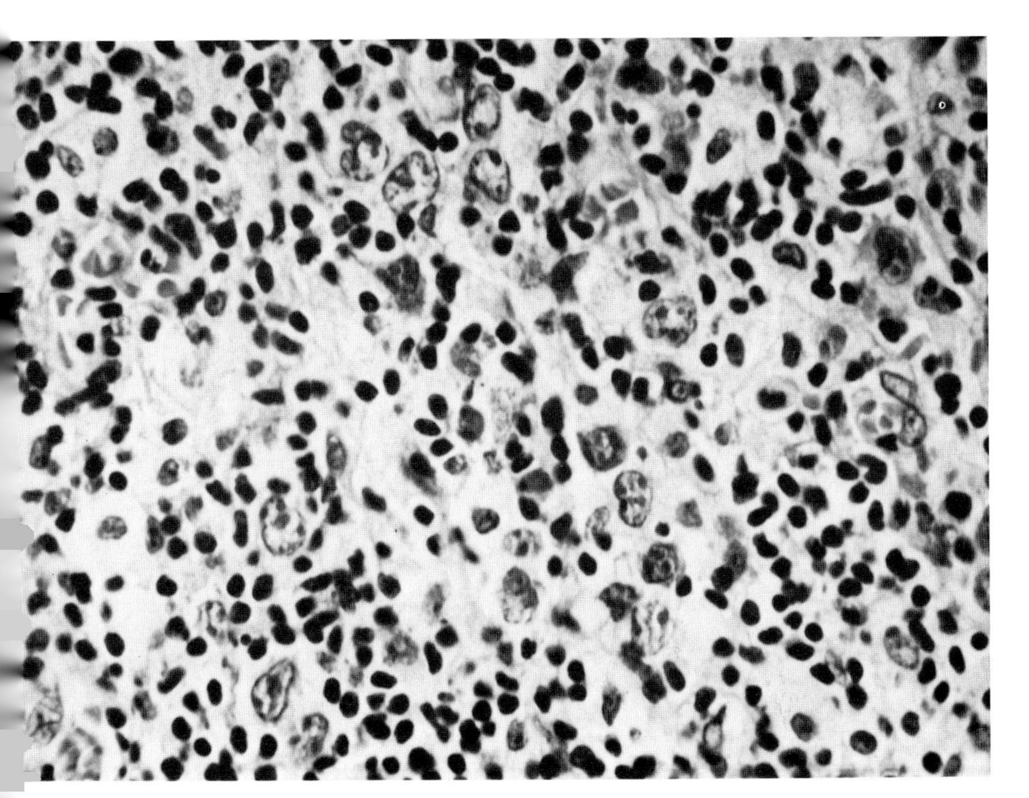

'igure 3-19. This photomicrograph (reduced 15% from 400×, H. & E.) represents a nixed cell type of non-Hodgkin's lymphoma that is characterized by a mixture of many mall, hyperchromatic lymphocytic cells and some larger, pale histiocytic cells with promi- ent nucleoli.

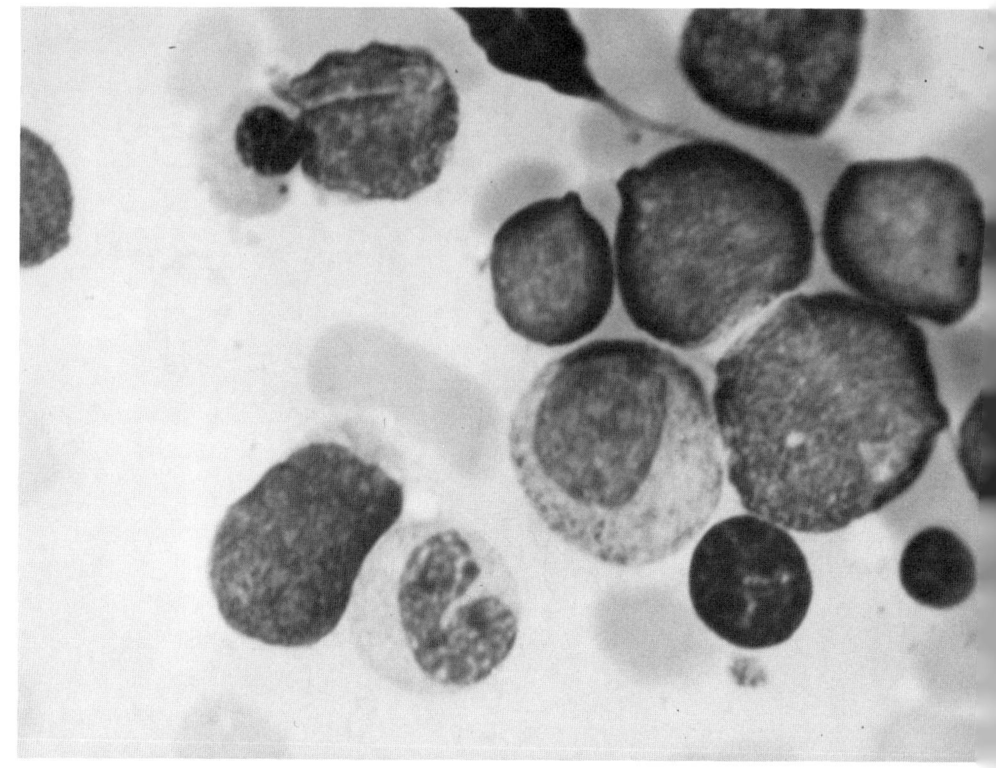

Figure 3-20. This photomicrograph (reduced 15% from 1100×, Wright stain) from bon marrow smear of a child with Burkitt's lymphoma shows a cluster of large lymphoblasts tha are commonly found in Burkitt's lymphoma.

usually the first treatment, as well as the treatment of choice, especially ir well localized, Stage I or II lymphomas with involvement above the di aphragm.

The doses of radiotherapy should be carefully calculated so that the minimal, but effective individual dose can be administered over a relative ly long period of time in order to avoid all the preventable radiation induced morbidities. Under favorable conditions, certain lymphoma were thought to be radiocurable by several authors,[189-191] and lymphoma induced neurological deficits had been successfully reversed to normal b means of radiotherapy. However, any lymphomas, especially the imma ture and pleomorphic varieties, that do not show satisfactory response t radiotherapy should be treated with chemotherapy.

Multidrug and multicycle chemotherapy is usually needed in treatin advanced stages and disseminated forms of lymphomas. When the centra nervous system is involved by lymphoma, radiotherapy and intratheca administration of proper chemotherapeutic agents should be instituted In addition, patients with advanced diffuse lymphomas and documente skeletal involvement and in complete clinical remission of their systemic disease are candidates for prophylactic treatment for central nervous system lymphoma.

Surgery is indicated when radiotherapy and chemotherapy are not able to reverse the neurological deficits caused by vertebral compression fracture with extrusion of bony elements into the spinal canal or by radioresistant epidural lymphomatous deposits. In addition to removing all the mechanical impingements of the spinal cord or nerves, surgery can also be employed to provide stability for any important structural damages of the spine brought about by the lymphomatous process.

PROGNOSIS

Many factors directly and indirectly influence the prognosis of malignant lymphomas:[192-213]

Stage of Lymphoma. The higher the stage, the worse the prognosis, and within the same stage, the Substage B with constitutional symptoms has a worse prognosis than Substage A with no constitutional symptoms.

Type of Lymphoma. In general, non-Hodgkin's lymphomas have a worse prognosis than Hodgkin's disease because of their wider body system involvements. Within the family of non-Hodgkin's lymphomas, histiocytic lymphoma, lymphoma with diffuse cellular pattern, and all lymphocytic predominance, nodular sclerosis, mixed cellularity, and lymphosis. Likewise, the prognosis of Hodgkin's disease in worsening order is lymphocytic predominance, nodular sclerosis, mixed cellularity, lymphocytic depletion. Furthermore, within the same histologic cell type, the less mature and more pleomorphic variety has a worse prognosis than the more mature and less pleomorphic type.

Age and Sex. Everything being equal, women and young children tend to fare lymphomas better than men and adults.

The Presence of Pruritis, Herpes Zoster and Abnormal Laboratory Studies. (Anemia, thrombocytopenia, hypercalcemia, elevated serum liver enzymes, BUN, creatinine, etc.) All are merely reflections of various systemic lymphomatous involvements and are poor prognostic signs.

The Presence of Lymphomatous Involvement of the Central Nervous System and Leukemia, carcinomas and sarcomas arising from the treatments of malignant lymphomas, are grave prognostic indicators.

Primary Lymphomas of the Bone have significantly better prognosis than the regular types of Hodgkin's disease and non-Hodgkin's lymphomas with secondary bone involvement and the same histologic appearance because of their limited intraosseous involvement.

Failure to Show Favorable Response to various modalities of lymphoma therapy indicates a poor prognosis.

REFERENCES

1. Block, J. B., Edgcomb, J., Eisen, A., and Van Scott, E. J.: Mycosis fungoides: Natural history and aspects of its relationship to other malignant lymphomas. *Am J Med, 34:*228-235, 1963.
2. Cohen, S. R., Stenn, K. S., Braverman, I. M., and Beck, G. J.: Mycosis fungoides: Clinicopathologic relationships, survival, and therapy in 59 patients with observations on occupation as a new prognostic factor. *Cancer, 46:*2654-2666, 1980.
3. Cry, D. P., Geokas, M. D., and Worsley, G. H.: Mycosis fungoides-hematologic findings and terminal course. *Arch Dermatol, 94:*558-573, 1966.
4. Epstein, E. H., Levin, D. L., Croft, J. D., and Lutzner, M. A.: Mycosis fungoides — survival, prognostic features, response to therapy and autopsy findings. *Medicine, 15:*61-72, 1972.
5. Hamminga, L., Mudler, J. D., Evans C., Scheffer, E., Meyer, C. J. L. M., and Van Vloten, W. A.: Staging lymphography with respect to lymph node histology, treatment, and follow-up in patients with mycosis fungoides. *Cancer, 47:*692-697, 1981.
6. Marglin, S. I., Soulen, R. L., Blank, V., and Castelino, R. A.: Mycosis fungoides. Radiographic manifestations of extracutaneous intrathoracic involvement. *Diagnostic Radiol, 180:*35-37, 1979.
7. Rappaport, H., and Thomas, L. B.: Mycosis fungoides: The pathology of extra cutaneous involvement. *Cancer, 34:*1198-1229, 1974.
8. Wolfe, J. D., Trevor, E. D., and Kjeldsberg, C. R.: Pulmonary manifestations of mycosis fungoides. *Cancer, 46:*2648-2653, 1980.
9. Worm, A. M., Hastrup, N., Hou-Jennsen, K., and Thomsen, K.: Bone marrow involvement in mycosis fungoides demonstrated by needle biopsy. *J Cutan Pathol, 5:*31-34, 1978.
10. Baroni, C. D., and Malchiodi, F.: Histology, age, sex distribution, and pathologic correlation of Hodgkin's disease. *Cancer, 95:*1549-1555, 1980.
11. Braunstein, E. M., and White, S. J.: Non-Hodgkin lymphoma of bone. *Radiology, 135:*59-63, 1980.
12. Coles, W. C., and Schulz, M. D.: Bone involvement in malignant lymphoma. *Radiology, 50:*458-462, 1948.
13. Freeman, C., Berg, J. W., and Cutler, S. J.: Occurrence and prognosis of extranodal lymphomas. *Cancer, 29:*252-260, 1972.
14. Sugarbaker, E. D., and Craver, L. F.: Lymphosarcoma. A study of 196 cases with biopsy. *JAMA, 115:*17-23, 1940.
15. Vieta, J. O., Friedell, H. L., and Craver, L. F.: A survey of Hodgkin's disease and lymphosarcoma in bone. *Radiology, 39:*1-15, 1942.
16. Steiner, P. E.: Hodgkin's disease: Incidence, distribution, nature and possible significance of lymphogranulomatous lesions in bone marrow; review with original data. *Arch Pathol, 36:*627-637, 1943.
17. Uehlinger, E.: Über Knochen-lymphogranulomatose. *Virchows Arch Pathol Anat, 288:*36-118, 1933.
18. Boston, H. D., Dahlin, D. C., Ivins, J. C., and Cupps, R. E.: Malignant lymphoma (so-called reticulum cell sarcoma) of bone. *Cancer, 34:*1131, 1974.
19. Coley, B. L., Higinbotham, N. L., and Grosbeck, H. P.: Primary reticulum-cell sarcoma of bone. Summary of 37 cases. *Radiology, 55:*641, 1950.
20. Dolan, P. A.: Reticulum cell sarcoma of bone. *Am J Roentgenol Radium Ther Nucl Med, 87:*121-127, 1962.
21. Dumont, J., Mazabraud, A.: Primary lymphomas of bone (so called "Parker and

Jackson's reticulum cell sarcoma"): Histological review of 75 cases according to the new classifications of non-Hodgkin's lymphomas. *Bio Medicine Express, 31:*271-275, 1979.
22. Edwards, J. E.: Primary reticulum cell sarcoma of the spine. Report of a case with autopsy. *Am J Pathol, 16:*835-844, 1940.
23. Francis, K. C., Higinbotham, N. L., and Coley, B. L.: Primary reticulum cell sarcoma of bone. Report of 44 cases. *Surg Gynecol Obstet, 99:*142, 1954.
24. Ivins, J. C., and Dahlin, D. C.: Reticulum-cell sarcoma of bone. *J Bone and Joint Surg, 35A:*835, 1953.
25. Ivins, J. C., and Dahlin, D. C.: Malignant lymphoma (reticulum cell sarcoma) of bone. *Mayo Clin Proc, 38:*375, 1963.
26. Jack, G. A.: Radiotherapy of reticulum cell sarcoma of bone. *Radiol Clin Biol, 40:*230-242, 1971.
27. Khanolkar, V. R.: Reticulum-cell sarcoma of bone. *Arch Pathol, 46:*467-476, 1948.
28. Mac Cormack, J. L., Ivins, J. C., Dahlin, D. C., and Johnson, E. W., Jr.: Primary reticulum cell sarcoma of bone. *Cancer, 5:*1182, 1952.
29. Mac Intosh, D. J., Price, C. H. G., and Jeffree, G. M.: Malignant lymphoma (reticulosarcoma) in bone. *Clin Oncol, 3:*287-300, 1977.
30. Magnus, H. A., and Wood, H. L. C.: Primary reticulosarcoma of bone. *J Bone & Joint Surg, 38-B:*258-278, 1956.
31. Mahoney, J. P., and Alexander, R. W.: Primary histiocytic lymphoma of bone: A light and ultrastructural study of four cases. *Am J Surg Pathol, 4:*149-161, 1980.
32. Medill, E. V.: Primary reticulum-cell sarcoma of bone. *J Fac Radiol Lond, 8:*102, 1956.
33. Mukadum, F. K., and Pinto, J. M.: Radiology in primary reticulum cell sarcoma of bone (a review of 53 cases). *Indian J Cancer, 12:*170-178, 1975.
34. Parker, F., Jr., and Jackson, H., Jr.: Primary reticulum-cell sarcoma of bone. *Surg Gynecol Obstet, 68:*45, 1939.
35. Potdar, G. G.: Primary reticulum-cell sarcoma of bone in western India. *Brit J Cancer, 24:*48-55, 1970.
36. Sherman, R. S., and Snyder, R. E.: The roentgen appearance of primary reticulum-cell sarcoma of bone. *Am J Roentgenol, 58:*291, 1947.
37. Shoji, H., and Miller, J. R.: Primary reticulum cell sarcoma of bone — significance of clinical features upon the prognosis. *Cancer, 28:*1234, 1971.
38. Short, J. H.: Malignant lymphoma (reticulum cell sarcoma) of bone. *Radiography, 43:*139-143, 1977.
39. Sweet, D. L., Mass, D. P., Simon, M. A., and Shapiro, C. M.: Histiocytic lymphoma (reticulum-cell sarcoma) of bone. *J Bone & Joint Surg, 63-A:*79-84, 1981.
40. Valls, J., Muscolo, D., and Schajowicz, F.: Reticulum-cell sarcoma of bone. *J Bone & Joint Surg, 34-B:*588, 1952.
41. Van Den Bout, A. H.: Malignant lymphoma (reticulum cell sarcoma) of bone. *S Afr Med J, 57:*193-195, 1980.
42. Wang, C. C., and Fleischli, D. J.: Primary reticulum cell sarcoma of bone with emphasis on radiation therapy. *Cancer, 22:*994-998, 1968.
43. Wilson, J. W., and Pugh, D. R.: Primary reticulum-cell sarcoma of bone, with emphasis on roentgen aspects. *Radiology, 65:*343, 1955.
44. Blount, W. P.: Hodgkin's Disease: An orthopaedic problem. *J Bone & Joint Surg, 11:*761-770, 1929.
45. Dyttert, V.: Primary osseous lymphogranuloma. A contribution. *Neoplasma, 13:*105-111, 1966.
46. Fucilla, I. S., and Hamann, A.: Hodgkin's disease in bone. *Radiology, 77:*53-60, 1961.

47. Inglesakis, J. A., Abbes, M., and Martin, E.: Maladie de Hodgkin a debut vertebral. *Soc Chir Marseille, 15:*77-84, 1963.
48. Kooreman, P. J., and Haex, A. J.: Hodgkin's disease of the sekeleton. *Acta Med Scand, 115:*177-196, 1943.
49. Livingston, S. K.: Hodgkin's disease of the skeleton without glandular involvement. A case report proven by autopsy. *J Bone & Joint Surg, 17:*189-194, 1935.
50. Spencer, J., and Dresser, R.: Lymphoblastoma (Hodgkin's and sarcoma type) of bone. With a report of three cases simulating primary malignant tumor of bone. *N Engl J Med, 214:*877-879, 1936.
51. Bluming, A. Z., Ziegler, J. L., and Carbone, P. P.: Bone marrow involvement in Burkitt's lymphoma: Results of a prospective study. *Brit J Haematol, 22:*369-376, 1972.
52. Burkitt, D.: Sarcoma involving jaw in African children. *Brit J Surg, 46:*218, 1958.
53. Carbone, P. P., Bernard, C. W., Bennett, T. M., Ziegler, J. L., Cohen, M. H., and Gerber, P.: NIH clinical staff conference. Burkitt's tumor. *Ann Intern Med, 70:*817, 1969.
54. Cockshott, W. P., and Evans, K. T.: Childhood paraplegia in lymphosarcoma (Burkitt's tumour). *Brit J Radiol, 36:*914, 1963.
55. Dunnick, N. R., Reaman, G. H., Head, G. C., Shawker, T. H., and Ziegler, J. L.: Radiographic manifestations of Burkitt's lymphoma in American patients. *Am J Roentgenol, 132:*1-6, 1979.
56. Whittaker, L. R.: The radiological appearance of Burkitt's tumour involving bone. *Aust Radiol, 13:*307-310, 1969.
57. Ziegler, J. L., and Bluming, A. Z.: Intrathecal chemotherapy in Burkitt's lymphoma. *Brit Med J, 3:*508-512, 1971.
58. Ziegler, J. L., Wright, D. H., and Kyalwazi, S. K.: Differential diagnosis of Burkitt's lymphoma of the face and jaws. *Cancer, 27:*503-514, 1971.
59. Acar, S., Tekinalp, G., Özsoyu, S., Cevik, N., and Yasar, H.: Burkitt's lymphoma cell leukemia. *Acta Haematol* (basel), *57:*188-192, 1977.
60. Cehreli, C., and Tosun, N.: Burkitt's lymphoma cell leukemia in a Turkish boy *Cancer, 36:*1444-1449, 1975.
61. Clift, R. A., Wright, D. H., and Clifford, P.: Leukemia in Burkitt's lymphoma. *Blood 22:*243-251, 1963.
62. Flandrin, G., Brouet, J. C., Daniel, M. T., and Preudhomme, J. L.: Acute leukemia with Burkitt's tumor cells: A study of six cases with special reference to lympho cyte surface markers. *Blood, 45:*183-188, 1975.
63. Gutterman, J., Rodrigues, V., and McMullan, G.: Remission induction of acute leukemia developing in Burkitt's lymphoma. *Cancer, 29:*626-629, 1972.
64. Heideman, R. L.: Acute leukemia in Burkitt's lymphoma. *Med Pediatr Oncol, 2:*215-222, 1976.
65. Jaiyesimi, F., Oluboyedo, D., Taylor, D., and Familuasi, J. B.: Burkitt's lymphom presenting as acute leukemia. *Acta Haematol* (basel), *54:*115-119, 1975.
66. Mathe, G., Pouillait, P., Schwarzenberg, L., Hayat, M., Amiel, J. L., Schlumberger J. R., Misset, J. L., Jasmin, C., and Vassal, F.: Leukemic conversion of non Hodgkin's malignant lymphomata. *Br J Cancer, 31:*96-101, 1975.
67. Prokocimer, M., Matzner, Y., Ben-Bassat, H., and Polliack, A.: Burkitt's lymphom presenting as acute leukemia (Burkitt's lymphoma cell leukemia). *Cancer 45:*2884-2889, 1980.
68. Stevens, D. A., O'Connor, G. T., Levine, P. H., and Rosen, R. B.: Acute leukemia wit "Burkitt's lymphoma cells" and Burkitt's lymphoma. *Ann Intern Med, 76:*967-97 1972.

69. Hancock, B. W., Huck, P., and Ross, B.: Avascular necrosis of the femoral head in patients receiving intermittent cytotoxic and corticosteroid therapy for Hodgkin's disease. *Postgrad Med J, 54:*545-546, 1978.
70. Hope-Stone, H. F.: The diagnosis of osteo-necrosis in Hodgkin's disease — active disease or infarction. *Br J Radiology, 52:*580-582, 1979.
71. Park, W. M., and Cannell, L. B.: Osteonecrosis in Hodgkin's disease. *Br J Radiol, 51:*328-332, 1978.
72. Timothy, A. R., Tucker, A. K., Malpas, J. S., Wrigley, P. F., and Sutcliffe, S. B.: Osteonecrosis after intensive chemotherapy for Hodgkin's disease. *Lancet, 1:*154, 1978.
73. Benfield, G. F.: Primary lymphosarcoma of lung associated with hypertrophic pulmonary osteoarthropathy. *Thorax, 34:*279-280, 1979.
74. Kay, J. C., Rosenberg, M. A., and Burd, R.: Hypertrophic osteoarthropathy and childhood Hodgkin's disease. *Pediatr Radiol, 112:*177-178, 1974.
75. Lofters, W. S., and Walker, T. M.: Hodgkin's disease and hypertrophic pulmonary osteoarthropathy. Complete clearing following radiotherapy. *West Indian Med J, 27:*227-230, 1978.
76. Aisenberg, A. C., Kaplan, M. M., Reider, S. U., and Goldman, J. M.: Serum alkaline phosphatase at the onset of Hodgkin's disease. *Cancer, 26:*318-326, 1970.
77. Belliveau, R. E., Wiernik, P. H., and Abt, A. B.: Liver enzymes and pathology in Hodgkin's disease. *Cancer, 34:*300-305, 1974.
78. Cerda, J. J., Toskes, P. P., Shopa, N. A., and Wilkinson, J. H.: The relationship of serum alkaline phosphatase to urinary hydroxyproline excretion in liver and bone diseases. *Clin Chem Acta, 27:*437-443, 1970.
79. Deeble, T. J., and Goldberg, D. M.: Assessment of biochemical tests for bone and liver involvement in malignant lymphoma patients. *Cancer, 45:*1451-1457, 1980.
80. Harris, J. M., Jr., Tang, D. B., and Weltz, M. D.: Diagnostic tests and Hodgkin's disease. A standard approach to their evaluation. *Cancer, 41:*2388-2392, 1978.
81. Johnson, R. E., Thomas, L. B., Johnson, S. K., and Johnston, G. S.: Correlation between abnormal baseline liver tests and long term clinical in Hodgkin's disease. *Cancer, 33:*1123-1126, 1974.
82. Kippen, D. A., and Freeman, J. B.: Isolated histiocytic lymphoma of the spleen causing fever and hypercalcemia. *Arch Surg, 112:*1233-1234, 1977.
83. McKenna, R. W., Bloomfield, C. D., and Brunning, R. D.: Nodular lymphoma: Bone marrow and blood manifestations. *Cancer, 36:*428-440, 1975.
84. Williamson, B. R., Carey, R. M., Innes, D. J., Teates, C. D., Bray, S. T., Lees, R. F., Sturgill, B. C.: Poorly differentiated lymphocytic lymphoma with ectopic parathormone production:Visualization of metastatic calcification by bone scan. *Clin Nucl Med, 3:*382-384, 1978.
85. Bucy, P. C., and Jerva, M. J.: Primary epidural spinal lymphosarcoma. *J Neurosurg, 19:*142, 1962.
86. Bunn, P. A., Schein, P. S., Banks, P. M., and Devita, V. T.: Central nervous system complications in patients with diffuse histiocytic and undifferentiated lymphoma: Leukemia revisited. *Blood, 47:*3-10, 1976.
87. Ervin, T., and Canellos, G. P.: Successful treatment of recurrent primary central nervous system lymphoma with high dose Methotrexate. *Cancer, 45:*1556-1557, 1980.
88. Herbst, K. D., Corder, M. P., and Justice, G. R.: Successful therapy with Methotrexate of a multicentric mixed lymphoma of the central nervous system. *Cancer, 38:*1476-1478, 1976.

89. Hunt, T. R., Roser, C. M., and Williamson, W. P.: Lymphoma of spinal nerve root. *J Neurosurg, 17:*342, 1960.
90. Levitt, L. J., Dawson, D. M., Rosenthal, D. S., and Moloney, W. C.: CNS involvement in the non-Hodgkin's lymphomas. *Cancer, 45:*545-552, 1980.
91. Mitsumoto, H., Breuer, A. C., and Lederman, R. J.: Malignant lymphoma of the central nervous system. *Cancer, 46:*1258-1262, 1980.
92. Murphy, W. T., and Bilge, N. C.: Compression of spinal cord in patients with malignant lymphoma. *Radiology, 82:*495, 1964.
93. Olson, M. E., Chernik, N. L., and Posner, J. B.: Infiltration of the leptomeninges by systemic cancer. *Arch Neurol, 30:*122, 1974.
94. Siegal, T., Or, R., Matzner, Y., and Samuels, L. D.: Spinal meningeal uptake of Technetium-99M Methylene Diphosphonate in meingeal seeding by malignant lymphoma. *Cancer, 46:*2413-2415, 1980.
95. Skarin, A. T., Zuckerman, K. S., Pitman, S. W., Rosenthal, D. S., Maloney, W., Frei, E., III, and Canellos, G. P.: High dose Methotrexate with folic acid rescue in the treatment of advnaced non-Hodgkin's lymphoma including CNS involvement. *Blood, 50:*1039, 1977.
96. Smith, M. J., and Stenstrom, K. W.: Compression of spinal cord caused by Hodgkin's disease. *Radiology, 51:*77, 1948.
97. Sparling, H. J., Jr., Adams, R. D., and Parker, F., Jr.: Involvement of the nervous system by malignant lymphoma. *Med* (Baltimore), *26:*285, 1947.
98. Van Allen, M. W., and Rahme, E. S.: Lymphosarcomatous infiltration of cauda equina. *Arch Neurol, 7:*476, 1962.
99. Verity, G. L.: Neurologic manifestations and complications of lymphoma. *Radiol Clin North Am, 6:*97, 1968.
100. Viets, H. R., and Hunter, F. T.: Lymphoblastomatous involvement of the nervous system. *Arch Neurol & Psychiat, 29:*1246, 1933.
101. Young, R. C., Howser, D. M., Anderson, T., Fisher, R. I., Jaffe, E., and Devita, V. T., Jr.: Central nervous system complications of non-Hodgkin's lymphoma. The potential role for prophylactic therapy. *Am J Med, 66:*435-443, 1979.
102. Castellino, R. A., Billingham, J., and Dorfman, R. F.: Lymphographic accuracy in Hodgkin's disease and malignant lymphoma with a note on the "reactive" lymph node as a cause of most false positive lymphogram. *Investigative Radiology, 9:*155, 1924.
103. Efremidis, S. C., Dan, S. J., Cohen, B. A., Mitty, H. A., and Rabinowitz, J. G.: Displaced paraspinal line: Role of CT and lymphography. *Am J Roentgenol, 136:*505-509, 1981.
104. Glees, J. P., Gazet, J. C., MacDonald, J. S., and Peckham, M. J.: The accuracy of lymphography in Hodgkin's disease. *Clin Radiol, 25:*5, 1974.
105. Heifetz, L. J., Fuller, L. M., Rodgers, R. W., Martin, R. G., Butler, J. J., North, L. B. Gamble, J. F., and Shullenberger, C. C.: Laparotomy findings in lymphangiogram-staged I and non-Hodgkin's lymphomas. *Cancer, 45:*2778-2786, 1980.
106. Sako, M., Kono, M., and Nishimine, M.: Lymphographic classification of malignant lymphoma. *Lymphology, 12:*23-25, 1979.
107. Tallroth, K., Wiljasalo, M., Valle, M., and Korhola, O.: Lymphography in the assessment of mycosis fungoides. *Lymphology, 10:*147-150, 1977.
108. Beyer, D., and Peters, P. E.: Real-time ultrasonography — an efficient screening method for abdominal and pelvic lymphadenopathy. *Lymphology, 13:*142-149 1980.
109. Carroll, B. A., and Ta, H. N.: The ultrasonic appearance of extranodal abdominal lymphoma. *Radiology, 136:*419-425, 1980.

110. Ginaldi, S., Bernardino, M. E., Jing, B. S., and Green, B.: Ultrasonographic patterns of hepatic lymphoma. *Radiology, 136:*427-431, 1980.
111. Glees, J. P., Taylor, K. J. W., Gazet, J. C., Peckham, M. J., and McCready, V. R.: Accuracy of gray scale ultrasonography of liver and spleen in Hodgkin's disease and the other lymphomas compared with isotope scans. *Clin Radiol, 28:*233, 1977.
112. Kaude, J. V., and Joyce, P. H.: Evaluation of abdominal lymphomas by ultrasound. *Gastrointest Radiol, 5:*249-254, 1980.
113. Kremer, H., and Grobner, W.: Sonography of polypoid gastric lesions by the fluid-filled stomach method. *JCU, 9:*51-54, 1981.
114. Miller, J. H., Hindman, B. W., and Lam, A. H.: Ultrasound in the evaluation of small bowel lymphoma in children. *Radiology, 135:*409-414, 1980.
115. Mittelstaedt, C. A.: Ultrasound as a useful imaging modality for tumor detection and staging. *Cancer Res, 40:*3072-3078, 1980.
116. Rabin, M. S., Funston, M. R., Kam, J., Goudie, E., Richter, I., Schmaman, I., and Butterworth, A.: Ultrasound and barium study in the evaluation of upper abdominal masses. *S Afr Med J, 57:*231-235, 1980.
117. Bryan, P. J., Dinn, W. M., Grossman, Z. D., Wistow, B. W., McAfee, J. G., and Kieffer, S. A.: Correlation of computed tomography, gray scale ultrasonography, and radionuclide imaging of the liver in detecting space-occupying processes. *Radiology, 124:*387-393, 1977.
118. Hauser, M. F., and Alderson, P. O.: Gallium-67 imaging in abdominal disease. *Semin Nucl Med, 8:*251-270, 1978.
119. Kreel, L.: The EMI whole body scanner in the demonstration of lymph node enlargement. *Clin Radiol, 27:*421-429, 1976.
120. Longo, D. L., Schilsky, R. L., Blei, L., Cano, R., Johnston, G. S., and Young, R. C.: Gallium-67 scanning: limited usefulness in staging patients with non-Hodgkin's lymphoma. *Am J Med, 68:*695-700, 1980.
121. Rudders, R. A., McCaffrey, J. A., and Kahn, P. C.: The relative roles of Gallium-67-citrate scanning and lymphangeography in the current management of malignant lymphoma. *Cancer, 40:*1439-1443, 1977.
122. Seabold, J. E., Votaw, M. L., Keyes, J. W., Jr., Foley, W. D., Balachandran, S., and Gill, S. P.: Gallium citrate Ga67 scanning: Clinical usefulness in lymphoma patients. *Arch Intern Med, 136:*1370-1374, 1976.
123. Shirkhoda, A., Staab, E. V., and Mittelstaedt, C. A.: Renal lymphoma imaged by ultrasound and Gallium-67. *Radiology, 137:*175-180, 1980.
124. Shreiner, D. P., and Hsu, Y.: Comparison of reticuloendothelial scans with bone scans in malignant disease. *Clin Nucl Med, 6:*101-104, 1981.
125. Siddiqui, A. R., Oseas, R. S., Wellman, H. N., Doerr, D. R., and Baehner, R. L.: Evaluation of bone-marrow scanning with Technetium-99M sulfur colloid in pediatric oncology. *J Nucl Med, 20:*379-386, 1979.
126. Weber, W. G., DeNardo, G. L., and Bergin, J. J.: Scintiscanning in malignant lymphomatous involvement of bone. *Arch Intern Med, 121:*433-437, 1968.
127. Alcorn, F. S., Metegrano, V. C., Petasnick, J. P., and Clark, J. W.: Contributions of computed tomography in staging and management of malignant lymphoma. *Radiology, 125:*717, 1977.
128. Best, J. K., Blackledge, G., Forbes, W. St. C., Todd, I. D. H., Eddleston, B., Crowther, D., and Isherwood, I.: Computed tomography of the abdomen in the staging and clinical management of lymphoma. *Br Med J, 2:*1675, 1978.
129. Crowther, D., Blackledge, G., and Best, J. K.: The role of computed tomography of the abdomen in the diagnosis and staging of patients with lymphoma. *Clin Hematology, 8:*567-591, 1979.

130. Ellert, J., and Kreel, L.: The role of computed tomography in the initial staging and subsequent management of the lymphomas. *J Comput Assist Tomogr, 4:*368-391, 1980.

131. Falappa, P., Trodella, L., and Maresca, G.: Lymphomatous involvement of the kidneys: Computed tomography and ultrasound demonstration. *Diagn Imaging, 49:*266-268, 1980.

132. Harell, G. S., Breiman, R. S., Gladstein, E. J., Marshall, W. H., Jr., and Castellino, R. A.: Computed tomography of the abdomen in the malignant lymphomas. *Radiol Clin North Am, 15:*391-400, 1977.

133. Jones, S. E., Tobias, D. A., and Waldman, R. S.: Computed tomographic scanning in patients with lymphoma. *Cancer, 41:*480-486, 1978.

134. Redman, H. C., Federal, W. A., Castellino, R. A., and Glastein, E.: Computerized tomography as an adjunct in the staging of Hodgkin's and non-Hodgkin's lymphoma. *Radiology, 124:*381, 1977.

135. Schaner, E. G., Head, G. L., Doppmann, J. L., and Young, R. C.: Computed tomography in the diagnosis, staging and management of abdominal lymphoma. *J Comput Assist Tomogr, 1:*176, 1977.

136. Bonadonna, G., Pizzetti, F., Musumeci, R., Valagussa, P., Banfi, A., and Veronesi, V.: Staging laparotomy in non-Hodgkin's lymphomata. *Br J Cancer, 31:*252-260, 1975.

137. Dorfman, R. F., and Kim, H.: Relationship of histology to site in the non-Hodgkin's lymphomata: A study based on surgical staging procedures. *Br J Cancer, 31:*217-220, 1975.

138. Dresser, R. K., Moran, E. M., and Ultmann, J. E.: Staging of Hodgkin's disease and lymphoma. Diagnostic procedures including staging laparotomy and splenectomy. *Med Clin North Am, 57:*479, 1978.

139. Ferguson, D. J., Allen, L. W., Griem, M. L., Rappaport, H., and Ultmann, J.: Surgical experience with staging laparotomy in 125 patients with lymphoma. *Arch Intern Med, 131:*356, 1973.

140. Gladstein, E., Guernsey, J. M., Rosenberg, S. A., and Kaplan, H. S.: The value of laparotomy and splenectomy in the staging of Hodgkin's disease. *Cancer, 24:*709-718, 1969.

141. Goffinet, D. R., Warnke, R., Dunnick, N. R., Castellino, R., Glastein, E. J., Nelson, T. S., Dorfman, R. F., Rosenberg, S. A., and Kaplan, H. S.: Clinical and surgical (laparotomy) evaluation of patients with non-Hodgkin's lymphomas. *Cancer Treat Rep, 61:*481, 1977.

142. Kaplan, H. S., Dorfman, R. F., Nelson, T. S., and Rosenberg, S. A.: Staging laparotomy and splenectomy in Hodgkin's disease: Analysis of indications and patterns of involvement in 285 consecutive patients. *Nat Cancer Inst Mon, 36:*291, 1973.

143. Nicholas, G. G., and Shochat, S. J.: Transabdominal bone biopsy during staging laparotomy for Hodgkin's disease. *Am J Surg, 135:*260-261, 1978.

144. Whittaker, J. A., Slater, A., Al-Ismail, S. A. D., Gough, J., Evans, K. T., Evans, I. H., and Crosby, D. L.: An assessment of laparotomy in the management of patients with Hodgkin's disease. *Q J Med, 47:*291, 1978.

145. Aisenberg, A. C.: The staging and treatment of Hodgkin's disease. *N Engl J Med, 299:*1288-1232, 1978.

146. Carbone, P. P., Kaplan, H. S., Musshoff, K., Smithers, D. W., and Tubiana, M.: Report of the committee on Hodgkin's disease staging classification. *Cancer Res, 31:*1860-1861, 1971.

147. Chabner, B. A., Fisher, R. I., Young, R. C., and DeVita, V. T.: Staging of non-Hodgkin's lymphoma. *Semin Oncol, 7:*285-291, 1980.
148. Chabner, B. A., Johnson, R. E., DeVita, V. T., Canellos, G. P., Hubbard, S. P., Johnson, S. K., and Young, R. C.: Sequential staging in non-Hodgkin's lymphoma. *Cancer Treat Rep, 61:*993-997, 1977.
149. Abrams, H. S.: The osseous system in Hodgkin's disease. *Ann Surg, 108:*296-304, 1938.
150. Beachley, M. C., Lau, B. P., and King, E. R.: Bone involvement in Hodgkin's disease. *Am J Roentgenol Radium Ther Nucl Med, 114:*559-563, 1972.
151. Brunning, R. D., Bloomfield, C. D., McKenna, R. W., and Peterson, L.: Bilateral trephine bone marrow biopsies in lymphoma and other neoplastic diseases. *Ann Intern Med, 82:*365-366, 1975.
152. Craver, L. F., and Copeland, M. M.: Changes in bone in Hodgkin's granuloma. *Arch Surg, 28:*1062-1086, 1934.
153. Falconer, E. H., and Leonard, M. E.: Skeletal lesions in Hodgkin's disease. *Ann Intern Med, 29:*1115, 1948.
154. Horan, F. T.: Bone involvement in Hodgkin's disease. A survey of 201 cases. *Br J Surg, 56:*277, 1969.
155. Jackson, H., Jr., and Parker, F., Jr.: Hodgkin's disease. II. Pathology. *N Engl J Med, 231:*35, 1944.
156. Jackson, H., Jr., and Parker, F., Jr.: Hodgkin's disease. IV. Involvement of certain organs. *N Engl J Med, 232:*547, 1945.
157. Jones, S. E., Rosenberg, S. A., and Kaplan, H. S.: Non-Hodgkin's lymphoma. I. Bone marrow involvement. *Cancer, 29:*954-960, 1972.
158. Moir, P. J., and Brockis, J. G.: Observations on bone lesions in Hodgkin's disease. *Br J Surg, 36:*414-417, 1949.
159. Montgomery, A. H.: Hodgkin's disease of bone. *Ann Surg, 87:*755-766, 1928.
160. Rosenberg, S. A.: Bone marrow involvement in the non-Hodgkin's lymphomata. *Br J Cancer, 31:*261-264, 1975.
161. Steiner, P. E.: Hodgkin's disease: The incidence, distribution, nature and possible significance of the lymphogranulomatous lesions in bone marrow; a review with original data. *Arch Path, 26:*627, 1943.
162. Stuhlbarg, J., and Ellis, F. W.: Hodgkin's disease of bone. Favorable prognostic significance? *Am J Roentgenol Radium Ther Nucl Med, 93:*568-572, 1965.
163. Vieta, J. O., Friedell, H. L., and Craver, L. F.: A survey of Hodgkin's disease and lymphosarcoma in bone. *Radiology, 39:*1, 1942.
164. Granger, W., and Whitaker, R.: Hodgkin's disease in bone, with special reference to periosteal reaction. *Br J Radiol, 40:*939-948, 1967.
165. Dennis, J. W.: The solitary dense vertebral body. *Radiology, 77:*618, 1962.
166. Hertz, M., Solomon, A., and Aghai, E.: 'Ivory vertebra' in Hodgkin's disease. Restoration of trabecular pattern after therapy. *JAMA, 238:*2402, 1977.
67. Martin, D. J., and Ash, J. M.: Diagnostic radiology in non-Hodgkin's lymphoma. *Semin Oncology, 4:*297-309, 1977.
68. Stein, R. S., and Flexner, J. M.: Ivory vertebra in Hodgkin's disease. *JAMA, 239:*2550, 1978.
69. Viola, M. V., Kovi, J., and Nukhopadhyay, M.: Reversal of myelofibrosis in Hodgkin's disease. *JAMA, 223:*1145, 1973.
70. Mandell, G. A.: Resolution of Hodgkin's induced ivory vertebrae. *Pediat Radiol, 7:*178-179, 1978.

171. Duncan, A. W.: Calcification of the anterior spinal longitudinal vertebral ligaments in Hodgkin's disease. *Clin Radiol, 24:*394, 1973.
172. Anderson, T., Bender, R. A., Fisher, R. I., Devita, V. T., Chabner, B. A., Berard, C. W., Norton, L., and Young, R. C.: Combination chermotherapy in non-Hodgkin's lymphoma: Results of long-term follow-up. *Cancer Treat Rep, 61:*1057-1066, 1977.
173. Andrieu, J. M., Montagnon, B., Asselain, B., Bayle-Weisgerber, C., Chastang, C., Teillet, F., and Bernard, J.: Chemotherapy-radiotherapy association in Hodgkin's disease, clinical stages IA II_2A: Results of a prospective clinical trial with 166 patients. *Cancer, 46:*2126-2130, 1980.
174. Cabanillas, F., Bodey, G. P., and Freireich, E. J.: Management with chemotherapy only of stage I and II malignant lymphoma of aggressive histologic types. *Cancer, 46:*2356-2359, 1980.
175. Chen, M. G., Prosnitz, L. R., Gonzalez-Serva, A., and Fischer, D. B.: Results of radiotherapy in control of stage I and II non-Hodgkin's lymphoma. *Cancer, 43:*1245-1254, 1979.
176. Cooper, M. R., Pajak, T. F., Nissen, N. I., Stutzman, L., Brunner, K., Cuttner, J., Falkson, G., Grunwald, H., Bank, A., Leone, L., Seligman, B. R., Silver, R. T., Weiss, R. B., Haurani, F., Blom, J., Spurr, C. L., Glidwell, O. J., Gottlieb, A. J., and Holland, J. F.: A new effective four drug combination of CCNU (1-[2-Chloroethyl]-3-Cyclohexyl-1-Nitrosourea) (NSC-79038), vinblastine, prednisone, and procarbazine for the treatment of advanced Hodgkin's disease. *Cancer, 46:*654-662, 1980.
177. Diggs, C. H., Wiernik, P. H., and Sutherland, J. C.: Treatment of advanced untreated Hodgkin's disease with SCAB an alternative to MOPP. *Cancer, 47:*224-228, 1981.
178. Ervin, T. J., Weichselbaum, R. R., and Greenberger, J. S.: Radiation therapy for non-Hodgkin's lymphoma. *Clin Haematol, 8:*657-666, 1979.
179. Ezdinli, E. Z., Costello, W. G., Silverstein, M. N., Berard, C., Hartsock, R. J., and Sokal, J. E.: Moderate versus intensive chemotherapy of prognostically favorable non-Hodgkin's lymphoma. *Cancer, 46:*29-33, 1980.
180. Goffinet, D. R., Glastein, E., Fuks, Z., and Kaplan, H. S.: Abdominal irradiation in non-Hodgkin's lymphomas. *Cancer, 37:*2297-2806, 1976.
181. Hansen, H. H., Selawry, O. S., Pajak, T. F., Spurr, C. L., Falkson, G., Brunner, K., Cuttner, J., Nissen, N. I., Holland, J. F.: The superiority of CCNU in the treatment of advanced Hodgkin's disease: Cancer and leukemia Group B study. *Cancer, 47:*14-18, 1981.
182. Mauch, P., Goodman, R., Rosenthal, D. S., Botnick, L., Piro, A. J., and Hellman, S.: An evaluation of total nodal irradiation as treatment for stage IIIA Hodgkin's disease. *Cancer, 43:*1255-1261, 1979.
183. Pene, F., Henry-Amar, M., LeBourgeois, J. P., Hayat, M., Gerard-Marchant, R., Laugier, A., Mathe, G., and Tubiana, M.: A study of relapse and course of 153 cases of Hodgkin's disease (clinical stages I and II) treated at the Institute Gustave-Roussy from 1963 to 1970 with radiotherapy alone or with adjuvant monochemotherapy. *Cancer, 46:*2131-2141, 1980.
184. Riddell, S., Weinerman, B., Kemel, S., Schipper, H., and Vadas, G.: The treatment resistance of lymphocyte depleted Hodgkin's disease. *Cancer, 46:*1503-1508, 1980.
185. Rodgers, R. W., Fuller, L. M., Hagemeister, F. B., Johnston, D. A., Sullivan, J. A., North, L. B., Butler, J. J., Velasquez, W. S., Conrad, F. G., and Schullenberger, C. C.: Reassessment of prognostic factors in stage IIIA and IIIB Hodgkin's disease treated with MOPP and radiotherapy. *Cancer, 47:*2196-2203, 1981.

186. Rosenberg, S. A., Kaplan, H. S., Gladstein, E. J., and Portlock, C. S.: Combined modality therapy of Hodgkin's disease. A report on the stanford trials. *Cancer, 42:*991-1000, 1978.
187. Straus, D. J., Myers, J., Passe, S., Young, C. W., Nisce, L. Z., Lee, B. J., Koziner, B., Arlin, Z., Kempin, S., Gee, T., and Clarkson, B. D.: The eight-drug radiation therapy program (MOPP/ABDV/RT) for advanced Hodgkin's disease. *Cancer, 46:*233-240, 1980.
188. Vander Werf-Messing, B.: Radiotherapy of extranodal non-Hodgkin's lymphoma. Recent results in cancer research, *65:*111-128, 1978.
189. Easson, E. C.: Possibilities for the cure of Hodgkin's disease. *Cancer, 19:*345-350, 1966.
190. Kaplan, H. S.: Evidence for a tumoricidal dose level in radiotherapy of Hodgkin's disease. *Cancer Res, 26:*1221-1224, 1966.
191. Smithers, D. W.: Factors influencing survival in patients with Hodgkin's disease. *Clin Radiol, 20:*124-132, 1969.
192. Andersen, A. P., Brinker, H., and Lass, F.: Prognosis in Hodgkin's disease with special reference to histologic type. *Acta Radiol, 9:*81-101, 1970.
193. Bearman, R. M., Pangalis, G. A., and Rappaport, H.: Hodgkin's disease, lymphocyte depletion type. *Cancer, 41:*293-302, 1978.
194. Berard, C. W., Thomas, L. B., Axtel, L. M., Kruse, M., Newell, E., and Kagan, R.: The relationship of histopathological subtype to clinical stage of Hodgkin's disease at diagnosis. *Cancer Res, 31:*1776-1785, 1971.
195. Bitran, J. D., Golomb, H. M., Ultmann, J. E., Sweet, D. L., Jr., Lester, E. P., Stein, R. S., Miller, J. B., Moran, E. M., Kinnealey, A. E., Vardiman, J. E., Kinzie, J., and Roth, N. O.: Non-Hodgkin's lymphoma, poorly differentiated lymphocytic and mixed cell types (results of sequential staging procedures, response to therapy, and survival of 100 patients), *Cancer, 42:*88-95, 1978.
196. Butler, J. J.: Relationship of histologic findings to survival in Hodgkin's disease. *Cancer Res, 31:*1770-1775, 1971.
197. Coggins, C. H.: Renal failure in lymphoma. *Kidney Int., 17:*847-855, 1980.
198. Come, S. E., and Chabner, B. A.: Staging in non-Hodgkin's lymphoma: Approach, results and relationship to histopathology. *Clin Haematology, 4:*645-656, 1979.
199. Hande, K. R., Reimer, R. P., and Fisher, R. I.: Comparison of nodal primary versus extranodal primary histiocytic lymphoma. *Cancer Treat Rep, 61:*999-1000, 1977.
200. Hauson, T. A. S.: Histological classification and survival in Hodgkin's disease. A study of 251 cases with special reference to nodular sclerosing Hodgkin's disease. *Cancer, 17:*1595-1603, 1964.
201. Hoppe, R. T., Rosenberg, S. A., Kaplan, H. S., and Cos, R. S.: Prognostic factor in pathological stage IIIA Hodgkin's disease. *Cancer, 46:*1240-1246, 1980.
202. Jones, S. E., Fuks, Z., Kaplan, H. S., and Rosenberg, S. A.: Non-Hodgkin's lymphoma. V. Results of radiotherapy. *Cancer, 32:*682-691, 1973.
203. Keller, A. R., Kaplan, H. S., Lukes, R. J., and Rappaport, H.: Correlation of histopathology with other prognostic indicators in Hodgkin's disease. *Cancer, 22:*487-499, 1968.
204. Mauch, P., Goodman, R., and Hellman, S.: The significance of mediastinal involvement in early stage Hodgkin's disease. *Cancer, 42:*1039-1045, 1978.
205. Musshoff, K.: Prognostic and therapeutic implications of staging in extranodal Hodgkin's disease. *Cancer Res, 31:*1814-1827, 1971.
206. Neiman, R. S., Rosen, P. S., and Lukes, R. J.: Lymphocyte depletion in Hodgkin's disease. *N Engl J Med, 288:*751, 1963.

207. Patchefsky, A. S., Brodovsky, H., Southard, M., Menduke, H., Gray, S., and Hoch, W. S.: Hodgkin's disease. A clinical and pathologic study of 235 cases. *Cancer, 32:*150-161, 1973.
208. Reddy, S., Pellettiere, E., Saxena, V., and Hendrickson, F. B.: Extranodal non-Hodgkin's lymphoma. *Cancer, 46:*1925-1931, 1980.
209. Schnitzer, B., Nishiyama, R. H., Heidelberger, K. P., and Weaver, D. K.: Hodgkin's disease in children. *Cancer, 31:*560-567, 1973.
210. Weinstein, H. J., and Link, M. P.: Non-Hodgkin's lymphoma in childhood. *Clin Haematol, 8:*699-716, 1979.
211. Whitcomb, M. E., Schwarz, M. I., Keller, A. R., Flannery, E. P., and Blom, J.: Hodgkin's disease of the lung. *Am Rev Respir Dis, 106:*79-85, 1972.
212. Wilimas, J., Thompson, E., and Smith, K. L.: Long-term results of treatment of children and adolescents with Hodgkin's disease. *Cancer, 46:*2123-2125, 1980.
213. Wilson, J. F., Marsa, G. W., and Johnson, R. E.: Herpes Zoster in Hodgkin's disease. *Cancer, 29:*461-465, 1972.
214. Baccarani, M., Bosi, A., Papa, G.: Second malignancy in patients treated for Hodgkin's disease. *Cancer, 46:*1735-1740, 1980.
215. Borum, K.: Increasing frequency of acute myeloid leukemia complicating Hodgkin's disease. *Cancer, 46:*1247-1252, 1980.
216. Bouroncle, B. A.: Sternberg-Reed cells in the peripheral blood of patients with Hodgkin's disease. *Blood, 27:*544-556, 1966.
217. Brody, R. S., Schottenfeld, D., and Reid, A.: Multiple primary cancer risk after therapy for Hodgkin's disease. *Cancer, 40:*1917-1926, 1977.
218. Canellos, G. P., DeVita, V. T., Arsenau, J. C., Whang-Peng, J., and Johnson, R. E. C.: Second malignancy complicating Hodgkin's disease. *Lancet, 1:*947-949, 1975.
219. Castro, G. A. M., Church, A., Pechet, L., and Snyder, L. M.: Leukemia after chemotherapy of Hodgkin's disease. *N Engl J Med, 289:*103-104, 1973.
220. Come, S. E., Jeffe, E. S., Anderson, J. C., Mann, R. B., Johnson, B. L., Devita, V. T., and Young, R. C.: Leukemic progression in non-Hodgkin's lymphoma: Clinicopathologic features and therapeutic implications. *Blood, 52:*273, 1979.
221. DeVita, V. T., Jr.: The consequences of chemotherapy of Hodgkin's disease: The 10th David A. Karnofsky memorial lecture. *Cancer, 47:*1-13, 1981.
222. Gendelman, S., Rizzo, F., and Mones, R. J.: Central nervous system complications of leukemic conversion of the lymphomas. *Cancer, 24:*676, 1969.
223. Gulati, S. C., Mertelsmann, R., Gee, T., Good, R. A., Clarkson, B., Moore, M. A. S., and Koziner, B.:Analysis of multiple cell markers in acute leukemia complicating Hodgkin's disease. *Cancer, 46:*725-729, 1980.
224. Hall, T. C.: Leukemia in patients treated for Hodgkin's disease. *N Engl J Med, 298:*853-854, 1978.
225. Ibbot, J. W., and Whitelaw, D. M.: The relation between lymphosarcoma and leukemia. *Canadian Med Assoc J, 94:*517, 1966.
226. Jacquillat, C., Auclerc, G., Weil, M., Boiron, M., and Bernard, J.: Acute leukemia, Kaposi sarcoma, epitheliomas complicating 30 observations of Hodgkin's disease. *Cancer Res, 46:*247, 1976.
227. Janet, J. D., Golomb, H. M., Vardiman, J.: Nonrandom chromosomal abnormality in acute nonlymphocytic leukemia in patients treated for Hodgkin's disease and non-Hodgkin's lymphoma. *Blood, 50:*759-769, 1977.
228. Krikorian, J. G., Burke, J. S., Rosenberg, S. A., and Kaplan, H. S.: Occurrence of non-Hodgkin's lymphoma after therapy for Hodgkin's disease. *N Engl J Med, 300:*452-458, 1979.

229. Larsen, J., and Brinker, H.: The incidence and characteristics of acute hyeloid leukemia arising in Hodgkin's disease. *Scand J Haematol, 18:*197-206, 1977.
230. Li, F. P., Corkery, J., Canellos, G., and Neitlich, H. W.: Breast cancer after Hodgkin's disease in two sisters. *Cancer, 47:*201-202, 1981.
231. Lowenbraun, S., Sutherland, J. C., Feldman, M. J., and Serpick, A. A.: Transformation of reticulum cell sarcoma to acute leukemia. *Cancer, 27:*579-585, 1971.
232. Newman, D. R., Maldonado, J. E., Harrison, E. G., Jr., Kiely, J. M., and Linman, J. W.: Myelomonocytic leukemia in Hodgkin's disease. *Cancer, 25:*128-134, 1970.
233. Rosner, F., and Grunwald, H.: Hodgkin's disease and acute leukemia. Report of eight cases and review of the literature. *Am J Med, 58:*339-353, 1975.
234. Rowley, J. D., Golomb, H. M. and Vardiman, J.: Non-random chromosomal abnormalities in acute non-lymphocytic leukemia in patients treated for Hodgkin's disease and non-Hodgkin's lymphoma. *Blood, 50:*759-769, 1977.
235. Scheerer, P. P., Pierce, R. V., Schwartz, D. L., and Linman, J. W.: Reed-Sternberg cell leukemia and lactic acidosis: Unusual manifestations of Hodgkin's disease. *N Engl J Med, 270:*274-278, 1964.
236. Smith, J., O'Connell, R. S., Huuos, A. G., and Woodard, H. Q.: Hodgkin's disease complicated by radiation sarcoma in bone. *Br J Radiol, 53:*314-321, 1980.
237. Toland, D. M., and Coltman, C. A., Jr.: Second malignancies complicating Hodgkin's disease. *Blood, 46:*1013, 1975.
238. Zeffren, J. L., and Ultmann, J. E.: Reticulum cell sarcoma terminating in acute leukemia. *Blood, 15:*277-284, 1960.

Chapter 4

Leukemia

CLASSIFICATION

LEUKEMIA IS A SYSTEMIC neoplastic disease characterized by abnormal proliferation of hematopoietic cells in the bone marrow and other organs. The hematopoietic cells can be expected to appear in the peripheral blood during the course of the disease. On a functional, morphologic, and pathophysiologic basis, leukemias and related diseases can be grouped into two main divisions: the lymphoproliferative (lymphoid tissue) and myeloproliferative (bone marrow tissue) diseases. Leukemia can also be classified according to the following: the duration of the disease; predominant cell type in blood and bone marrow; and leukocyte count in the peripheral blood. On the basis of duration of the disease, leukemia can be subdivided into acute (life expectancy six months or less), subacute (life expectancy six to twelve months), and chronic (life expectancy twelve months or more) types. Needless to say, with continuous improvement of the treatments of leukemias, the life expectancy of leukemic patients is ever increasing. Consequently, the time-based classification of leukemias is becoming obsolete.

Classification of leukemias can be based on leukocyte count in the peripheral blood: *leukemic leukemia* — the leukocyte count is greater than 15,000 per MM^3; *subleukemic leukemia* — the leukocyte count is less than normal, but there are enough abnormal cells to suggest the presence of leukemia; and *aleukemic leukemia* — the leukocyte count is less than normal and the blood contains very few or no abnormal cells, unless the smears of the buffy coats are diligently scrutinized. On the other hand, when the cell type found on blood and bone marrow examination and the course of the disease are considered together, a comprehensive and generally accepted classification of leukemias results and is presented in Table 4-I.

TABLE 4-I
CLASSIFICATION OF LEUKEMIA

	Type of Leukemia	Predominant Cell
Acute leukemia	Lymphoblastic (lymphocytic) 1-21	Lymphoblasts
	Myeloblastic (granulocytic, myelocytic) 22-38	Myeloblasts
	Promyelocytic 39-51	Promyelocytes
	Myelomonocytic 52-63	Myeloblasts and monoblasts
	Monocytic 64-81	Monoblasts
Chronic leukemia	Lymphocytic (lymphatic) 82-109	Lymphocytes
	Myelocytic (granulocytic) 110-138	Myelocytes (granulocytes)
Rare types of leukemia in either acute or chronic form	Erythroleukemia (Di Guglielmo's syndrome) 139-157	Myeloblasts and abnormal erythroblasts
	Eosinophilic 158-170	Eosinophils and precursors
	Basophilic 171-176	Basophils and precursors
	Neutrophilic 177-179	Neutrophils and precursors
	Hairy cell (leukemic reticuloendotheliosis) 180-185	Hairy cells (lymphocytes or histiocytes)
	Plasma cell 186-192	Plasma cells
	Mast cell 193-198	Mast cells
	Megakaryocytic 199-205	Megakaryocytes
	Reed-Sternberg cell 206	Reed-Sternberg cells

ETIOLOGY

There are many direct and indirect causes of leukemias:

- *Ionizing radiation* — Radiation from atomic bombs,[207-213] occupational exposure,[214-218] radiotherapy for ankylosing spondylitis,[219-222] irradiation for hyperthyroidism,[223-224] x-ray treatment for thymic enlargement,[225-226] excessive diagnostic x-ray exposure,[227-230] radioisotopes,[142, 231] etc., are the examples.
- *Chronic exposure to leukemogenic chemicals* — They include Benzene,[232-237] ethylene oxide,[238] petroleum products,[239] and chlordane and heptachlor.[240]
- Cytotoxic drugs[241-255]
- Chromosomal abnormalities[256-276]
- Viruses[277-288]
- Leukemic transformation of transplanted human bone marrow cells[289-290]
- Hereditary or familial factors[291-301]

INCIDENCE

Although various forms of leukemias occur throughout life, they do show a definite pattern of predilection. For examples, leukemias affect twice as many male patients as female patients. Acute lymphocytic leukemia is the most common form of leukemia in children and is also the most common malignant disease of children and the leading medical cause of death in young children. In contrast, acute myelocytic leukemia shows strong predilection for adults and chronic lymphocytic leukemia tends to affect the oldest patients. Gunz and Baikie (1974)[302] reported the incidence of various forms of leukemias in the United States in the following proportion: chronic leukemia 50 percent (approximately, lymphocytic 25%, granulocytic 22%, and myelomonocytic 3%) and acute leukemia 50 percent (approximately, lymphoblastic 20%, myeloblastic 20% and myelomonoblastic 10%). In 1960, the overall yearly death rate from leukemia in twenty-five countries with roughly 20% of the world's population was estimated as 5.8 per 100,000 population, and leukemias and malignant lymphomas accounted for about 10 percent of all cancer deaths and approximately 1.5 percent of deaths from all causes.[302-303]

It should be emphasized that the different forms of myeloproliferative and lymphoproliferative diseases are dynamic and related pathologic processes in which one entity can be transformed into one or more other forms under suitable and favorable circumstances. For examples, multiple myeloma can develop into plasma cell leukemia[186-192] and various types of leukemias also originate in malignant lymphomas,[304-316] Waldenstron's macroglobulinemia,[317-318] and polycythemia vera.[319-326] On the other hand, leukemia can terminate in malignant histiocytosis,[327-328] and chronic leukemia can be transformed into acute leukemia in its terminal stage.[329-335]

CLINICAL SYMPTOMS AND SIGNS

The wide spectrum of symptoms and signs of leukemia is caused by infiltration of various organs by the leukemic process which interferes with the normal functions of these involved organs. The following is a list of affected organs and their associated symptoms and signs.

- *Constitutional symptoms and signs* — pallor, lethargy, weakness, anorexia, weight loss, night sweats, low-grade fever, ease of fatigue, malaise, etc.
- *Lymphnodes* — lymphadenopathy
- *Visceral organs* — splenomegaly, hepatomegaly, and renomegaly associated with abdominal and flank discomforts, obstipation, melena, hematuria, and oliguria
- *Bones and joints* — bone pain, especially in the metaphyseal regions of long tubular bones, joint effusion and tenderness, mimicking pyarthrosis, osteomyelitis, rheumatic fever, and scurvy. Spinal pain caused by destruction and compression fracture of the vertebrae or

by leukemic infiltration of the spinal cord or nerves resulting in dysesthesia, paresis, paralysis, bladder and bowel disturbances, etc. Neurological symptoms can also be caused by direct extension of the greatly enlarged leukemic paraspinal lymph nodes into spinal canal through the intervertebral foramina.

- *Central nervous system* — headache, nausea, vomiting, blurred vision, and cranial nerve palsies
- *Cutaneous tissue* — ecchymoses, pyoderm, and masses in subcutaneous tissue
- *Gum* – hemorrhage and hypertrophy

Generally speaking, the acute leukemias and chronic leukemias in blastic crises tend to have much more acute onset and severity of symptoms than the chronic leukemias, which can be very insidious and even asymptomatic.

LABORATORY STUDIES

The abnormal laboratory findings are the manifestations of dysfunctions of various organs affected by leukemia.

- Leukemic cells in different stages of maturation and differentiation in the peripheral blood, bone marrow, and lymphoid organs.
- Thrombocytopenia, anemia, leukopenia, and loss of bone marrow fat caused by replacement of the normal bone marrow elements by the proliferating leukemic cells.
- Elevated SGOT, SGPT, alkaline phosphatase, etc., due to liver damage by leukemia.
- Hyperuricemia and hyperuricosuria brought about by increased nucleic acid catabolism.[336-340]
- Elevated BUN and creatinine, hematuria, and concentrated urine from renal damage by leukemia and uric acid nephropathy secondary to leukemia.
- Hypercalcemia caused by bone destruction by the leukemic process.[341-343]
- Hypocalcemia, hypomagnesemia, and hyperphosphatemia produced by release of phosphates, sulfate, and other organic anions from leukemic cells that bind these two cations[344-346] or induced by systemic glucocorticoid administration.
- Reduction of serum fibrinogen, plasminogen, and coagulation factors V, VIII, X, and XIII, further encouraging hemorrhagic diathesis.[41, 49-50, 347-351]
- Release of procoagulants from leukemic blast cells initiating intravascular coagulation and producing hemorrhage.[43-45, 47, 352]

- High serum Vitamin B12[353-356] muramidase (lysozyme)[357-362] from degradation of leukemic granulocytes.
- Reduced CSF sugar, increased CSF protein and spinal fluid pleocytosis in the presence of central nervous system leukemia.

ROENTGENOGRAPHIC MANIFESTATIONS

Many articles have been written on the wide spectrum of the roentgenographic manifestations of leukemia.[363-384] The most consistent radiological finding in acute leukemia in children is a transverse zone of increased radiolucency through the metaphyseal region of the most rapidly growing bones. It is in this region that the presence of leukemic cells depresses endochondral ossification and can eventually produce roundish radiolucencies and even pathologic fracture. Periosteal new bone formation can also occur in the involved regions. In contrast, roentgenographically detectable bone changes are less common in chronic leukemia, which may show generalized osteoporosis, foci of rarefaction or radiopacity, and periosteal new bone formation.

Spinal manifestations of leukemia resemble those of long tubular bones. They include radiolucent zones at the superior and inferior margins of the vertebrae or severe osteoporosis (Figure 4-1) in acute leukemia of childhood. In addition, osteolytic vertebral lesions, generalized osteoporosis, compression fractures of vertebral bodies, expanding intervertebral disks, and varying degrees of vertebral radiopacity are the other roentgenographic features produced by various types of leukemias in the spine (Figures 4-2 through 4-4). In addition, leukemia-infiltrated paraspinal lymph nodes can cause erosion of the adjacent vertebral bodies and can even extend into the spinal canal through the intervertebral formina to cause different kinds of vertebral destruction.

PATHOLOGIC FEATURES

Gross Pathology. The leukemic, osteoporotic spine shows thinning and reduction of trabeculae and erosion of the vertebral cortex from the medullary cavity. Bone marrow with leukemic infiltration has a grayish-red color and large osteolytic lesions frequently contain foci of hemorrhage and necrosis (Figures 4-5 through 4-7). Osteosclerotic lesions are usually hard and yellowish-white in color due to calcification and ossification. Collapsed vertebral bodies, expanded intervertebral disks and extravertebral extension of leukemic tissue, when present, are readily visible (Figure 4-8).

Microscopic Pathology. The predominant cell types present in the bone marrow and blood smears enable the pathologists and hematologist to differentiate one type of leukemia from the rest. A representativ

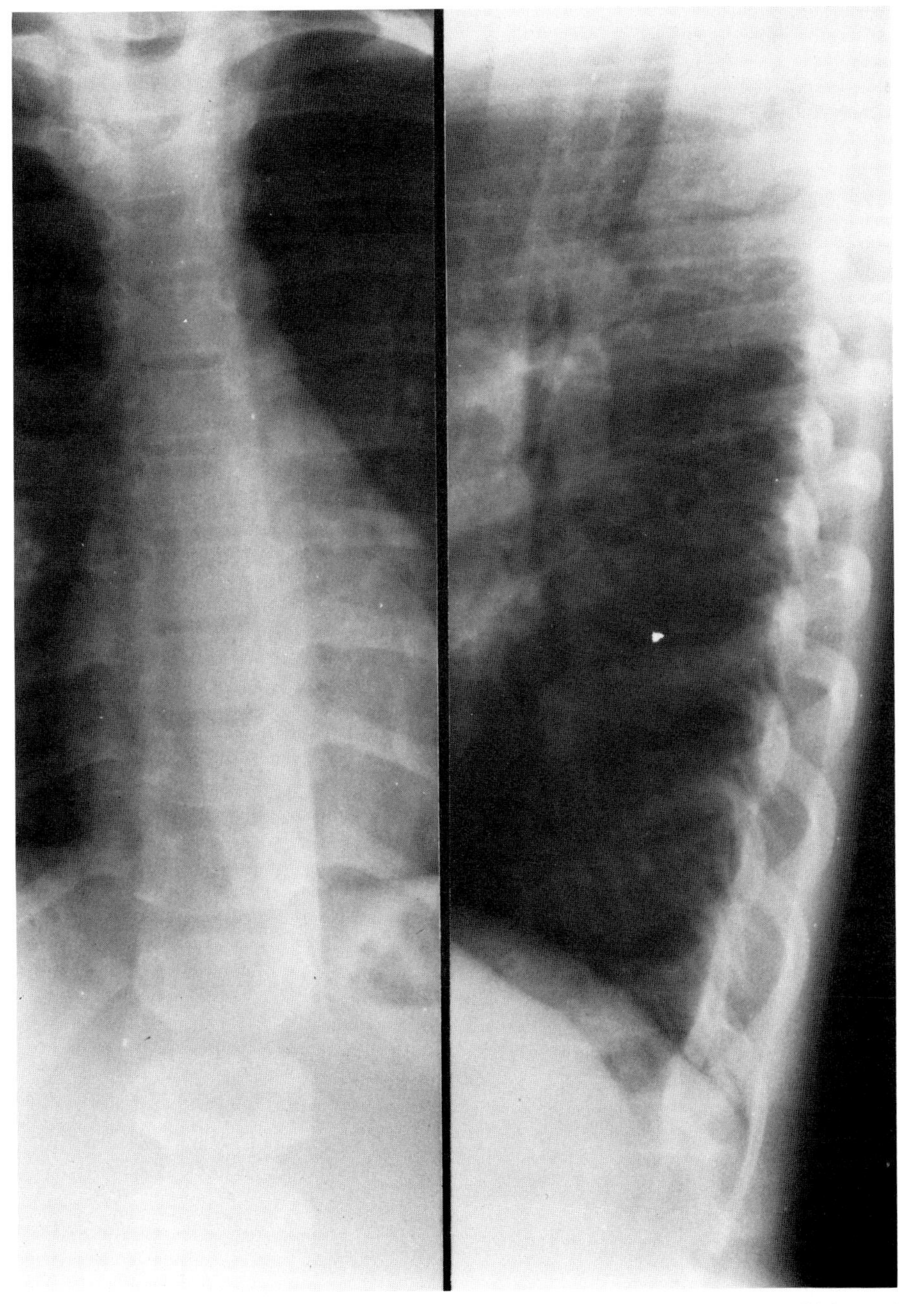

Figure 4-1. Roentgenographs of the thoracolumbar spine of an eight-year-old boy with acute lymphocytic leukemia show an extreme degree of osteoporosis of the thoracolumbar spine caused by thorough infiltration and trabecular destruction by the leukemic cells.

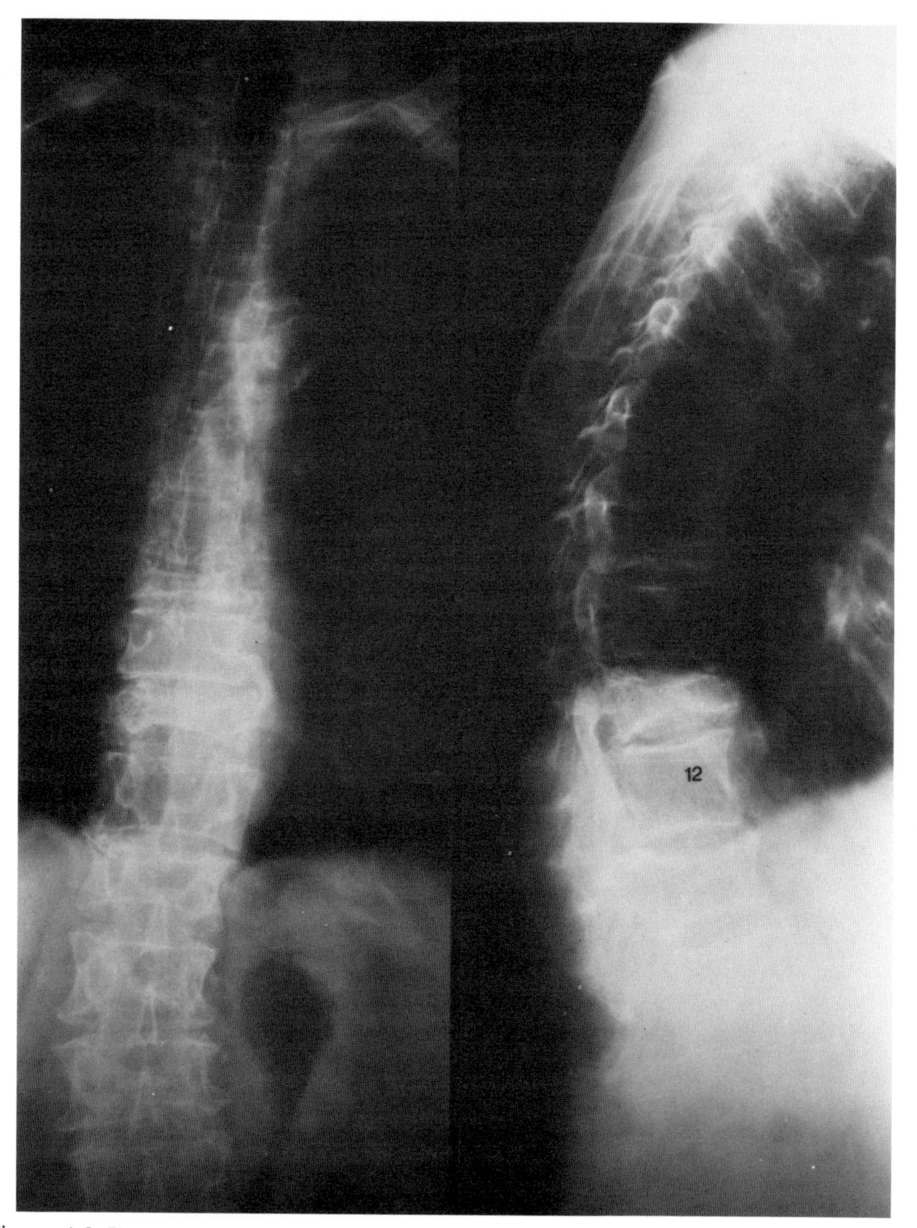

Figure 4-2. X-rays of the thoracolumbar spine belonging to a sixty-nine-year-old female patient with chronic lymphocytic leukemia show generalized osteoporosis and several compression fractures caused by leukemic involvement of the spine and the osteoporotic effect of prolonged systemic corticosteroid administration.

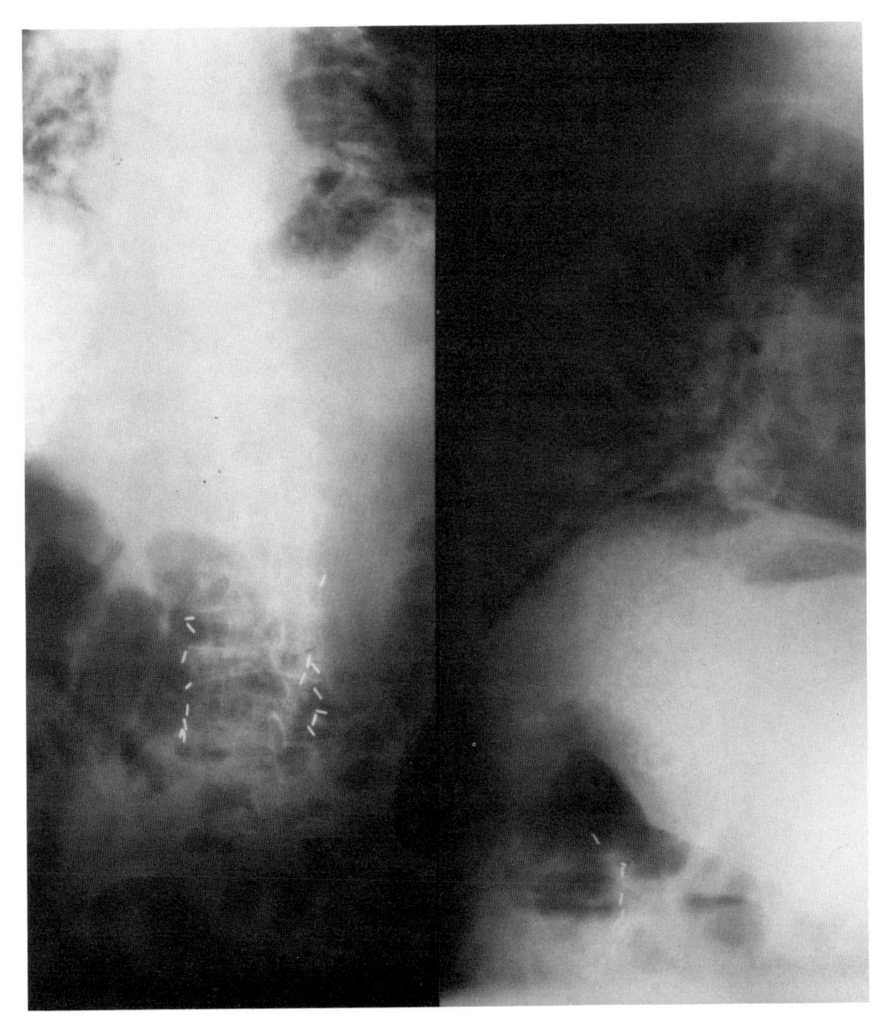

Figure 4-3. Thoracolumbar spine x-rays of a fifty-five-year-old man with mast cell leukemia show extreme osteoporosis, compression fracture of every vertebral body, and expansion of intervertebral disks into the collapsed vertebral bodies.

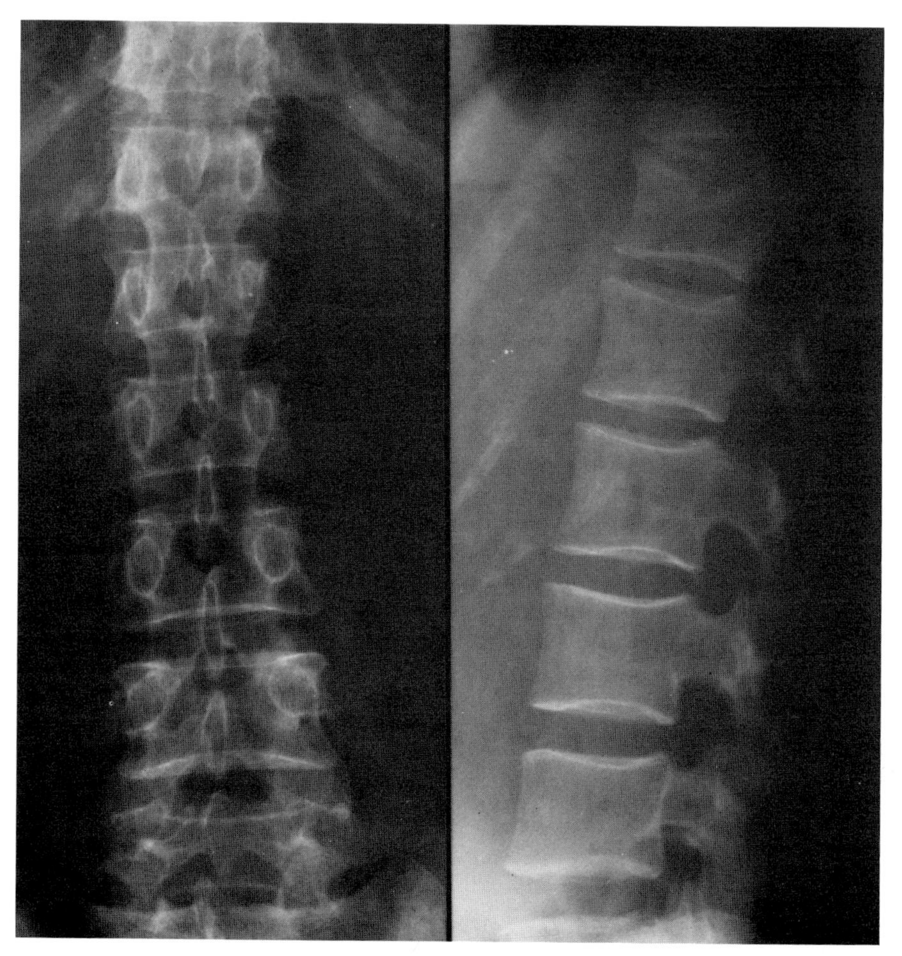

Figure 4-4. Lumbar spine x-rays of a fifty-seven-year-old man with chronic myelocytic (granulocytic) leukemia show moderate degree of osteoporosis plus a compression fracture of the first lumbar vertebral body. Note the faint horizontal osteosclerotic lines through the midportion of the vertebral bodies.

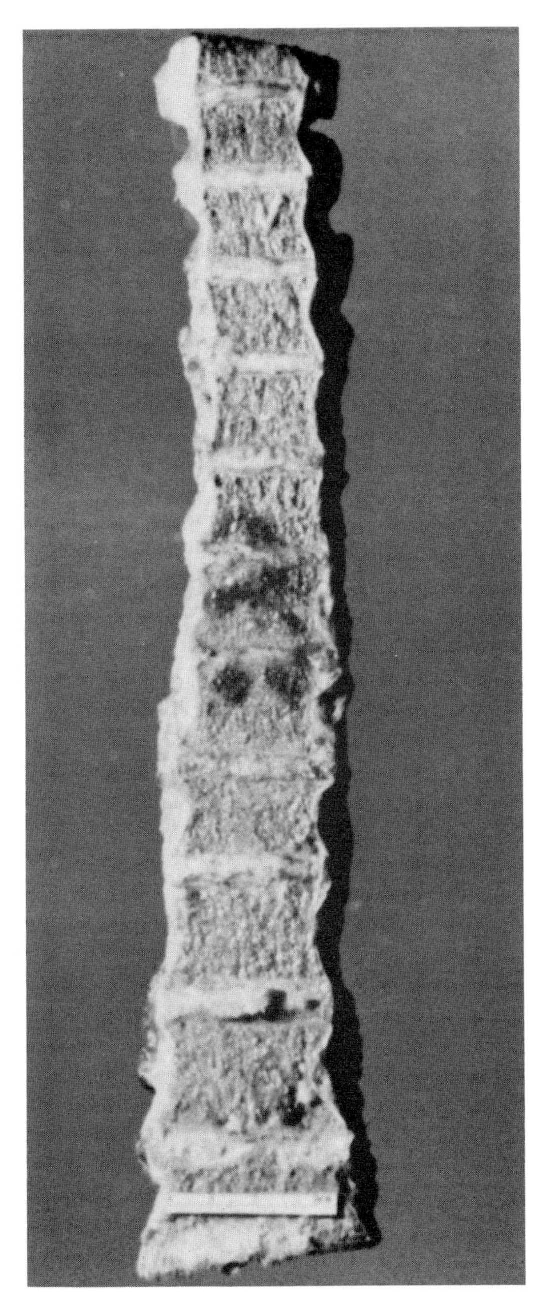

Figure 4-5. Longitudinal section of the thoracolumbar spine belonging to a victim of acute granulocytic leukemia shows foci of hemorrhage in the eleventh, twelfth thoracic, and first lumbar vertebral bodies.

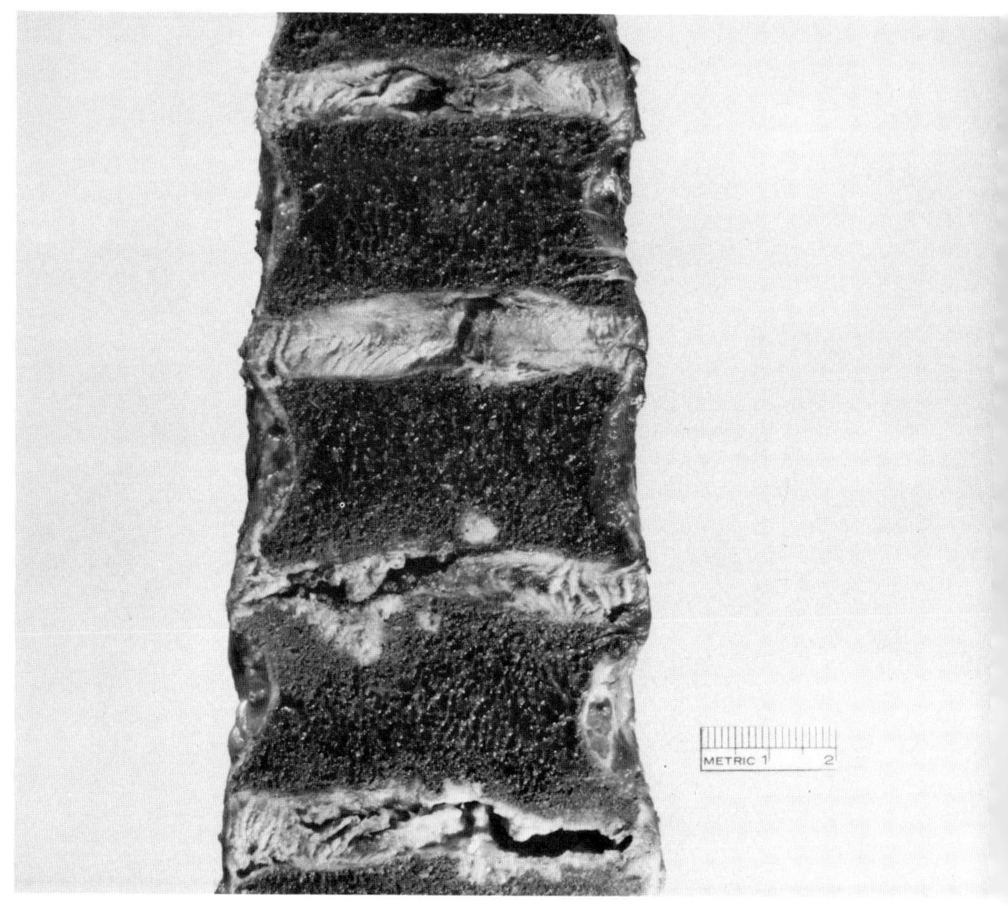

Figure 4-6. Longitudinal section of the lower thoracic spine from a patient who died of acute erythroleukemia shows some trabecular destruction plus a small focus of necrosis in the middle vertebral body.

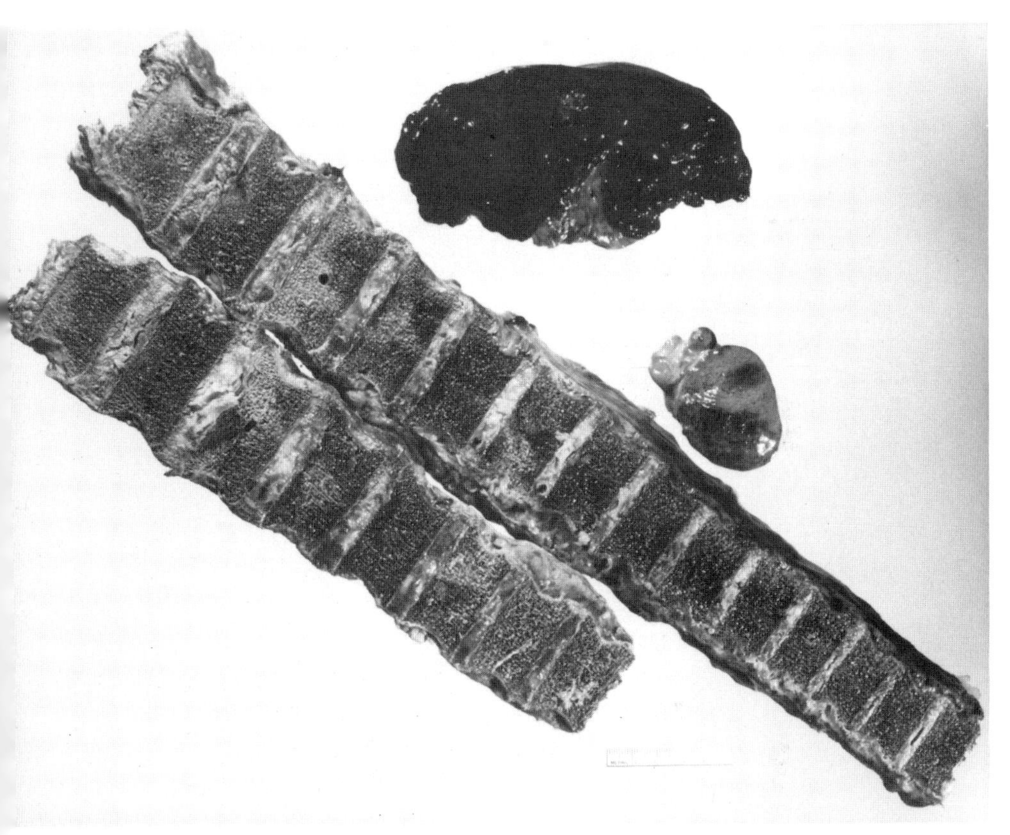

Figure 4-7. Longitudinal section of the entire thoracolumbar spine from a victim of acute monocytic leukemia shows the grossly intact vertebral bodies and intervertebral disks in spite of the fact that microscopic examination revealed diffuse vertebral infiltration by the leukemic process. Note the greatly enlarged lymph node and a portion of the patient's spleen with several light foci visible to the naked eyes.

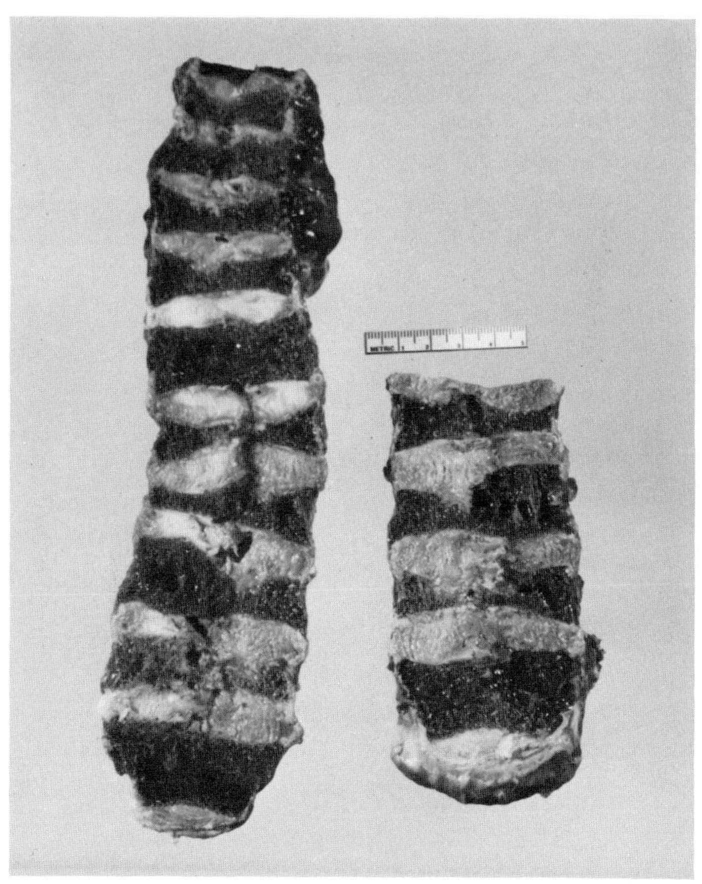

Figure 4-8. Longitudinal section through the thoracolumbar spine of the same patient with mast cell leukemia, whose x-rays were shown in Figure 4-3, shows compression fracture of every vertebral body and expansion of intervertebral disks into the deformed vertebral bodies. The mast cell leukemia process had thoroughly infiltrated the entire thoracolumbar spine.

photomicrograph of each type of leukemia is presented in Figures 4-9 to 4-21.

Acute lymphoblastic leukemia (Figure 4-9)
Acute myeloblastic leukemia (Figure 4-10)
Acute promyelocytic leukemia (Figure 4-11)
Acute myelomonocytic leukemia (Figure 4-12)
Acute monocytic leukemia (Figure 4-13)
Chronic lymphocytic leukemia (Figure 4-14)
Chronic myelocytic leukemia (Figure 4-15)
Erythroleukemia (Figure 4-16)
Basophilic leukemia (Figure 4-17)
Hairy cell leukemia (Figure 4-18)
Plasma cell leukemia (Figure 4-19)
Mast cell leukemia (Figure 4-20)
Megakaryocytic leukemia (Figure 4-21)

Needless to say, bone marrow aspiration frequently yields more reliable and diagnostic leukemic features than simple peripheral blood smears,

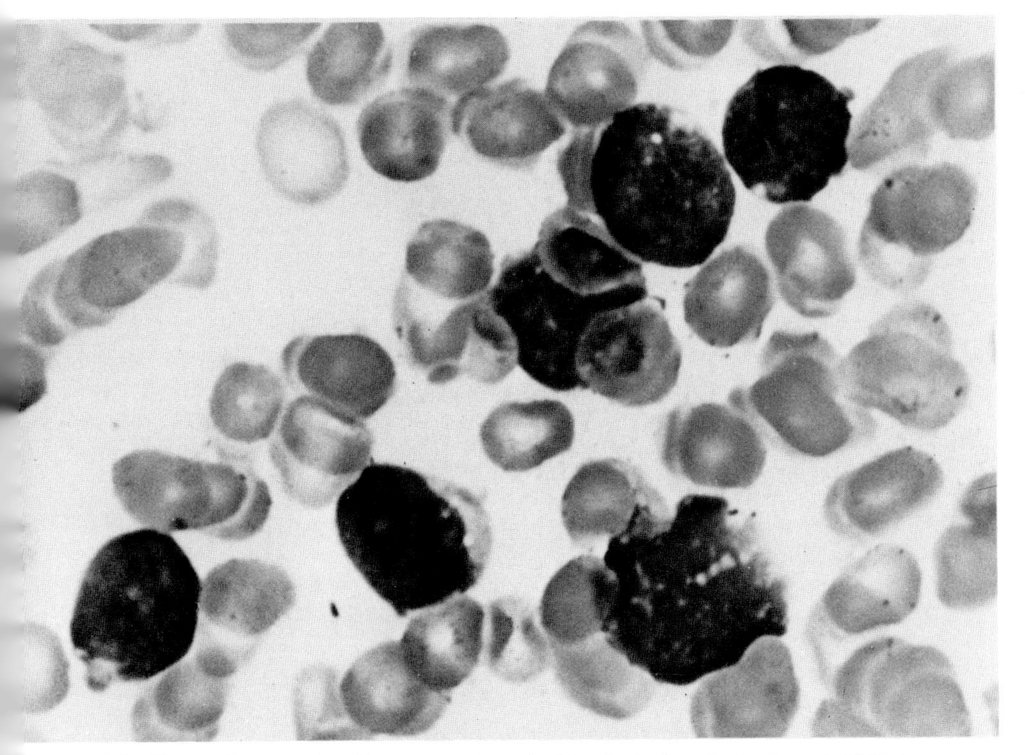

igure 4-9. Photomicrograph of an acute lymphoblastic leukemia (reduced 18% from 100 ×, Leishman Stain) shows several lymphoblasts whose nuclei nearly occupy the entire ell, leaving very little room for the basophilic cytoplasm.

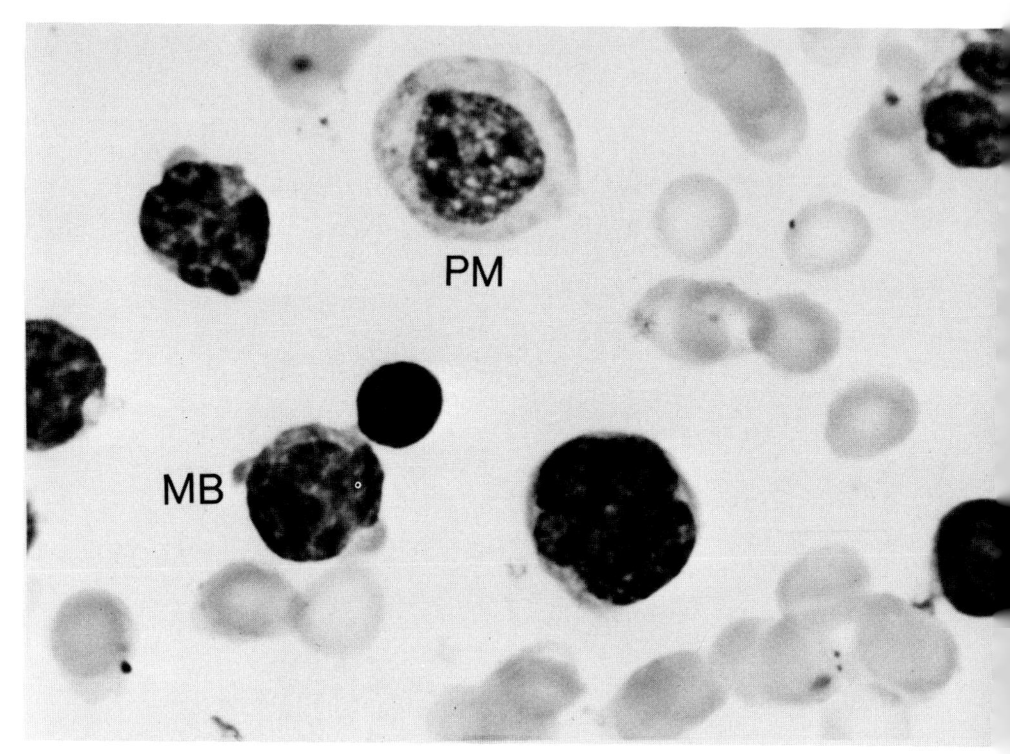

Figure 4-10. Photomicrograph of an acute myeloblastic leukemia (reduced 18% from 1100×, Leishman Stain) showing several myeloblasts (MB) and a promyelocyte (PM).

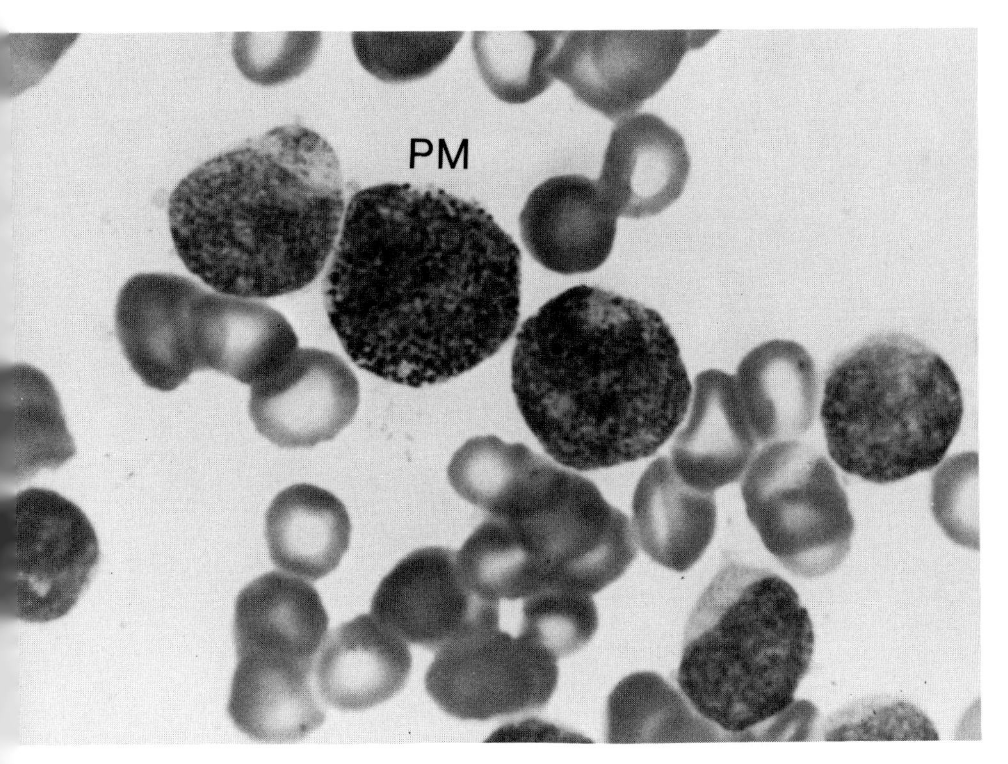

'igure 4-11. Photomicrograph of an acute promyelocytic leukemia (reduced 18% from 100×, Leishman Stain) showing three promyelocytes (PM) in the center of the picture.

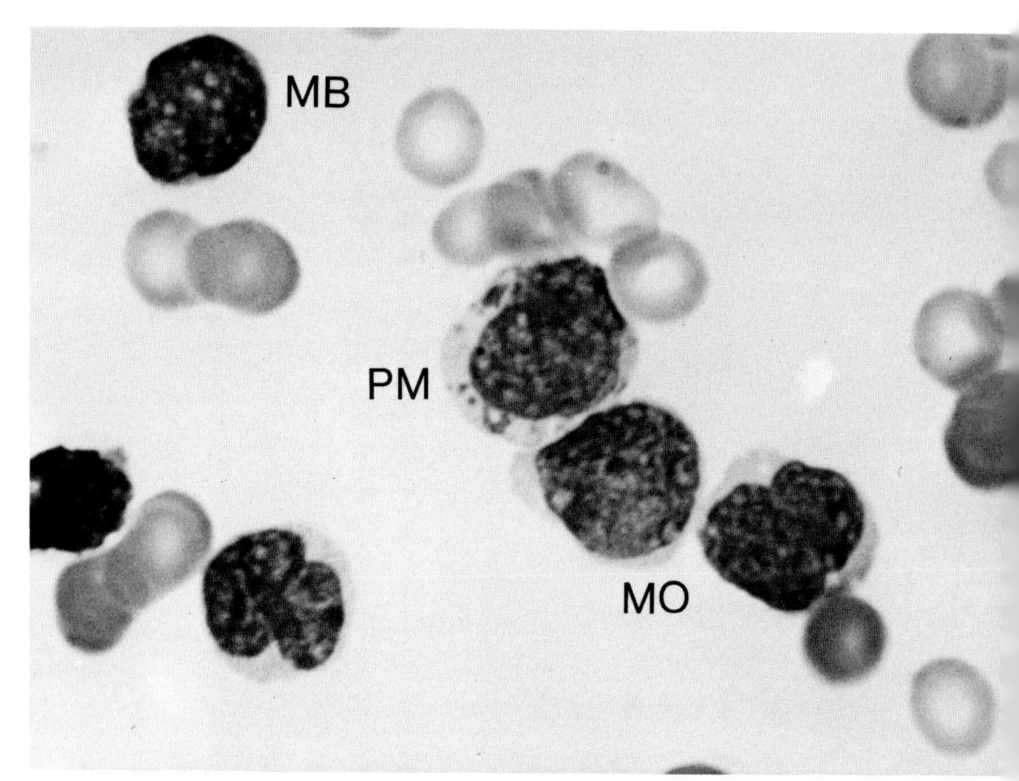

Figure 4-12. Photomicrograph of an acute myelomonocytic leukemia (reduced 15% from 1100 ×, Leishman Stain) showing a mixture of myeloblastic, promyelocytic, and monoblastic cells — myeloblast (MB), promyelocyte (PM), monoblast (MO).

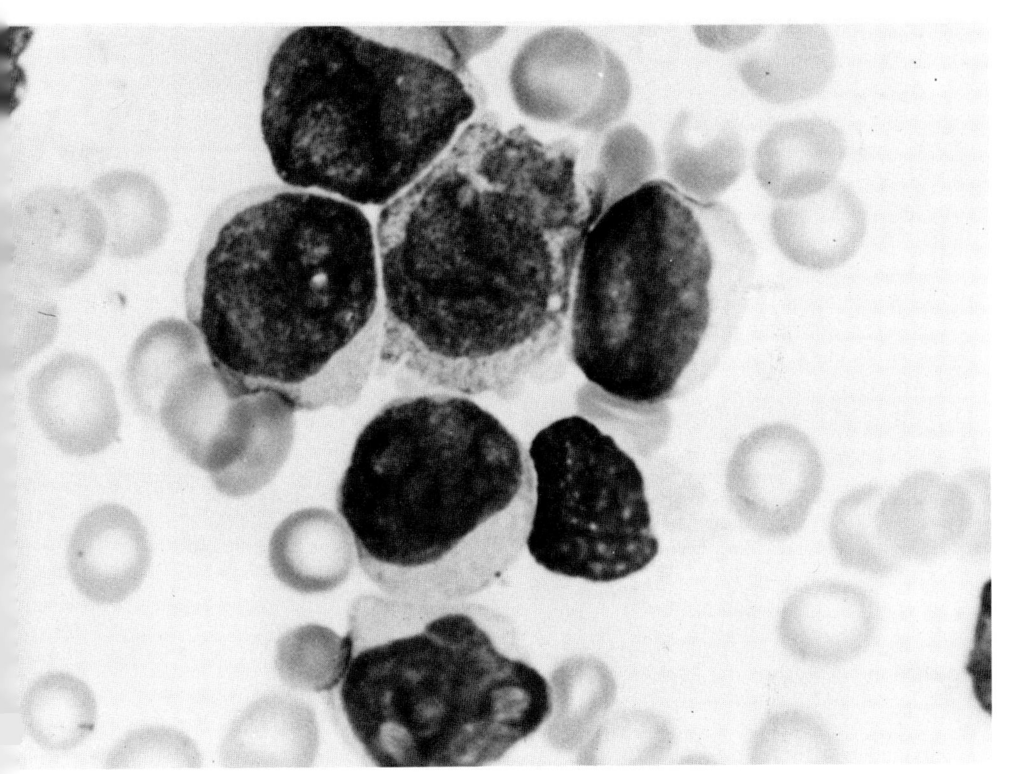

Figure 4-13. Photomicrograph of an acute monocytic leukemia (reduced 15% from 1100×, Leishman Stain) shows a cluster of monoblasts with a nodular nucleus and pale blue cytoplasm.

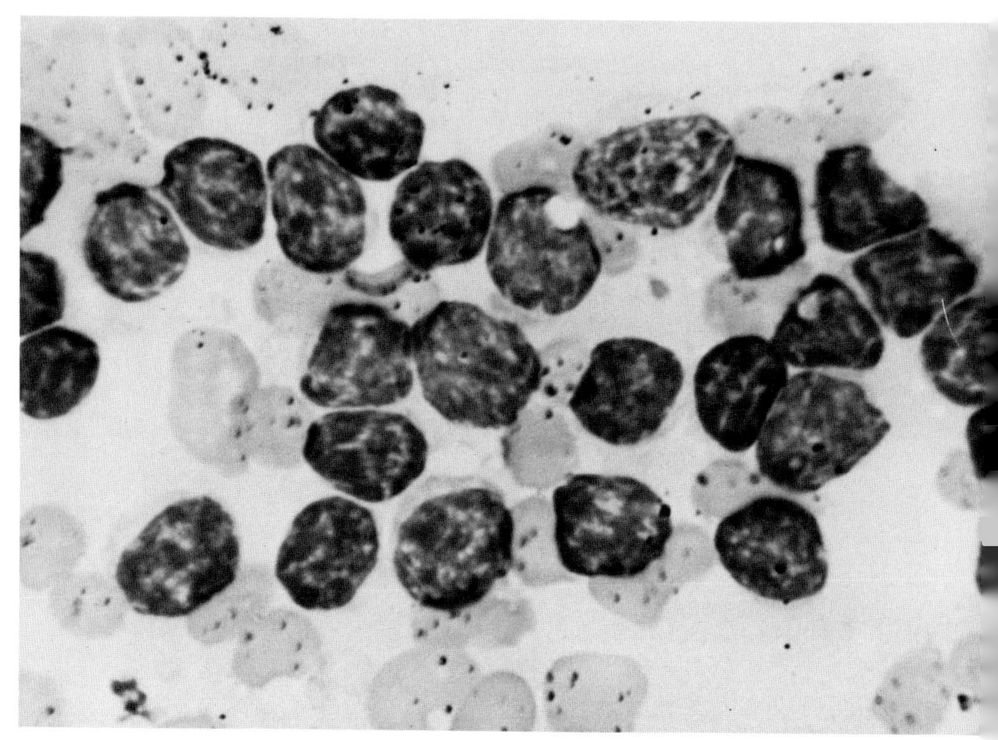

Figure 4-14. Photomicrograph of a chronic lymphocytic leukemia (reduced 18% from 1100×, Leishman Stain) shows many somewhat atypical lymphocytes with some variation in nuclear size and shape.

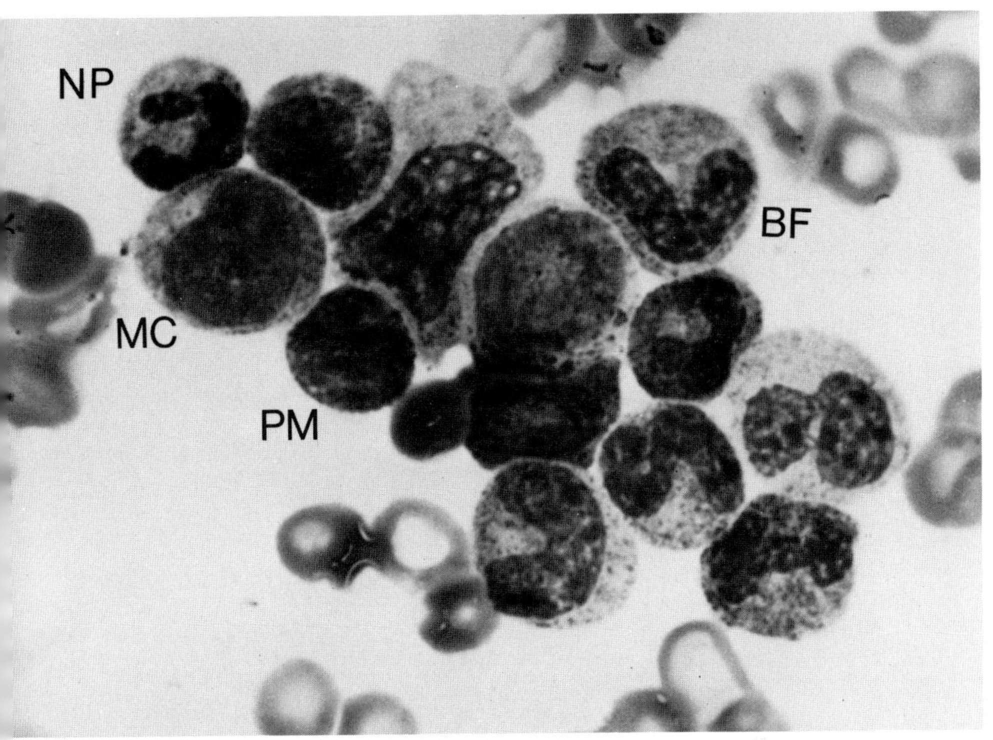

Figure 4-15. Photomicrograph of a chronic myelocytic leukemia (reduced 17% from 1100×, Leishman Stain) shows myelocytic cells in different stages of maturity — PM (promyelocyte), MC (myelocyte), BF (band form), NP (neutrophil).

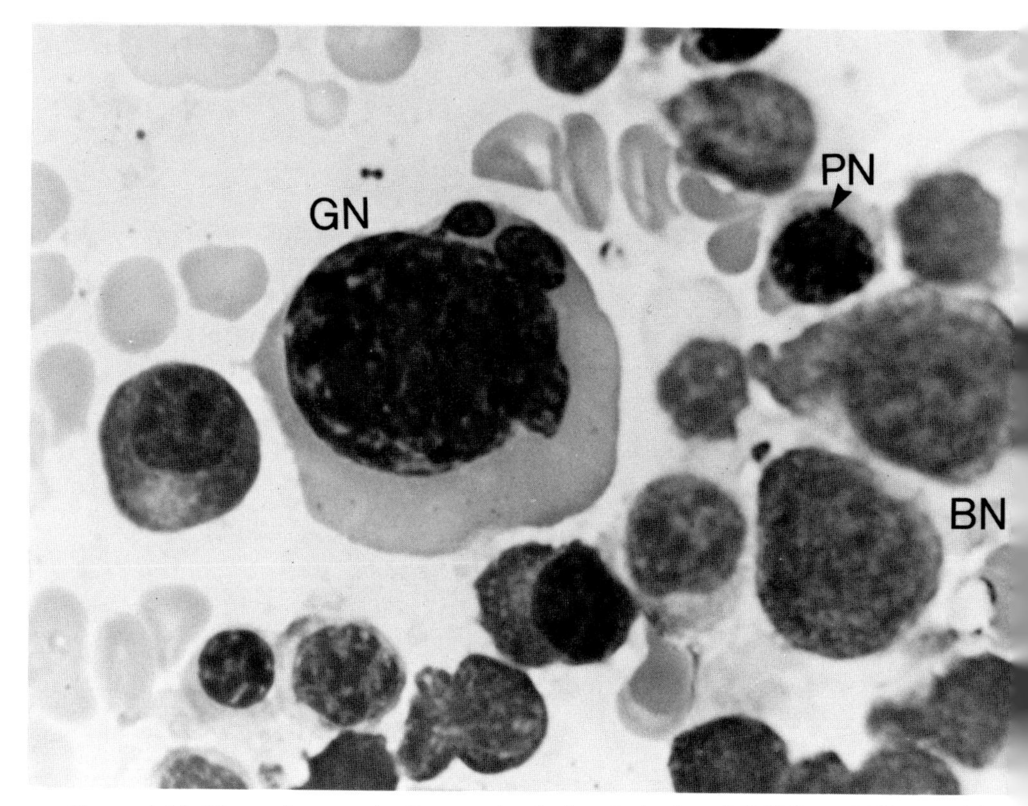

Figure 4-16. Photomicrograph of an erythroleukemia (reduced 15% from 1100×, Leishman Stain) shows erythrocytic cells in different stages of maturation. GN (giant normoblast), BN (basophilic normoblast), PN (polychromic normoblast). Courtesy of Dr. John W. Rebuck, Department of Hematology, Henry Ford Hospital, Detroit, Michigan.

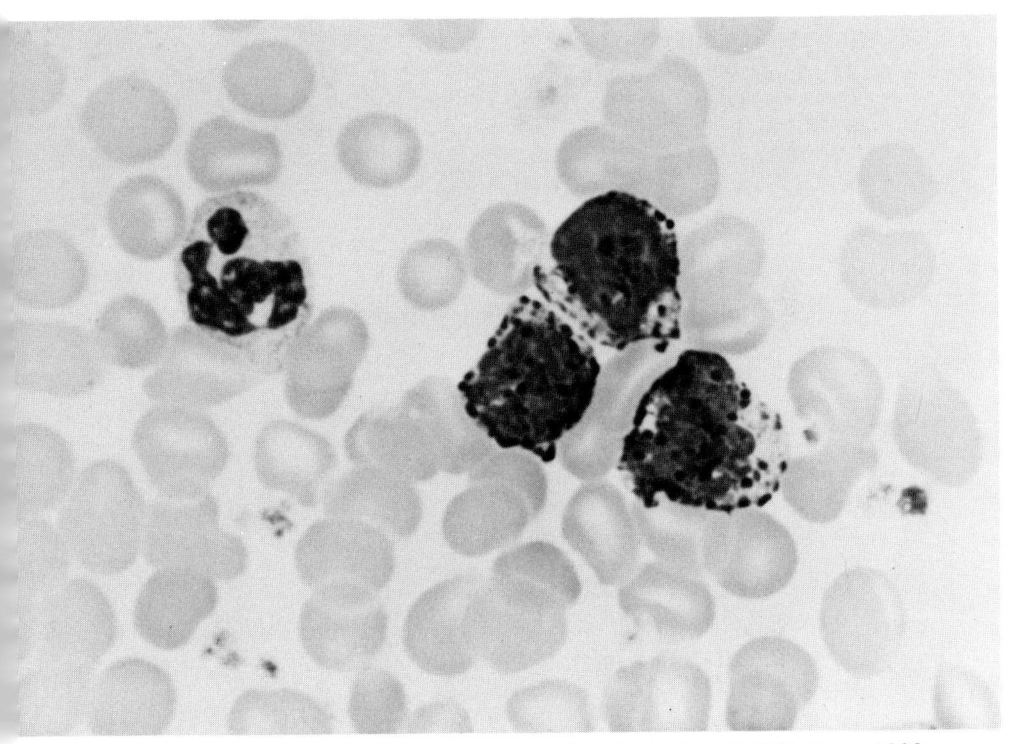

Figure 4-17. Photomicrograph of a basophilic leukemia (reduced 18% from 1000×, Leishman Stain) shows three basophils with their typical round basophilic granules in a pale blue cytoplasm.

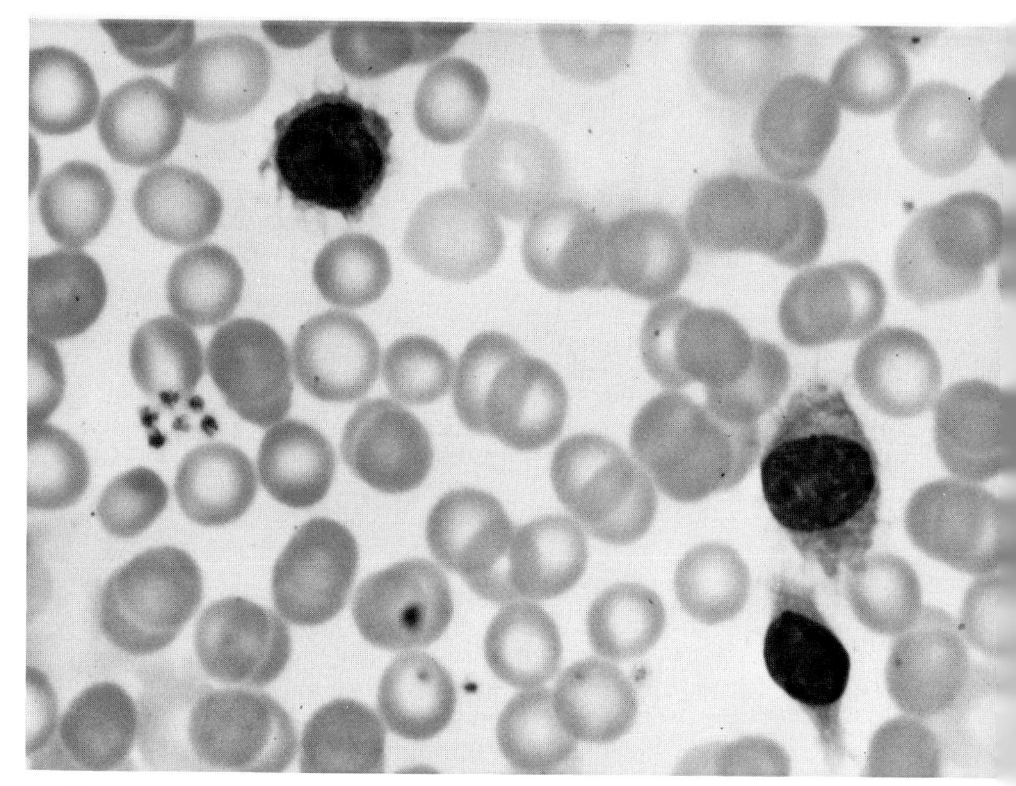

Figure 4-18. Photomicrograph of a hairy cell leukemia (reduced 15% from 1000× Leishman Stain) shows three hairy cells with their typical hairlike cytoplasmic processes.

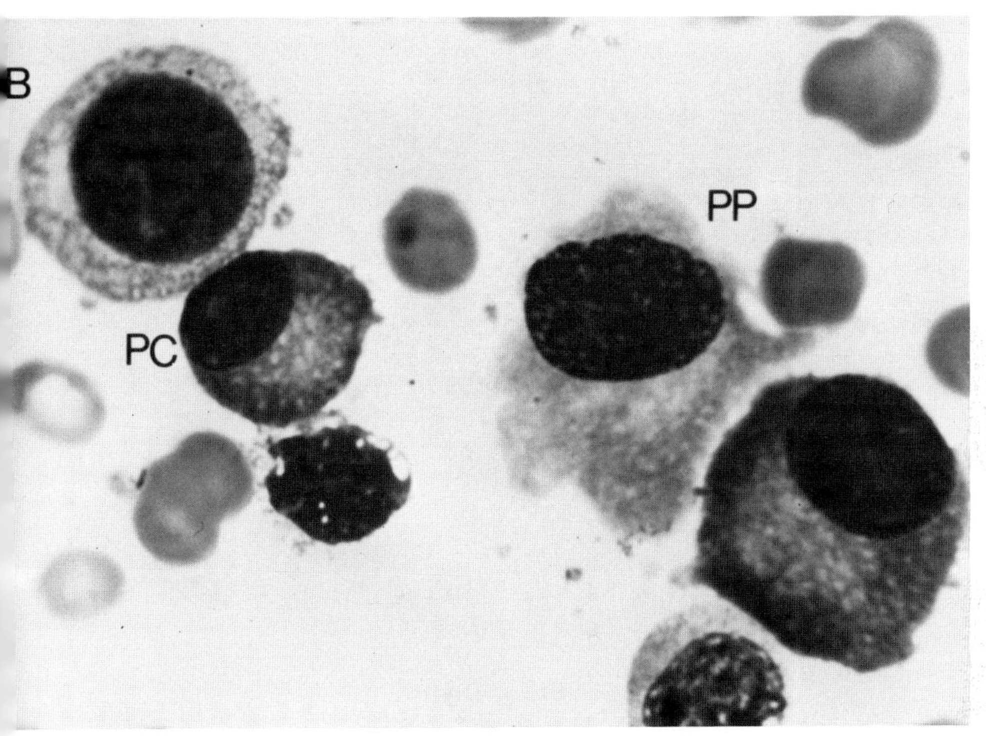

'igure 4-19. Photomicrograph (reduced 17% from 1300×, Leishman Stain) of the ·eripheral blood smear of a case of plasma leukemia showing plasma cells in different tages of differentiation and maturation — PB (plasmoblast), PP (proplasma cell), PC plasma cell).

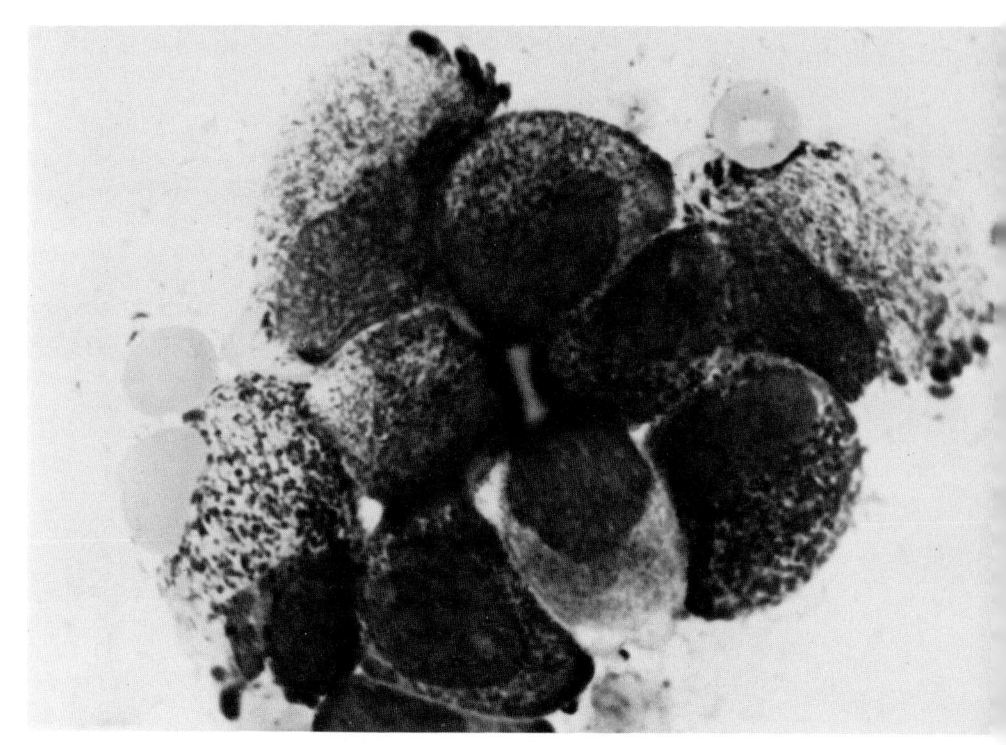

Figure 4-20. Photomicrograph of a mast cell leukemia (reduced 18% from 1300×, Leishman Stain) shows a cluster of mast cells with deeply eosinophilic cytoplasmic granules.

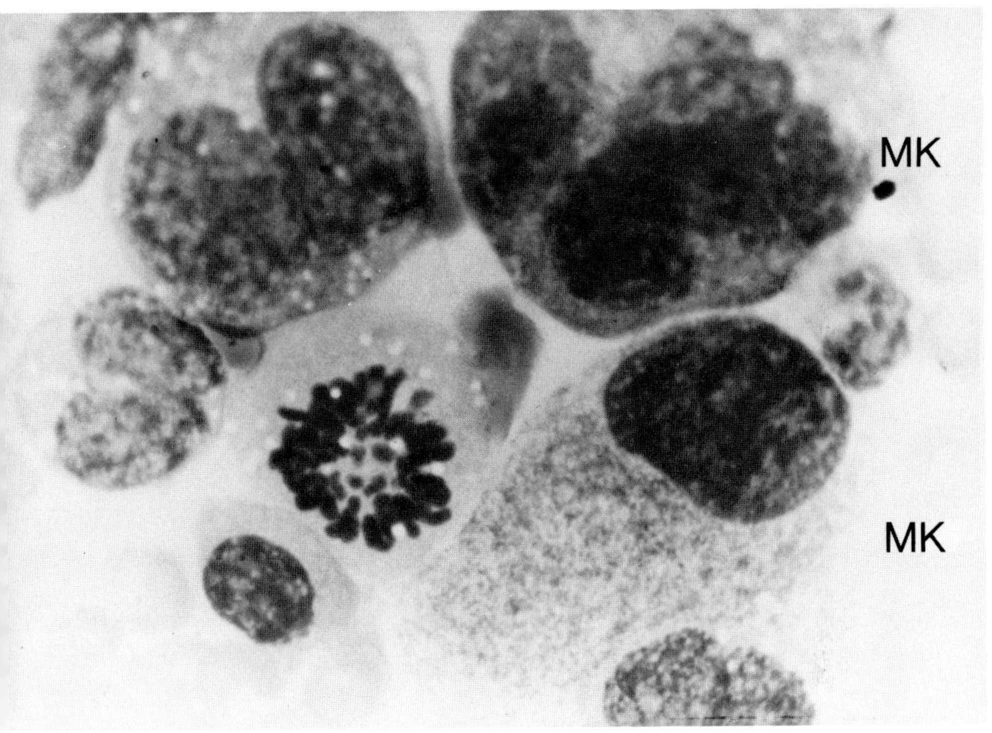

Figure 4-21. Photomicrograph of a megakaryocytic leukemia (reduced 18% from 1000×, Leishman Stain) shows the presence of two large megakaryocytes (MK) next to a cell in mitosis. Courtesy of Dr. John W. Rebuck, Department of Hematology, Henry Ford Hospital, Detroit, Michigan.

especially in aleukemic leukemia and rare and atypical forms of leukemia. In addition, demonstration of leukemic cells in spinal fluid obtained by spinal puncture strongly suggests the presence of leukemic involvement of the central nervous system.

In spite of the fact that most forms of leukemia can be identified on the basis of their distinctive cellular morphology, poorly differentiated and very immature types of acute leukemia and blastic transformation of different myeloproliferative and lymphoproliferative diseases can sometimes present a very difficult diagnostic problem. In addition, leukemoid reaction of severe infections, polycythemia rubra vera, and myelofibrosis with myeloid metaplasia can be mistaken for chronic granulocytic leukemia. Under these circumstances, ultrastructural studies by means of electron microscopy and special cytochemical staining techniques are valuable tools in differentiating one type of leukemia from the others. The following is a list of useful cytochemical stains and a brief description of their practical applications.

- *Leukocyte Peroxidase* — Cells of neutrophilic, eosinophilic, and monocytic origins show positive staining reaction for leukocyte peroxidase. It is also useful in differentiating these cells from cells of lymphoid or erythroid series, which are peroxidase negative.[385-388]
- *Leukocyte Alkaline Phosphatase* — Chronic granulocytic leukemia has a very low level of leukocyte alkaline phosphatase, whereas leukemoid reaction of infections, polycythemia rubra vera, and myelofibrosis with myeloid metaplasia has a high normal or significantly elevated level of the same enzyme.[389-390]
- *Sudan Black B Stain* — Cells of acute granulocytic leukemia are usually sudan black B stain positive whereas cells of acute lymphocytic leukemia are frequently sudan black B stain negative.[391-392]
- *Periodic Acid Schiff (PAS) Stain* — Cells of acute erythroleukemia and acute lymphocytic leukemia contain a significant amount of cytoplasmic glycogen granules that show positive staining reaction to PAS stain. In contrast, cells of acute granulocytic leukemia are usually not stained by PAS stain.[153, 393-398]
- *Leukocyte Acid Phosphatase* — The presence of tartrate-resistant acid phosphatase in reticuloendothelial cells is useful in identifying cells of leukemic reticuloendotheliosis (hairy cell leukemia).[185, 399-402]
- *Leukocyte Esterases* — When a-naphthyl acetate or a-naphthyl butyrate is used as substrate, cytochemical staining for leukocyte esterases is strongly positive in monocytes and weak or negative in neutrophils whereas the reverse is true when the substrate, naphthol AS-D chloroacetate, is used.[403-407]
- *Serum and Urine Lysozyme (Muramidase)* — In the absence of renal

disease (renal tissue has a high concentration of muramidase), serum and urine muramidase is derived from degradation of granulocytes. Consequently, this lysozyme is of diagnostic and prognostic importance in measuring the turnover of cells of granulocytic and monocytic series because lymphocytes, erythrocytes, and platelets are practically devoid of this lysozyme.[357-362, 408-409]

The above-mentioned cytochemical stains and their clinical applications are summarized in Table 4-II.

TABLE 4-II
CYTOCHEMICAL STAINS AND CLINICAL APPLICATIONS

Cytochemical Stain	*Clinical Application*
Leukocyte peroxidase	Differentiate neutrophilic, eosinophilic, and monocytic leukemia from lymphocytic leukemia and erythroleukemia
Leukocyte alkaline phosphatase	Differentiate leukemoid reaction of infections, polycythemia rubra vera, and myelofibrosis with myeloid metaplasia from chronic lymphocytic leukemia
Sudan black B stain	Differentiate acute granulocytic leukemia from acute lymphocytic leukemia
Periodic acid Schiff (PAS) stain	Differentiate acute erythroleukemia and acute lymphocytic leukemia from acute granulocytic leukemia
Leukocyte acid phosphatase	Differentiate leukemic reticuloendotheliosis (hairy cell leukemia) from other leukemias
Leukocyte esterases	Differentiate monocytic leukemia from neutrophilic leukemia
Serum and urine lysozyme (Muramidase)	Monitor the cellular turnover of granulocytic and monocytic leukemia

Table 4-II indicates that several cytochemical stains can be used simultaneously and independently to achieve a positive identification of a highly atypical leukemia which lacks the distinctive morphology for diagnosis by routine methods.

TREATMENT

Infection, hemorrhages, severe dysfunctions of leukemia-infiltrated vital organs, and central nervous system leukemia are the main causes of death in leukemia. Anemia, cytotoxic effects of chemotherapy, radiation treatment,[410-411] and an impaired cellular and immunological defense mechanism[412-416] make leukemic patients prone to succumb to bacterial, e.g. Staphylococcus aureus, Pseudomonas aeruginosa, Escherichia coli, Klebsiella Aerobacter, Proteus valgaris, Bacteroides, etc.; fungal, e.g. Candida, Aspergillus, Phycomycetes, etc.; protozoan, e.g. Pneumocystitis carinii, Toxoplasma gondii, etc.; and viral infections, e.g. herpes zoster, varicella virus, cytomegalo virus, etc.[417-442]

Obviously, these potentially life-threatening infections should be vigorously prevented or treated with appropriate immunizations and antibiotics.[443-454] Protective isolation[455-461] can also be utilized for high risk patients with acute leukemia or in immunosuppressed patients who have previously undergone total body irradiation prior to bone marrow transplantation.[462-465] The following should be meticulously integrated in order to prolong life and minimize morbidity of leukemic victims: systemic chemotherapy with corticosteroids and cytotoxic drugs,[466-489] immunotherapy,[490-496] bone marrow transplantation,[497-506] etc., to control the relentless leukemic process; blood, platelet, and leukocyte transfusions to combat anemia, thrombocytopenia, leukopenia, and the associated hemorrhagic diathesis and susceptibility to infections;[507-511] splenectomy for thrombocytopenia, hypersplenism, and prevention of splenic origin of blastic transformation;[512-520] adequate hydration and various medical means to correct hypercalcemia, hyperuricemia and other serum electrolyte and biochemical imbalance; and radiotherapy and intrathecal chemotherapy to treat central nervous system leukemia.[521-545]

PROGNOSIS

Many factors directly or indirectly influence the prognosis of various kinds of leukemias.[2-3, 12, 22, 35, 38, 100, 546-560]

AGE. When acute leukemias (especially acute lymphocytic leukemia) appear in patients between two and ten years of age, they carry a better prognosis than the same diseases occurring in teenagers, young adults, and children under two years of age.

SEX. Since leukemias affect twice as many male patients as female patients, leukemia-related deaths naturally show definite predilection for male patients.

RACE. Under the same treatment regimes, Caucasian children show higher survival rate than the comparable black children.

CONSTITUTIONAL SYMPTOMS. Persistent and severe constitutional symptoms, such as weight loss, anorexia, fever, malaise, generalized weakness, night sweats, ease of fatigue, etc., are unfavorable prognostic signs.

OVERTLY ABNORMAL LABORATORY STUDIES. Anemia; thrombocytopenia; elevated SGOT, SGPT, alkaline phosphatase, BUN, creatinine, vitamin B12, and muramidase; hematuria; hyperuricemia; hypercalcemia; hyperphosphatemia; reduction of blood clotting factors; reduced CSF sugar, increased CSF protein and spinal fluid pleocytosis; etc., which are the reflections of dysfunctions of the various leukemia-infiltrated organs, are poor prognostic indicators.

EXTENT OF LEUKEMIC INVOLVEMENT OF DIFFERENT ORGANS. Since leukemia can involve lymph nodes, liver, spleen, kidneys, bone and joint, lungs, gastrointestinal tract, central nervous system, heart, mediastinum, skin, etc., severe impairment of function of some of these vital organs will inevitably bring about the victims' demise.

TYPE OF LEUKEMIA. Chronic leukemia has a more favorable prognosis than acute leukemia of the same cell type and the same chronic leukemia in blastic crisis. In addition, everything being equal, patients with acute lymphocytic leukemia tend to survive longer than patients with acute granulocytic leukemia.

PHYSICAL AND IMMUNOLOGIC CHARACTERISTICS OF LEUKEMIC CELLS. The presence of a large population of extremely immature and bizarre leukemic cells and leukemic cells with atypical immunologic markers (B and T cell markers) indicates a poor prognosis for long-term survival.

CONCURRENT PRESENCE OF INFECTIOUS, METABOLIC, CARDIOVASCULAR, PULMONARY, RENAL, AND OTHER MALIGNANT DISEASES. Tuberculosis, diabetes mellitus, myocardial infarct, heart failure, uremia, emphysema, carcinomas, sarcomas, etc., when coupled with leukemia, make the prognosis for long-term survival very poor indeed.

PATIENTS' RESPONSE TO TREATMENT AND THE DURATION OF THEIR REMISSION. Favorable response to treatment depends on susceptibility of leukemic cells to cytotoxic drugs and the patients' ability to withstand aggressive treatments. Failure to show favorable response to antileukemic therapy will allow acute leukemia to run a relatively short fatal course.

REFERENCES

1. Back, E. H.: Death after intrathecal methotrexate. *Lancet, 2:*1005, 1969.
2. Bennett, J. M., Klemperer, M. R., and Segal, G. B.: Survival prediction based on morphology of lymphoblasts. *Recent Results Cancer Res, 43:*23, 1974.
3. Boggs, D. R., Wintrobe, M. M., and Cartwright, G. E.: The acute leukemias. Analysis of 322 cases and review of the literature. *Medicine, 41:*163-225, 1962.
4. Catovsky, D., Goldman, S. M., Okos, A., Frisch, B., and Galton, D. A. G.: T-lymphoblastic leukemia: A distinct variant of acute leukemia. *Br Med J, 2:*642, 1974.
5. Cutler, S. J., Axtell, H., and Heise, H.: Ten thousand cases of leukemia: 1940-1962. *J Natl Cancer Inst, 39:*993, 1967.
6. Falleta, J. M., Mukhopadhyay, N., Starling, K. A., and Fernbach, D. J.: Leukemic blasts with membrane characteristics of either T or B cells. *Pediatr Res, 8:*400, 1974.
7. George, S. L., Fernbach, D. J., and Lee, E. T.: Early deaths in newly diagnosed cases of pediatric acute leukemia: A southwest oncology group study. *Cancer, 42:*781-786, 1978.
8. Greaves, M. F., Brown, G., Rapson, N. T., and Lister, T. A.: Antisera to acute lymphoblastic leukemia cells. *Clin Immunol Immunopathol, 4:*67, 1975.
9. Hagbin, M., Tan, C. T., Clarkson, B. D., Mikie, V., Burchenal, J. H., and Murphy, H. L.: Treatment of acute lymphoblastic leukemia in children with prophylactic "intrathecal methotrexate and intensive systemic chemotherapy. *Cancer Res, 35:*807, 1975.

10. Hendin, B., Devivo, D. C., Torack, R., Lell, M. E., Ragab, A. H., and Vietti, T. J.: Parenchymatous degeneration of the central nervous system in childhood leukemia. *Cancer, 33:*468, 1974.
11. Holland, J. F., and Glidewell, O. J.: Survival expectancy in acute lymphocytic leukemia. *N Engl J Med, 287:*769, 1972.
12. Kawashima, K., Suzuki, H., Yamada, K., Kato, Y., Watanabe, E., Morishima, Y., Takeyama, H., and Kobayashi, M.: Long-term survival in acute leukemia in Japan. A study of 304 cases. *Cancer, 45:*2181-2187, 1980.
13. Kim, T., Nesbitt, M. E., D'angio, G. D., and Levitt, S.: The role of central nervous system irradiation in children with acute lymphoblastic leukemia. *Radiology, 104:*635, 1972.
14. Leventhal, B. G., Levine, A. S., Graw, R. G., Jr., Simon, R., Freireich, E. J., and Henderson, E. S.: Long term second remissions in acute lymphatic leukemia. *Cancer, 35:*1136, 1975.
15. Mathe, G., Pouillart, P., Sterescu, M., Amiel, J. L., Schwarzenberg, L., Schneider, M., Hayat, M., DeVassal, F., DeJasmin, D., and LaFleur, M.: Subdivision of classical varieties of acute lymphoblastic leukemia: A correlation with prognosis and cure expectancy. *Eur J Clin Biol Res, 16:*554, 1971.
16. Saiki, J. H., Thompson, S., Smith, F., and Atkinson, R.: Paraplegia following intrathecal chemotherapy. *Cancer, 29:*370, 1972.
17. Simone, J.: Acute lymphocytic leukemia in children. *Semin Hematol, 11:*28, 1974.
18. Sullivan, M. P., Humphrey, G. B., Vietti, T. J., Haggard, M. E., and Lee, E.: Superiority of conventional intrathecal methotrexate therapy, unmaintained, or radiotherapy (2000-2500 rads tumor dose) in treatment for meningeal leukemia. *Cancer, 35:*1066, 1975.
19. Tsukimoto, I., Wong, K. Y., and Lampkin, B. C.: Surface markers and prognostic factors in acute lymphoblastic leukemia. *N Engl J Med, 294:*245, 1976.
20. Whang-Peng, J., and Knutsen, T.: Lymphocytic leukemias, acute and chronic. *Clin Haematol, 9:*87-127, 1980.
21. Zuelzer, W. W., and Flatz, G.: Acute childhood leukemia: A ten year study. *Am J Dis Child, 100:*886, 1960.
22. Beard, M. E. J., and Fairley, G. H.: Acute leukemias in adults. *Semin Hematol, 11:*5, 1974.
23. Bierman, H. R., Cohen, P., McClelland, J. N., and Shimkin, M. B.: The effect of transfusion and antibiotics upon the duration of life in children with lymphogenous leukemia. *J Pediatr, 37:*455, 1950.
24. Bodey, G. P., Coltman, C. A., Freireich, E. J., Bonnet, J. D., Gehan, E. A., Hart, A. B., Hewlett, J. S., McCredie, K. B., Saika, J. H., and Wilson, H. E.: Chemotherapy of acute leukemia: Comparison of cytarabine along and in combination with vincristine, prednisone, and cyclophosphamide. *Arch Intern Med, 133:*260, 1974.
25. Bull, J. M., Duttera, M. J., Northrup, J. D., Henderson, E. S., Stashick, E. D., and Carbone, P. P.: Serial *in vitro* bone marrow culture in acute myelocytic leukemia. *Blood, 42:*679, 1973.
26. Clarkson, B. D.: Acute myelocytic leukemia in adults. *Cancer, 30:*1572, 1972.
27. Cline, M. J., and Rosenbaum, E.: Prediction of *in vivo* cytotoxicity of chemotherapeutic agents by their *in vitro* effect on leukocytes from patients with acute leukemia. *Cancer Res, 28:*2516, 1958.
28. Crosby, W. H.: To treat or not to treat acute granulocytic leukemia. *Arch Intern Med, 122:*79, 1968.
29. Crowther, D., Powles, R. L., Bateman, C. J. T., Beard, H. E. J., Gauci, G. L., Wrigley,

P. F. M., Malpas, J. S., Fairley, G. H., and Scott, R. B.: Management of adult acute myelogenous leukemia. *Br Med J, 1:*101, 1973.

30. Dameshek, W., Necheles, T. F., and Finkel, H. E.: Survival in myeloblastic leukemia of adults. *N Engl J Med, 275:*700, 1966.
31. Fairley, G. H.: The treatment of acute myeloblastic leukemia. *Br J Haematol, 20:*567, 1971.
32. Fleming, I., Simone, J., Jackson, R., Johnson, T., and Walters, M. C.: Splenectomy and chemotherapy in acute myelocytic leukemia of childhood. *Cancer, 33:*427, 1974.
33. Glucksberg, H., Buckner, C. D., Fefer, A., DeMarsh, Q., Coleman, D. Dobrow, R. B., Huff, J., Kjobech, C., Hill, A. S., Dittman, W., Neiman, P. E., Cheerer, M. A., Einstein, A. B., Jr., and Thomas, E. D.: Combination chemotherapy for acute non-lymphoblastic leukemia in adults. *Cancer Chemother Rep, 59:*1131, 1975.
34. Gutterman, J. V., Rodriguez, V., Mavligit, G., Burgess, M. A., Gehan, E., Hersh, E. M., McCredie, K. B., Reed, R., Smith, T., Bodey, G. P., Sr., and Freireich, E. J.: Chemo-immunotherapy of adult acute leukemia: Prolongation of remission in myeloblastic leukemia with BCG. *Lancet, 2:*1405, 1974.
35. Henderson, E. S., Wallace, H. J., Yates, J., Scharlau, C., Rakowski, I., Ellison, R. R., and Holland, J. F.: Factors influencing prognosis in adult acute myelocytic leukemia. *Adv Biosci, 14:*72, 1975.
36. Pizzo, P. A., Henderson, E. S., and Leventhal, B. G.: Acute myelogenous leukemia in children: A preliminary report of combination chemotherapy. *J Pediatr, 88:*125, 1976.
37. Rheingold, J. J., Kaufman, R., Adelson, E., and Lear, A.: Smoldering acute leukemia. *N Engl J Med, 268:*812, 1963.
38. Wiernik, P. N., and Serpick, A. A.: Factors affecting remission and survival in adult acute non-lymphocytic leukemia (ANLL). *Medicine* (Baltimore), *49:*505, 1970.
39. Bernard, J., Lasneret, Chome, J., Levy, J. P., and Boiron, M.: A cytological and histological study of acute promyelocytic leukemia. *J Clin Path, 13:*628, 1963.
40. Bernard, J., Weil, M., Boiron, M., Jacquillate, C., Flandrin, G., and Gemon, M. F.: Acute promyelocytic leukemia: Results of treatment by Daunorubicin. *Blood, 41:*489, 1973.
41. Didisheim, P., Trombold, J. S., Vandervoot, R. L. E., and Songin, M. R.: Acute promyelocytic leukemia with fibrinogen and factor V deficiencies. *Blood, 23:*717, 1964.
42. Ghitis, J.: Acute promyelocytic leukemia. *Blood, 21:*237, 1963.
43. Gralnick, H. R., and Abrell, E.: Studies of the pro-coagulant and fibrinolytic activity of promyelocytes in acute promyelocytic leukaemia. *Br J Haematol, 24:*89-99, 1973.
44. Gralnick, H. R., Bagley, J., and Abrell, E.: Heparin treatment for hemorrhagic diseases of acute promyelocytic leukemia. *Am J Med, 52:*167-174, 1972.
45. Gralnick, H. R., and Sultan, C.: Acute promyelocytic leukemia: Hemorrhagic manifestation and morphologic criteria. *Br J Haematol, 29:*373, 1975.
46. Hillestead, L. K.: Acute promyelocytic leukemia. *Acta Med Scandinav, 159:*189, 1957.
47. Pitney, W. R.: Disseminated intravascular coagulation. *Sem Hematol, 8:*65, 1971.
48. Rachmilewitz, D., Rachmilewitz, E. A., Polliack, A., and Hershko, C.: Acute promyelocytic leukemia: A report of five cases with a comment on the diagnostic significance of serum vitamin B12 determination. *Br J Haematol, 22:*87, 1972.
49. Rand, J. J., Moloney, W. C., Sise, H. S.: Coagulation defects in acute promyelocytic leukemia. *Arch Intern Med, 123:*39, 1969.

50. Rosenthal, L. L.: Acute promyelocytic leukemia associated with hypofibrinogenemia. *Blood, 21:*495, 1963.
51. Tan, H. K., Wages, B., and Gralnick, H. R.: Ultrastructural studies in acute promyelocytic leukemia. *Blood, 39:*628-636, 1972.
52. Geary, C. G., Catovsky, D., Wiltshaw, E., Milner, G. R., Schole, M. C., Van Noorden, S., Wadsworth, L. D., Muldal, S., Mac Iver, J. E., and Galton, D. A. I.: Chronic myelomonocytic leukemia. *Br J Haematol, 50:*289, 1975.
53. Law, I. P., Koch, F. J., Cannon, G. B., Heberman, R. B., and Oldham, R. K.: Acute myelomonocytic leukemia associated with paraproteinemia. *Cancer, 37:*1359, 1976.
54. Linman, J. W.: Myelomonocytic leukemia and its preleukemic phase. *J Chron Dis, 22:*713, 1970.
55. Miescher, P. A., and Farquet, J. J.: Chronic myelomonocytic leukemia in adults. *Semin Haematol, 11:*129, 1974.
56. Muggia, F. M., Heinemann, H. O., Farhangi, M., and Osserman, E. F.: Lysozymuria and renal tubular dysfunction in monocytic and myelomonocytic leukemia. *Am J Med, 47:*351, 1969.
57. Osgood, E. F.: Acute monocytic leukemia as an explanation for "Hiatus Leukemicus" and "Myelo-monocytic leukemia." *Blood, 33:*268, 1969.
58. Osserman, E. F., and Lawlor, D. P.: Serum and urinary lysozyme (Muramidase) in monocytic and monomyelocytic leukemia. *J Exp Med, 124:*94, 1966.
59. Polliack, A., McKenzie, S., Gee, T., Lampen, N., DeHarven, E., and Clarkson, B. D.: A scanning electron microscopic study of 34 cases of acute granulocytic, myelomonocytic monoblastic and histiocytic leukemia. *Am J Med, 59:*308, 1975.
60. Pruzanski, W., and Platts, M. E.: Serum and urinary proteins, lysozyme (muramidase), and renal dysfunction in mono- and myelomonocytic leukemia. *J Clin Invest, 49:*1694, 1970.
61. Saarni, M. I., and Linman, J. W.: Myelomonocytic leukemia: Disorderly proliferation of all marrow cells. *Cancer, 27:*1221, 1971.
62. Sexauer, J., Kass, L., and Schnitzer, B.: Subacute myelomonocytic leukemia. *Am J Med, 57:*853, 1974.
63. Zittoun, R.: Subacute and chronic myelomonocytic leukemia: A distinct haematological entity. *Br J Haematol, 32:*1, 1976.
64. Belding, H. W., Daland, G. A., and Parker, F., Jr.: Histiocytic and monocytic leukemia: A clinical, hematological and pathological differentiation. *Cancer, 8:*237, 1955.
65. Clough, P. W.: Monocytic leukemia. *Bull Johns Hopkins Hosp, 51:*148, 1932.
66. Dameshek, W.: Acute monocytic (histiocytic) leukemia: Review of literature and case reports. *Arch Intern Med, 46:*718, 1930.
67. Evans, F. J., and Hilton, J. H. B.: Polymyositis associated with acute monocytic leukemia. Case report and review of the literature. *Canad Med Assoc J, 91:*1272, 1964.
68. Evans, T. S.: Monocytic leukemia. *Medicine, 21:*421, 1942.
69. Forkner, C. E.: Clinical and pathologic differentiation of acute leukemias with special reference to acute monocytic leukemia. *Arch Intern Med, 53:*1, 1934.
70. Freeman, A. I., and Journey, L. J.: Ultrastructural studies on monocytic leukemia. *Br J Haematol, 20:*225, 1971.
71. Glick, A. D., and Horn, R. G.: Identification of promonocytes and monocytoid precursors in acute leukaemia of adults: Ultrastructural and cytochemical observations. *Br J Haematol, 26:*395, 1974.

72. Herbut, P. A., and Miller, F. R.: Histopathology of monocytic leukemia. *Am J Pathol, 23:*93, 1947.
73. Lichtman, M. A., and Weed, R. I.: Peripheral cytoplasmic characteristics of leukocytes in monocytic leukemia: Relationship to clinical manifestations. *Blood, 40:*52, 1972.
74. McKenna, R. W., Bloomfield, C. D., Dick, F., Nesbit, M. E., and Brunning, R. D.: Acute monoblastic leukemia: Diagnosis and treatment of ten cases. *Blood, 46:*481, 1975.
75. Montgomery, H., and Watkins, C. H.: Exfoliative dermatitis as a manifestation of monocytic leukemia (Schilling). *Min Med, 21:*636, 1938.
76. Osgood, E. E.: Monocytic leukemia: Report of six cases and review of one hundred and twenty-seven cases. *Arch Intern Med, 59:*931, 1937.
77. Poulik, M. D., Berman, L., and Prasad, A. S.: "Myeloma protein" in patient with monocytic leukemia. *Blood, 33:*246, 1969.
78. Schumacher, H. R., Szekely, I. E., and Park, S. A.: Monoblasts of acute monoblastic leukemia. *Cancer, 31:*209, 1973.
79. Shaw, M. T., and Nordquist, R. E.: "Pure" monocytic or histiomonocytic leukemia: A revised concept. *Cancer, 35:*208, 1975.
80. Sinn, C. M., and Dick, F. W.: Monocytic leukemia. *Amer J Med, 20:*588, 1956.
81. Watkins, C. H., and Hall, B. E.: Monocytic leukemia of the Naegeli and Schilling types. *Am J Clin Pathol, 10:*387, 1940.
82. Astrom, K. E., Mancall, E. L., and Richardson, E. P., Jr.: Progressive multifocal leuko-encephalopathy: A hitherto unrecognized complication of chronic lymphatic leukaemia and Hodgkin's disease. *Brain, 81:*93, 1958.
83. Brody, J. I., Burningham, R. A., Nowell, P. C., Rowlands, D. T., Freiburg, P., and Daniele, R. P.: Persistent lymphocytosis with chromosomal evidence of malignancy. *Am J Med, 58:*547, 1975.
84. Brown, G. M., Elliott, S. M., and Young, W. A.: The hemolytic factor in the anemia of lymphatic leukemia. *J Clin Invest, 30:*130, 1951.
85. Damesher, W.: Chronic lymphocytic leukemia — an accumulative disease of immunologically incompetent lymphocytes. *Blood, 29:*566, 1967.
86. Diamond, H. D., and Miller, D. G.: Chronic lymphocytic leukemia. *Med Clin N Amer, 45:*601, 1961.
87. Douglas, S. D., Cohen, G., Konig, E., and Bittinger, G.: Lymphocyte lysosomes and lysosomal enzymes in chronic lymphocytic leukemia. *Blood, 41:*511, 1973.
88. Durant, J. R., and Finkbeiner, J. A.: "Spontaneous" remission in chronic lymphatic leukemia? *Cancer, 17:*105, 1964.
89. Field, E. O., Dawson, K. B., Peckham, M. J., Hammersley, P. A., Cooling, C. I., Morgan, R. L., and Smithers, D. W.: The response of chronic lymphocytic leukemia to treatment by extracorporal irradiation of blood, assessed by isotope-labeling procedures. *Blood, 36:*87, 1970.
90. Galton, D. A. G.: The pathogenesis of chronic lymphocytic leukemia. *Can Med Assoc J, 94:*1005, 1966.
91. Gray, J. L., Jacobs, A., and Block, M.: Bone marrow and peripheral blood lymphocytosis in the prognosis of chronic lymphocytic leukemia. *Cancer, 33:*1169, 1974.
92. Green, R. A., and Dixon, H.: Expectancy for life in chronic lymphatic leukemia. *Blood, 25:*23, 1965.
93. Gunz, F. W., Gunz, J. P., Veale, A. M. O., Chapman, C. J., and Houston, I. B.: Familial leukaemia: A study of 909 families. *Scand J Haematol, 15:*117, 1975.
94. Holowach, J.: Chronic lymphoid leukemia in children. *J Pediat, 32:*84, 1949.

95. Jim, R. T. S., and Reinhard, E. H.: Agammaglobulinemia and chronic lymphocyti leukemia. *Ann Intern Med, 44:*790, 1956.
96. Liepman, M. K.: The chronic leukemias. *Med Clin North Am, 64:*705-727, 1980.
97. McPhedran, P., and Heath, C. W., Jr.: Acute leukemia occurring during chroni lymphocytic leukemia. *Blood, 35:*7, 1970.
98. Miller, D. G., Budinger, J. M., and Karnofsky, D. A.: A clinical and pathologic stud of resistance to infection in chronic lymphatic leukemia. *Cancer, 15:*307, 1962.
99. Minot, G. R., and Isaacs, R.: Lymphatic leukemia: Age, incidence, duration an benefit derived from irradiation. *Boston Med Surg J, 191:*1, 1924.
100. Peterson, L., Bloomfield, C. D., Sundberg, R. D., Gajlpeczalska, K. J., and Brunning R. D.: Morphology of chronic lymphocytic leukemia and its relationship to surviv al. *Am J Med, 59:*315, 1975.
101. Rai, K. R., Sawitsky, A., Cronkite, E. P., Chanana, A. D., Levy, R. N., and Pasternack B. S.: Clinical staging of chronic lymphocytic leukemia. *Blood, 46:*219, 1979.
102. Rosenthal, M. C., Pisciotta, A. V., Komninos, Z. D., Goldenberg, H., and Dameshek W.: The auto-immune hemolytic anemia of malignant lymphocytic disease. *Blood 10:*197, 1955.
103. Rubinstein, L., Herman, M. M., Long, T. F., and Wilbur, J. R.: Disseminated necrotiz ing leukoencephalopathy: A complication of treated central nervous systen leukemia and lymphoma. *Cancer, 35:*291, 1975.
104. Schumacher, H. R., Maugel, T. K., and Davis, K. D.: The lymphocyte of chroni lymphatic leukemia. 1. Electron microscopy: Onset. *Cancer, 26:*895, 1970.
105. Shimkin, M. B., Lucia, E. L., Oppermann, K. C., and Mettier, S. R.: Lymphocyti leukemia: An analysis of frequency, distribution and mortality at the University o California Hospital, 1913-1947. *Ann Intern Med, 39:*1254, 1953.
106. Spiers, A. S. D.: Chronic granulocytic leukaemia and chronic lymphocytic leukemia *Br Med J, 4:*460, 1974.
107. Wasi, P., and Block, M.: The mechanism of the development of anemia in untreatec chronic lymphatic leukemia. *Blood, 17:*597, 1961.
108. Wilson, J. D., and Nossal, G. J. V.: Identification of human T and B lymphocytes ir normal peripheral blood and in chronic lymphocytic leukemia. *Lancet, 2:*788 1971.
109. Yam, L. T., and Crosby, W. H.: Early splenectomy in lymphoproliferative disorders *Arch Intern Med, 133:*270, 1974.
110. Barrett, O. N., Jr., Conrad, M., and Crosby, W. H.: Chronic granulocytic leukemia ir childhood. *Am J Med Sci, 240:*587, 1960.
111. Bauke, J.: Chronic myelocytic leukemia. *Cancer, 24:*643, 1969.
112. Chabner, B. A., Haskell, C. M., and Cannellos, G. P.: Destructive bone lesions ir chronic granulocytic leukemia. *Medicine, 48:*401, 1969.
113. Conrad, M., Rappaport, H., and Crosby, W.: Chronic granulocytic leukemia: The aged. *Arch Intern Med, 116:*765, 1965.
114. Cooke, J. V.: Chronic myelogenous leukemia in children. *J Pediat, 42:*537, 1953.
115. Engel, E., McGee, B. J., Flexner, J. M., and Krantz, N. B.: Translocation of the Philadelphia chromosome onto the 17 short arm in chronic myeloid leukemia: A second example. *N Engl J Med, 293:*666, 1975.
116. Gomez, G. A., Sokal, J. E., Mittelman, A., and Aungst, C. W.: Splenectomy for palliation of chronic myelocytic leukemia. *Am J Med, 61:*14, 1976.
117. Gralinick, H. R., Harbor, J., and Vogel, C.: Myelofibrosis in chronic granulocytic leukemia. *Blood, 37:*152, 1971.
118. Green, T. W., Conley, C. L., Ashburn, L. I. and Peters, H. R.: Splenectomy for myeloid metaplasia of the spleen. *N Engl J Med, 248:*211, 1953.

119. Hadlock, D. C., Fortuny, I. E., McCullough, J., and Kennedy, B. J.: Continuous flow centrifuge leucopheresis in the management of chronic myelogenous leukemia. *Br J Haematol, 29:*443, 1975.
120. Hardisty, R. M., Speed, D. E., and Till, M.: Granulocytic leukaemia in childhood. *Br J Haemat, 10:*551, 1965.
121. Karanas, A., and Silver, R. T.: Characteristic of the terminal phase of chronic granulocytic leukemia. *Blood, 32:*445, 1968.
122. Kardinal, C. G., Bateman, J. R., and Weiner, J.: Chronic granulocytic leukemia. *Arch Intern Med, 136:*305, 1976.
123. Krakoff, I. H.: Studies of uric acid biosynthesis in the chronic leukemias. *Arthritis Rheum, 8:*772, 1965.
124. Kwaan, H. C., Pierre, R. V., and Long, D. L.: Meningeal involvement as first manifestation of acute myeloblastic transformation in chronic granulocytic leukemia. *Blood, 33:*348, 1969.
125. Liu, P. I., Ishimaru, T., McGregor, D. H., Okada, H., and Steer, A.: Autopsy study of granulocytic sarcoma (chloroma) in patients with myelogenous leukemia, Hiroshima-Nagasaki 1949-1969. *Cancer, 32:*948, 1973.
126. Monfardini, S., Gee, T., Fried, J., and Clarkson, B.: Survival in chronic myelogenous leukemia: Influence of treatment and extent of disease at diagnosis. *Cancer, 31:*492, 1973.
127. Nowell, P. C., and Hungerford, D. A.: Chromosome studies in human leukemia. II. Chronic granulocytic leukemia. *J Natl Cancer Inst, 27:*1013, 1961.
128. Odeberg, H., Olofsson, T., and Olsson, I.: Granulocyte function in chronic granulocytic leukemia. I. Bactericidal and metabolic capacities during phagocytosis in isolated granulocytes. *Br J Haematol, 29:*427, 1975.
129. Reisman, L. E., and Trujillo, J. M.: Chronic granulocytic leukemia of childhood. *J Pediat, 62:*710, 1963.
130. Richards, H. G. H., and Spiers, A. S. D.: Chronic granulocytic leukemia in pregnancy. *Br J Radiol, 48:*261, 1975.
131. Shaw, M. T., Bottomley, R. H., Grozea, P. N., and Nordquist, R. E.: Heterogeneity of morphological, cytochemical, and cytogenetic features in blastic phase of chronic granulocytic leukemia. *Cancer, 35:*199, 1975.
132. Shimkin, M. B., Mettier, S. R., and Bierman, H. R.: Myelocytic leukemia: An analysis of incidence, distribution and fatality, 1910-1948. *Ann Intern Med, 35:*194, 1951.
133. Sokal, J. E., Aungst, C. W., and Grace, J. T., Jr.: Immunotherapy in well-controlled chronic myelocytic leukemia. *N Y J Med, 73:*1180, 1973.
134. Spiers, A. S. D.: The treatment of chronic granulocytic leukemia. *Br J Haematol, 32:*291, 1976.
135. Spiers, A. S. D., Costello, C., Catovsky, D., Galton, D. A. G., and Goldman, J. M.: Chronic granulocytic leukemia: Multiple-drug chemotherapy for acute transformation. *Br Med J, 3:*77, 1974.
136. Stryckmans, P. A.: Current concepts in chronic myelogenous leukemia. *Semin Haemat, 11:*101, 1974.
137. Theologides, A.: Unfavorable signs in patients with chronic myelocytic leukemia. *Ann Intern Med, 76:*95, 1972.
138. Vallejos, C. S., Trujillo, J. M., Cork, A., Bodey, G. P., McCredie, K. B., and Freireich, E. J.: Blastic crisis in chronic granulocytic leukemia: Experience in 39 patients. *Cancer, 34:*1806, 1974.
139. Adamson, J. W., and Finch, C. A.: Erythropoietin and the regulation of erythropoiesis in Diguglielmo's syndrome. *Blood, 36:*590, 1970.

140. Baldni, M., Fudenberg, H. H., Fukutake, K., and Dameshek, W.: The anemia of the DiGuglielmo's syndrome. *Blood, 14:*334, 1959.
141. Bank, A., Larsen, P. R., and Anderson, H. M.: DiGuglielmo's syndrome after polycythemia. *N Engl J Med, 275:*489, 1966.
142. Bastrup-Madsen, P., Nielsen, K., and Mose, C. B.: Acute erythraemia (DiGuglielmo's syndrome) after thorotrast injection. *Acta Med Scand, 189:*349, 1971.
143. Bloomfield, C. D., Brunning, R. D., and Kennedy, B. J.: Daunorubicin-prednisone treatment of erythroleukemia. *Ann Intern Med, 81:*746, 1974.
144. Crossen, P. E., Fitzgerald, P. H., Menzies, R. C., and Brehaut, L. A.: Chromosomal abnormality, megaloblastosis and arrested DNA synthesis in erythroleukemia. *J Med Genet, 6:*95, 1969.
145. DiGuglielmo, G.: Un caso di eritroleucemia. *Folia Med, 13:*386, 1917.
146. DiGuglielmo, G.: Eritremia acute. *Boll Soc Med Clin Pavia, 40:*665, 1926.
147. Durant, J. R., and Tassoni, Em. M.: Coexistent DiGuglielmo's leukemia and Hodgkin's disease. *Am J Med Sci, 254:*824, 1967.
148. Eastman, P., Wallerstein, R. O., and Schrier, S. I.: Polycythemia converted to DiGuglielmo's syndrome. *JAMA, 204:*1141, 1968.
149. Finkle, H. E., and Brauer, M. J.: Giant eosinophilic granules in chronic DiGuglielmo syndrome. *N Engl J Med, 274:*209, 1966.
150. Gabuzda, T. G., Shute, H. E., and Erslev, A. J.: Regulation of erythropoiesis in erythroleukemia. *Arch Intern Med, 123:*60, 1969.
151. Heath, C. W., Jr., Bennett, J. M., Whang-peng, J., Berry, E. W., and Wiernick, P. H.: Cytogenetic findings in erythroleukemia. *Blood, 33:*453, 1969.
152. Necheles, T. F., and Dameshek, W.: The DiGuglielmo syndrome: Studies in hemoglobin synthesis. *Blood, 29:*550, 1967.
153. Quaglino, D., and Hayhoe, F. G. J.: Periodic-Acid-Schiff positivity in erythroblasts with special reference to DiGuglielmo's syndrome. *Br J Haematol, 6:*26, 1960.
154. Schwartz, S. O., and Critchlow, J.: Erythremic myelosis (DiGuglielmo's disease) critical review with report of four cases and comment on erythroleukemia. *Blood, 7:*765, 1952.
155. Scott, R. B., Ellison, R. R., and Ley, A. B.: A clinical study of twenty cases of erythroleukemia (DiGuglielmo's syndrome). *Am J Med, 37:*162, 1964.
156. Sheets, R. F., Drevets, C. C., and Hamilton, H. E.: Erythroleukemia (DiGuglielmo Syndrome): A report of clinical observations and experimental studies in seven patients. *Arch Intern Med, 111:*295, 1963.
157. Thurm, R. H., Casey, M. J., and Emerson, C. P.: Chronic DiGuglielmo syndrome. *Am J Med Sci, 253:*399, 1967.
158. Anteunis, A., Audebert, A. A., Krulik, M., DeBray, J., and Robineaux, R.: Acute eosinophilic leukemia. An ultrastructural study. *Virchows Arch Cell Pathol, 27:*237-248, 1978.
159. Bentley, H. P., Jr., Reardon, A. F., Knoedler, J. P., and Krivit, W. K.: Eosinophilic leukemia. Report of a case with review and classification. *Am J Med, 30:*310, 1961.
160. Benvenisti, D. S., and Ultmann, J. E.: Eosinophilic leukemia. *Ann Intern Med, 71:*731, 1969.
161. Bousser, J.: Eosinophilie et leucemie. *Sangre, 28:*553, 1957.
162. Chusid, M. J., and Dale, D. C.: Eosinophilic leukemia: Remission with vincristine and hydroxyurea. *Am J Med, 59:*297, 1975.
163. Evans, T. S., and Nesbit, R. R.: Eosinophilic leukemia; report of a case with autopsy confirmation; review of literature. *Blood, 4:*603, 1947.
164. Flannery, E. P., Dillon, D. E., Freeman, M. V. R., Levy, J. D., D'Ambrosio, U., and

Bedyner, J. L.: Eosinophilic leukemia with fibrosing endocarditis and short Y chromosome. *Cancer, 29:*660, 1972.

65. Goh, D., Swisher, S. N., and Rosenberg, C. A.: Cytogenic study in eosinophilic leukemia. *Ann Intern Med, 62:*80, 1975.
66. Gruenwald, H., Kiossoglou, K. A., Mitus, W. J., and Damishek, W.: Philadelphia chromosome in eosinophilic leukemia. *Am J Med, 39:*1003, 1965.
67. Hardy, W. R., and Anderson, R. E.: The hypereosinophilic syndromes. *Ann Intern Med, 68:*1220, 1968.
68. Kauer, G. L., and Eagle, R. L., Jr.: Eosinophilic leukemia with ph^1-positive cells. *Lancet, 2:*1340, 1964.
69. Presentey, B., Jerushalmy, Z., and Minti, U.: Eosinophilic leukemia: Morphological cytochemical and electron microscopic studies. *J Clin Pathol, 32:*261-271, 1979.
70. Stephens, D. J.: Acute eosinophilic leukemia. *Am J Med Sci, 189:*387, 1935.
71. Jennings, C. V., Dannaher, C. L., and Yam, L. T.: Basophilic leukemia. *South Med J, 73:*934-936, 1980.
72. Kyle, R. A., and Pease, G. L.: Basophilic leukemia. *Arch Intern Med, 118:*205, 1966.
73. Liso, V., Troccoli, G., and Specchia, G.: Mast cell leukemia and acute basophilic leukemia. Cytochemical studies. *Bibl Haematol, 45:*142-146, 1978.
74. Quattrin, N.: Follow-up of sixty-two cases of acute basophilic leukemia. *Biomedicine, 28:*72-79, 1978.
75. Swisher, R. W., Mueller, J. M., and Halloran, G.: Basophilic leukemia presenting as gastroduodenal ulceration: Effect of H-2-receptor blockade. *Am J Dig Dis, 23:*952-955, 1978.
76. Youman, J. D., Taddeini, L., and Cooper, T.: Histamine excess symptoms in basophilic chronic granulocytic leukemia. *Arch Int Med, 131:*560, 1963.
77. Jackson, I. M. D., and Clark, R. M.: A case of neutrophilic leukemia. *Am J Med Sci, 249:*72, 1965.
78. Rubin, H.: Chronic neutrophilic leukemia. *Ann Intern Med, 66:*93, 1966.
79. Tanzer, J., Harel, P., Boiron, M., and Bernard, J.: Cytochemical and cytogenetic findings in a case of chronic neutrophilic leukemia of mature cell type. *Lancet, 1:*397-388, 1964.
80. Bouroncle, B. A., Wiseman, B. K., and Doan, C. A.: Leukemic reticuloendotheliosis. *Blood, 13:*609, 1958.
81. Burke, J. S., Byrne, G. E., Jr., and Rappaport, H.: Hairy cell leukemia (leukemic reticuloendotheliosis). I. A clinical pathologic study of 21 patients. *Cancer, 33:*1399-1410, 1973.
82. Catovsky, D., Pettit, J. E., Galton, D. A. G., Spiers, A. S. D., and Harrison, C. V.: Leukemic reticuloendotheliosis ("Hairy" cell leukemia): A distinct clinicopathological entity. *Br J Haematol, 26:*9, 1964.
83. Ghadially, F. N., and Skinnider, L. F.: Ultrastructure of hairy cell leukemia. *Cancer, 29:*444-452, 1972.
84. King, G. W., Hurtubise, P. E., Sagone, A. L., Lobuglio, A. F., and Metz, E. N.: Leukemic reticuloendotheliosis: Study of the origin of the malignant cell. *Am J Med, 59:*411, 1975.
85. Yam, L. T., Li, C. Y., and Lam, K. W.: Tartrate-resistant acid phosphatase isoenzyme in the reticulum cells of leukemic reticuloendotheliosis. *N Engl J Med, 284:*357, 1971.
86. Kyle, R. A., Maldonado, J. E., and Bayrd, E. D.: Plasma cell leukemia. *Ann Intern Med, 133:*813, 1974.
87. Moss, W. T., and Ackerman, L. V.: Plasma cell leukemia. *Blood, 1:*396-406, 1946.

188. Muller, G. L., and McNaughton, E.: Multiple myeloma (plasmacytoma) with blood picture of plasma cell leukemia. *Folia Maemat, 46:*17, 1931.
189. Newman, W., Diefenbach, W. C. L., Quinn, M., and Meyer, L. M.: A case of acute plasma-cell leukemia supporting the concept of unity of plasma cellular neoplasia. *Cancer, 5:*514-520, 1952.
190. Patek, A. J., Jr., and Castle, W. B.: Plasma cell leukemia. *Am J M Sc, 191:*788, 1936.
191. Piney, A., and Riach, J. S.: Multiple myeloma. Aleukaemic and leukaemic. *Folia Haemat, 46:*37, 1931.
192. Rubinstein, M. A.: Multiple myeloma as a form of leukemia. *Blood, 4:*1049, 1949.
193. Caplan, R. M.: Urticaria pigmentosa and mastocytosis. *JAMA, 194:*1077, 1965.
194. Efrati, P., Klajman, A., and Spitz, H.: Mast cell leukemia? Malignant mastocytosis with leukemia-like manifestations. *Blood, 12:*869, 1957.
195. Friedman, B. I., Well, J. J., Frieman, D. C., and Braunstein, H.: Tissue mast cell leukemia. *Blood, 13:*70, 1958.
196. Mutter, R. D., Tannenbaum, M., and Ultmann, J. E.: Systemic mast cell disease. *Ann Intern Med, 59:*887, 1963.
197. Ono, S., Zompetti, L., Hagen, P., and Furth, J.: Relation of mastocytoma to mast-cell leukemia, and of heparin, histamine and serotonin to mast cells. *Blood, 14:*770, 1959.
198. Waters, W. J., and Lacson, P. S.: Mast cell leukemia presenting as urticaria pigmentosa: Report of a case. *Pediat, 19:*1033, 1957.
199. Allegra, S. R., and Broderick, P. A.: Acute aleukemic megakaryocytic leukemia: Report of a case. *Am J Clin Pathol, 55:*197, 1971.
200. Breton-Gorius, J., Reyes, F., Duhamel, G., Najman, A., and Gorin, N. C.: Megakaryoblastic acute leukemia: Identification by the ultrastructural demonstration of platelet peroxidase. *Blood, 51:*45-60, 1978.
201. Demmler, K., Burkhardt, R., Prechtel, K.: Megakaryoblastische myelose. *Klin Wochenschr, 48:*1168, 1970.
202. Garfield, D. H.: Acute erythromegakaryocytic leukemia after treatment with cytostatic agents. *Lancet, 2:*1037, 1970.
203. Gelin, G., and Wasserman, L. R.: Consideration on malignant megakaryocytes. *Sang, 30:*829, 1959.
204. Hansen, K. B., and Aabo, K.: Megakaryocytes in pulmonary blood vessels. 2. Relations to malignant haematological diseases, especially leukemia. *Acta Pathol Microbiol Scand, 86:*286-291, 1978.
205. Von Boros, J., and Karenyi, A.: Uber einen fall von akuter megakaryoblastenleukaemie zugleich einige bemerkungen zum problem der akuten leukaemie. *I. Klin Med, 118:*697, 1931.
206. Scheerer, P. P., Pierce, R. V., Schwartz, D. L., and Linman, J. W.: Reed-Sternberg cell leukemia and lactic acidosis: Unusual manifestations of Hodgkin's disease. *N Engl J Med, 270:*274-278, 1964.
207. Brill, A. B., Tomonaga, M., and Heyssel, R. M.: Leukemia in man following exposure to ionizing radiation: A summary of the findings in Hiroshima and Nagasaki, and a comparison with other human experience. *Ann Intern Med, 56:*590, 1962.
208. Folley, J. H., Borges, W., and Yamawaki, T.: Incidence of leukemia in survivors of atomic bomb in Hiroshima and Nagasaki, Japan. *Am J Med, 13:*311, 1952.
209. Heyssel, R., Brill, A. M., Woodbury, L. A., Nishimura, E. T., Ghose, T., Hoshino, T. and Yamasaki, M.: Leukemia in Hiroshima atomic bomb survivors. *Blood, 15:*313 1960.
210. Lange, R. D., Moloney, W. C., and Yamawaki, T.: Leukemia in atomic bomb survivors. *Blood, 9:*575, 1954.

211. Moloney, W. C.: Leukemia in survivors of atomic bombing. *N Engl J Med, 253*:88, 1955.
212. Moloney, W. C., and Kastenbaum, M. A.: Leukemogenic effects of ionizing radiation on atomic bomb survivors in Hiroshima city. *Science, 121*:308, 1955.
213. Moloney, W. C., and Lange, R. D.: Cytologic and biochemical studies on the granulocytes in early leukemia among atomic bomb survivors. *Texas Rep Biol Med, 12*:887, 1954.
214. Henshaw, P. S., and Hawkins, J. W.: Incidence of leukemia in physicians. *J Natl Cancer Inst, 4*:339, 1944.
215. March, H. C.: Leukemia in radiologists. *Radiology, 43*:275, 1944.
216. March, H. C.: Leukemia in radiologists in a 20 year period. *Am J Med Sci, 220*:282, 1950.
217. March, H. C.: Leukemia in radiologists. Ten years later. *Am J Med Sci, 242*:137, 1961.
218. Peller, S., and Pick, P.: Leukemia and other malignant disease in physicians. *JAMA, 147*:893, 1951.
219. Buckton, K. E., Jacobs, P. A., Court-Brown, W. M., and Doll, R.: A study of the chromosome damage persisting after x-ray therapy for ankylosing spondylitis. *Lancet, 2*:676, 1962.
220. Court-Brown, W. M., and Abbatt, J. D.: The incidence of leukemia in ankylosing spondylitis treated with x-rays: A preliminary report. *Lancet, 1*:1283, 1955.
221. Graham, D. C.: Leukemia following x-ray therapy for ankylosing spondylitis. *Arch Intern Med, 105*:51, 1960.
222. Silberberg, D. H., Frohman, L. A., and Duff, I. F.: The incidence of leukemia and related diseases in patients with rheumatoid (ankylosing) spondylitis treated with x-ray therapy. *Arthritis Rheum, 3*:64, 1960.
223. Pochin, E. E.: Leukemia following radio-iodine treatment of thyrotoxicosis. *Br Med J, 2*:1545-1550, 1960.
224. Saenger, E. L., Thomas, G. E., and Tompkins, E. A.: Incidence of leukemia following treatment of hyperthyroidism. *JAMA, 205*:855, 1968.
225. LaTourette, H. B., and Hodges, F. J.: Incidence of neoplasia after irradiation of thymic region. *Am J Roentgenol, 82*:667, 1959
226. Simpson, C. L., Hempelmann, L. H., and Fuller, L. M.: Neoplasia in children treated with x-rays in infancy for thymic enlargement. *Radiology, 64*:840, 1955.
227. Boice, J. D., and Land, C. E.: Adult leukemia following diagnostic x-rays? (Review of report by Bross, Ball, and Falen on a tri-state leukemia survey). *Am J Public Health, 69*:137-145, 1979.
228. Incidence of leukaemia after exposure to diagnostic radiation in utero. *Br Med J, 2*:1539-1545, 1960.
229. Dameshek, W., and Gunz, F. W.: Diagnostic and therapeutic x-ray exposure and leukemia. *JAMA, 163*:838-840, 1957.
230. Gunz, F. W., Borthwick, R. A., and Rolleston, G. I.: Acute leukemia in an infant following excessive intrauterine irradiation. *Lancet, 2*:190, 1958.
231. Rodriguez, V., Bodey, G. P., Trujillo, J. M., and Freireich, E. J.: Previous radiation exposure in patients with leukemia. *Arch Intern Med, 132*:874, 1973.
232. Aksoy, M., Dincol, K., Erdem, S., and Dincol, G.: Acute leukemia due to chronic exposure to benzene. *Am J Med, 52*:160-166, 1972.
233. Bowditch, M., Elkins, H. B., Hunter, F. T., Mallory, T. B., Gall, E. A., and Buckley, W. J.: Chronic exposure to benzene (Benzol). *J Industr Hyg Toxicol, 21*:321, 1939.
234. DeGowin, R. L.: Benzene exposure and aplastic anemia followed by leukemia 15 years later. *JAMA, 185*:748-751, 1963.

235. Rawson, R., Parker, F., Jr., and Jackson, H., Jr.: Industrial solvents as possible etiologic agents in myeloid metaplasia. *Science, 93:*541, 1941.
236. Tough, I. M., and Court-Brown, W. M.: Chromosome aberrations and exposure to ambient benzene. *Lancet, 1:*684, 1965.
237. Vigliani, E. C., and Saita, G.: Benzene and leukemia. *N Engl J Med, 271:*872, 1964.
238. Hogstedt, C., Malmqvist, N., Wadman, B.: Leukemia in workers exposed to ethylene oxide. *JAMA, 241:*1132-1133, 1979.
239. Brandt, L., Nilsson, P. G., and Mitelman, F.: Occupational exposure to petroleum products in men with acute non-lymphocytic leukemia. *Brit Med J, 1:*553, 1978.
240. Infante, P. F., Epstein, S. S., and Newton, W. A., Jr.: Blood dyscrasias and childhood tumors and exposure to Chlordane and Haptachlor. *Scand J Work Environ Health, 4:*137-150, 1978.
241. Bergsagel, D. E., Bailey, A. J., Langley, G. R., Macdonald, R. N., White, D. F., and Miller, A. B.: The chemotherapy on plasma-cell myeloma and the incidence of acute leukemia. *N Engl J Med, 301:*743-748, 1979.
242. Blythe, J. C.: Acute leukemia after Melphalan treatment for ovarian carcinoma. *J Med Assoc State Ala, 47:*42-43, 1977.
243. Brauer, M. J., and Dameshek, W.: Hypoplastic anemia and myeloblastic leukemia following chloramphenicol therapy. *N Engl J Med, 277:*1003, 1967.
244. Casciato, D. A., and Scott, J. L.: Acute leukemia following prolonged cytotoxic agent therapy. *Medicine, 58:*32-47, 1979.
245. Cohen, T., and Greger, W. P.: Acute myeloid leukemia following seven years of aplastic anemia induced by Chloramphenicol. *Am J Med, 43:*762-770, 1967.
246. Dougan, L., and Woodliff, A. J.: Acute leukemia associated with phenylbutazone treatment: A review of the literature and report of a further case. *Med J Aust, 1:*217, 1965.
247. Einhorn, N.: Acute leukemia after chemotherapy (Melphalan). *Cancer, 41:*444-447, 1978.
248. Greenspan, E. M., and Tung, B. G.: Acute myeloblastic leukemia after cure of ovarian cancer. *JAMA, 230:*418, 1974.
249. Kapadia, S. B., Krause, J. R., Ellis, L. D., Pan, S. F., and Wald, N.: Induced acute non-lymphocytic leukemia following long-term chemotherapy. A study of 2C cases. *Cancer, 45:*1315-1321, 1980.
250. Kaslow, R. A., Wisch, N., and Glass, J. I.: Acute leukemia following cytotoxic chem- otherapy. *JAMA, 219:*75, 1972.
251. Lawler, S. D., and Lele, K. P.: Chromosomal damage induced by chlorambucil ir chronic lymphocytic leukemia. *Scand J Haematol, 9:*603-612, 1972.
252. Morrison, J., and Yon, J. L.: Acute leukemia following chlorambucil therapy o advanced ovarian and fallopian tube carcinoma. *Gynecol Onchol, 6:*115-120, 1978
253. Penn, I.: Leukemias and lymphomas associated with the use of cytotoxic and im- munosuppressive drugs. *Recent Results Cancer Res, 69:*7-13, 1979.
254. Rosner, F., Grunwald, H. W., and Zarrabi, M. H.: Acute leukemia as a complication o cytotoxic chemotherapy. *Int J Radiat Oncol Biol Phys, 5:*1705-1707, 1979.
255. Stott, H., Fox, W., Girling, D. J., Stephens, R. J., and Galton, D. A.: Acute leukemi after Busulphan. *Br Med J, 2:*1513-1517, 1977.
256. Baikie, A. G., Court-Brown, W. M., Buckton, K. E., Harnden, D. G., Jacobs, P. A., anc Tough, I. M.: A possible specific chromosome abnormality in human chroni myeloid leukaemia. *Nature, 188:*1165, 1960.
257. Fitzgerald, P. F., Pickering, A. F., and Elby, J. R.: Clonal origin of the Philadelphi chromosome and chronic myeloid leukemia: Evidence from a sex chromosom mosaic. *Br J Haematol, 21:*473-480, 1971.

258. Forrester, R. H., and Louro, J. M.: Philadelphia chromosome abnormality in agnogenic myeloid metaplasia. *Ann Intern Med, 64:*622-627, 1966.
259. Goh, K., and Swisher, S. N.: Specificity of the Philadelphia chromosome: Cytogenic studies in cases of chronic myelocytic leukemia and myeloid metaplasia. *Ann Intern Med, 61:*609, 1964.
260. Goh, K. O., Swisher, S. N., and Herman, E. C., Jr.: Chronic myelocytic leukemia and identical twins. Additional evidence of the Philadelphia chromosome as postzygotic abnormality. *Arch Intern Med, 120:*214-219, 1967.
261. Goh, K. O., Lee, H., and Miller, G.: Down's syndrome and leukemia: Mechanism of additional chromosomal abnormalities. *Am J Ment Defic, 82:*542-548, 1978.
262. Hayata, I., Sakuraz, M., Kakati, S., and Sandberg, A. A.: Chromosomes and causation of human cancer and leukemia. XVI. Banding studies of chronic myelocytic leukemia, including five unusual ph[1]translocations, *Cancer, 36:*1177, 1975.
263. Hoshino, T., Kato, H., Finch, S. S., and Hrubec, Z.: Leukemia in offspring of atomic bomb survivors. *Blood, 30:*719-730, 1967.
264. Jacobs, E. M., Luce, J. K., and Cailleau, R.: Chromosome abnormalities in human cancer: Report of patient with chronic myelocytic leukemia and his non-leukemic monozygotic twin. *Cancer, 19:*869, 1966.
265. Kamada, N., Okada, K., Ito, T., Nakatsui, T., and Tomanaga, M.: Chromosome aberrations and neutrophile alkaline phosphatase in forty-three cases of leukemia, including fourteen cases of leukemia in atomic bomb survivors. *J Kyushu Hematol Soc, 17:*116-143, 1967.
266. Kiossoglou, K. A., Rosenbaum, E. H., Mitus, W. J., and Dameshek, W.: Multiple chromosomal aberrations in a Down's syndrome and twinning. Study of a family with a possible tendency to nondisjunction. *Blood, 24:*134-159, 1964.
267. Krauss, S., Sokal, J. E., and Sandberg, A. A.: Comparison of Philadelphia chromosome-positive and negative patients with chronic myelocytic leukemia. *Ann Intern Med, 61:*625, 1964.
268. Prigogina, E. L., Fleischman, E. W., Puchkova, G. P., Kulagina, O. E., Majakova, S. A., Balakirev, S. A., Frenkel, M. A., Khvatova, N. V., and Peterson, I. S.: Chromosomes in acute leukemia. *Hum Genet, 53:*5-16, 1979.
269. Rowley, J. D.: A new consistent chromosomal abnormality in chronic myelogenous leukaemia identified by quinacrine fluorescence and giemsa staining. *Nature, 243:*290-293, 1973.
270. Rowley, J. D.: Chromosome changes in acute leukemia. *Br J Haematol, 44:*339-346, 1980.
271. Sandberg, A. A., Ishihara, T., Crosswhite, L. H., and Hauschka, T. S.: Comparison of chromosome constitution in chronic myelocytic leukemia and other myeloproliferative disorders. *Blood, 20:*393, 1962.
272. Sandberg, A. A., Ishihara, T., Kikuchi, Y., and Crosswhite, L. H.: Chromosome differences among the acute leukemias. *Ann N Y Acad Sci, 113:*663, 1974.
273. Sandberg, A. A., Takagi, N., Sofuni, T., and Crosswhite, L. H.: Chromosome and causation of human cancer and leukemia. Karyotypic aspects of acute leukemia. *Cancer, 22:*1268-1282, 1968.
274. Tijo, J. H., Carbone, P., Whang, J., and Frei, E.: The Philadelphia chromosome and chronic myelogenous leukemia. *J Natl Cancer Inst, 36:*567, 1966.
275. Weinstein, H. J.: Congenital leukemia and the neonatal myeloproliferative disorders associated with Down's syndrome. *Clin Haematol, 7:*147-154, 1978.
276. Whang, J., Frei, E., III, Tijo, J. H., Carbone, P. P., and Brecker, G.: The distribution of the Philadelphia chromosome in patients with chronic myelogenic leukemia. *Blood, 22:*664, 1963.

277. Baxt, W., Hehlman, R., and Spiegelman, S.: Human leukemic cells contain reverse transcriptase associated with a high molecular weight virus-related RNA. *Nature, 244:*72, 1972.
278. Bryan, W. R., Moloney, J. B., O'Connor, T. E., Fink, M. A., and Dalton, A. J.: Viral etiology of leukemia. *Ann Intern Med, 62:*376-399, 1965.
279. Burger, C. L., Harris, W. N., Anderson, N. G., Bartlett, T. W., and Kniseley, R. M.: Virus-like particles in human leukemic plasma. *Proc Soc Exp Biol Med, 115:*151, 1964.
280. Gallagher, R. E., and Gallo, R. C.: Type C RNA tumor virus isolated from cultured human acute myelogenous leukemia cells. *Science, 187:*350, 1975.
281. Gross, L.: Viral etiology of leukemia and lymphomas. *Blood, 25:*377-381, 1965.
282. Henle, W.: Evidence for viruses in acute leukemia and Burkitt's tumor. *Cancer, 21:*580-586, 1968.
283. Jarrett, W. F. H.: Viruses and leukemia. *Br J Haematol, 25:*287, 1973.
284. Maduros, B. P., and Schwartz, S. O.: Viral etiology of leukemia. *Adv Intern Med, 11:*107, 1962.
285. Mak, T. W., Kurtz, S., Manaster, J., and Houseman, D.: Viral-related information on oncho-RNA virus-like particles isolated from cultures of marrow cells from leukemic patients in relapse and remission. *Proc Natl Acad Sci, 72:*623, 1975.
286. Meyskens, F. L., Jr., Jones, S. E., and Thoeny, R. H.: Tumor viruses and human cancer. Leukemia and RNA tumor viruses. *Ariz Med, 34:*763-766, 1977.
287. Newell, G. R., Harris, W. W., Bowman, K. O., Boone, C. W., and Anderson, N. G.: Evaluation of "virus-like" particles in the plasma of 255 patients with leukemia and related diseases. *N Engl J Med, 278:*1185-1191, 1968.
288. Cherr, C. J., and Todaro, C. J.: Primate type-C virus P30 antigen in cells from humans with acute leukemia. *Science, 187:*855, 1975.
289. Fialkow, P. J., Thomas, E. D., Bryant, J. I., and Neiman, P. E.: Leukaemic transformation of engrafted human marrow cells *in vivo. Lancet, 1:*251, 1971.
290. Thomas, E. D., Bryant, J. I., and Buckner, C. D.: Leukemic transformation of human marrow cells *in vivo. Lancet, 1:*1310, 1972.
291. Anderson, R. C.: Familial leukemia: A report of leukemia in five siblings, with a brief review of the genetic aspects of this disease. *Am J Dis Child, 81:*313, 1951.
292. Fitzgerald, P. H., Crossen, P. E., Adams, A. C., Sharman, C. V., and Gunz, F. W.: Chromosome studies in familial leukemia. *J Med Genet, 3:*96, 1966.
293. Gunz, F. W., and Dameshek, W.: Chronic lymphocytic leukemia in a family, including twin brothers and a son. *JAMA, 164:*1323, 1957.
294. Gunz, F. W., Fitzgerald, P. H., Crossen, P. H., Crossen, P. E., Mackenzie, I. S., Powles, C. P., and Jensen, G. R.: Multiple cases of leukemia in a sibship. *Blood, 27:*482, 1966.
295. Gunz, F. W., and Veale, A. M. O.: Leukemia in close relatives — accident or predisposition? *J Natl Cancer Inst, 42:*517, 1969.
296. Hornbaker, J. H.: Chronic leukemia in three sisters. *Am J Med Sci, 203:*322,1942.
297. MacMahon, B., and Levy, M. A.: Prenatal origin of childhood leukemia: Evidence from twins. *N Engl J Med, 270:*1082, 1964.
298. McPhedran, P., Heath, C. W., Jr., and Lee, J.: Patterns of familial leukemia. *Cancer, 24:*403, 1969.
299. Miller, R. W.: Deaths from childhood cancer in sibs. *N Engl J Med, 279:*122, 1968.
300. Reilly, E. B., Rappaport, S. I., Karr, N. W., Mills, H., and Carpenter, G. E.: Familial chronic lymphatic leukemia. *Arch Intern Med, 90:*87, 1952.
301. Rigby, P. G., Pratt, P. T., Rosenlof, R. C., and Lemon, H. M.: Genetic relationships in familial leukemia and lymphoma. *Arch Intern Med, 121:*67, 1968.

302. Gunz, F. W., and Baikie, A. G.: *Leukemia,* 3rd ed. New York, Grune and Stratton, 1974.
303. Cutler, S. J., and Young, J. L. (Eds.): *Third National Cancer Survey: Incidence Data.* Department of Health, Education, and Welfare, Bethesda, Md., 1975.
304. Lowenbraun, S., Sutherland, J. C., Feldman, M. J., and Serpick, A. A.: Transformation of reticulum cell sarcoma to acute leukemia. *Cancer, 27:*579-585, 1971.
305. Lynfield, V. L., Esseesse, I., Dorf, B., and Paltzik, R.: Mycosis fungoides terminating in acute myelomonocytic leukemia. *N Y State J Med, 80:*798-800, 1980.
306. Newmann, D. R., Maldonado, J. E., Harrison, E. G., Jr., Kiely, J. M., and Linman, J. W.: Myelomonocytic leukemia in Hodgkin's disease. *Cancer, 25:*128-134, 1970.
307. Powers, J. S., Lee, J. S., Nosanchuk, J. S., and Lee, J. C.: Acute leukemia complicating Hodgkin's disease. *J Pediat, 93:*323-324, 1978.
308. Prokocimer, M., Matzner, Y., Ben-Bassat, H., and Polliack, A.: Burkitt's lymphoma presenting as acute leukemia (Burkitt's lymphoma cell leukemia): Report of two cases in Israel. *Cancer, 45:*2884-2889, 1980.
309. Sahaxian, G. J., Al-Mondhiry, H., Lacher, M. J., and Connolly, C. E.: Acute leukemia in Hodgkin's disease. *Cancer, 33:*1369, 1974.
310. Schrek, R., and Donnelly, W. J.: Cytology in lymphosarcoma cell leukemia. *Am J Clin Pathol, 55:*646, 1971.
311. Schwartz, D. L., Pierre, R. V., Scheerer, P. P., Reed, E. C., and Linman, J. W.: Lymphosarcoma cell leukemia. *Am J Med, 38:*778, 1972.
312. Saleem, A., and Johnston, R. L.: Acute lymphoblastic leukemia following Hodgkin's disease. *Ann Clin Lab Sci, 10:*100-104, 1980.
313. Sternberg, M. H., Geary, C. G., and Crosby, W. H.: Acute granulocytic leukemia complicating Hodgkin's disease. *Arch Intern Med, 125:*496, 1970.
314. Sullivan, M. P.: Leukemic transformation on lymphosarcoma of childhood. *Pediatrics, 29:*589, 1962.
315. Zaccaria, A., Baccarani, M., Lauria, F., Fiachini, M., Mazza, P., and Tura, S.: Acute leukemia in patients treated for Hodgkin's disease: Report of two cases. *Haematologica* (Pravia), *64:*455-462, 1979.
316. Zeffren, J. L., and Ultmann, J. E.: Reticulum cell sarcoma terminating in acute leukemia. *Blood, 15:*277-284, 1960.
317. Forbes, I. J.: Development of acute leukemia in Waldenstrom's macroglobulinaemia after prolonged treatment with chlorambucil. *Med J Aust, 1:*918, 1972.
318. Rosner, F., and Grunwald, H. W.: Multiple myeloma and Waldenstrom's macroglobulinemia terminating in acute leukemia. Review with emphasis on karyotypic and ultrastructural abnormalities. *N Y State J Med, 80:*558-570, 1980.
319. Landaw, S. A.: Acute leukemia in polycythemia vera. *Semin Hematol, 13:*33, 1976.
320. Lawrence, J. H., Winchell, H. S., and Donald, W. G.: Leukemia in polycythemia vera: Relationship to splenic myeloid metaplasia and therapeutic radiation dose. *Ann Intern Med, 70:*763, 1969.
321. Masouredis, S. P., and Lawrence, J. H.: The problem of leukemia in polycythemia vera. *Am J Med Sci, 233:*268, 1957.
322. Modan, B., and Lilienfeld, A. M.: Polycythemia vera and leukemia — The role of radiation treatment. *Medicine, 44:*305, 1965.
323. Osgood, E. E.: Contrasting incidence of acute monocytic and granulocytic leukemias in P32 treated patients with polycythemia vera and chronic lymphocytic leukemia. *J Lab Clin Med, 64:*560, 1964.
324. Schwartz, S. O., and Ehrich, L.: The relationship of polycythemia vera to leukemia: A critical review. *Acta Hematol, 4:*129, 1950.

325. Walsh, J. R.: Polycythemia vera: Diagnosis, treatment, and relationship to leukemia. *Geriatrics, 33:*66-69, 1978.
326. Weinfeld, A., Westin, J., Ridell, B., and Swolin, B.: Polycythemia vera terminating in acute leukemia. A clinical, cytogenetic and morphologic study in 8 patients treated with alkylating agents. *Scand J Haematol, 19:*255-272, 1977.
327. Heaton, A., and Kahn, L. B.: Acute lymphocytic leukemia terminating in malignant histocytosis. A case report and literature review. *S Afr Med J, 57:*502-507, 1980.
328. Wick, M. R., Li, C. Y., Ludwig, J., Levitt, R., and Pierre, R. V.: Malignant histocytosis as a terminal condition in chronic lymphocytic leukemia. *Mayo Clin Proc, 55:*108-112, 1980.
329. Beard, M., Gauci, C., Sikora, R., Kirk, B., and Fairley, G. H.: Blast crisis of chronic myeloid leukaemia: The effect of intensive chemotherapy. *Scand J Haematol, 16:*258, 1976.
330. Bornstein, R. S., Nesbit, M., and Kennedy, B. J.: Chronic myelogenous leukemia presenting in blastic crisis. *Cancer, 30:*939, 1972.
331. Canellos, G. P., Devita, V. T., Wang-Peng, J., Chabner, B. A., Schein, P. S., and Young, R. C.: Chemotherapy of the blastic phase of chronic granulocytic leukemia: Hypodiploidy and response to therapy. *Blood, 47:*1003, 1976.
332. Hayes, D. M., Ellison, R. R., Glidewell, O., Holland, J. F., and Silver, R. T.: Chemotherapy for the terminal phase of chronic myelocytic leukemia. *Cancer Chemother Rep, 58:*233, 1974.
333. Peterson, L. C., Bloomfield, C. D., and Bruming, R. D.: Blast crisis as an initial or terminal manifestation of chronic myeloid leukemia: A study of 28 patients. *Am J Med, 60:*209, 1976.
334. Pretlow, T. G.: Chronic monocytic dyscrasia culminating in acute leukemia. *Am J Med, 46:*130, 1969.
335. Spiers, A. S. D., Costello, C., Catovsky, D., Galton, D. A. G., and Goldman, J. M.: Chronic granulocytic leukemia: Multiple-drug chemotherapy for acute transformation. *Br Med J, 3:*77, 1974.
336. Krakoff, I. H., and Balis, M. E.: Abnormalities of purine metabolism in human leukemia. *Ann N Y Acad Sci, 113:*1043, 1964.
337. Muggia, F. M., Ball, T. T., Jr., and Ultmann, J. E.: Allopurinol in the treatment of neoplastic disease complicated by hypercalcemia. *Arch Intern Med, 120:*12-18 1967.
338. Rundles, R. W.: Uric acid metabolism in leukemia and lymphoma. In Zarofonetis C. J. D. (Ed.): *Proceedings of the International Conference on Leukemia-Lymphoma* Philadelphia, Lea & Febiger, 1968, p. 385.
339. Sandberg, A. A., Cartwright, C. E., and Wintrobe, M. M.: Study on leukemia. I. Uric acid excretion. *Blood, 11:*154, 1956.
340. Yu, T.: Secondary gout associated with myeloproliferative diseases. *Arthritis Rheum 8:*765, 1965.
341. Benvenisti, D. S., Sherwood, L. M., and Heinemann, H. O.: Hypercalcemic crisis in acute leukemia. *Am J Med, 46:*979, 1969.
342. Burt, M. E., and Brennan, M. F.: Incidence of hypercalcemia and malignant neoplasm. *Arch Surg, 115:*704-707, 1980.
343. Haskell, C. M., Devita, V. T., and Canellos, G. P.: Hypercalcemia in chronic granulocytic leukemia. *Cancer, 27:*872-880, 1971.
344. Clarkson, D. R., Blondin, J., and Cryer, P. E.: Phosphate depletion and glucocorticoid induced hyperphosphatemia in lymphoblastic leukemia. *Metabolism, 22:*611 1973.

345. Jaffe, N., Kim, B. S., and Vawter, G. F.: Hypocalcemia: A complication of childhood leukemia. *Cancer, 29:*392, 1972.
346. Zusman, J., Brown, B. M., and Nesbitt, M. E.: Hyperphosphatemia, hyperphosphaturia, and hypocalcemia in acute lymphoblastic leukemia. *N Engl J Med, 289:*1335, 1973.
347. Brakman, P., Snyder, J., Henderson, E. S., and Astrup, T.: Blood coagulation and fibrinolysis in acute leukemia. *Br J Haematol, 18:*135, 1970.
348. Dietrich, M., Rasche, H., and Kubanek, B.: Coagulation disorder in acute leukemia as a prognostic factor. *Adv Biosci, 14:*175, 1975.
349. Gralnick, H., and Henderson, E. S.: Acquired coagulation factor deficiencies in leukemia. *Cancer, 26:*1097, 1970.
350. Rand, J. J., Moloney, W. C., and Sise, H. S.: Coagulation defects in acute promyelocytic leukemia. *Arch Intern Med, 123:*39-47, 1969.
351. Rasche, H., Dietrich, M., Gaus, W., and Schleyer, M.: Factor XIII activity and fibrin subunit structure in acute leukemia. *Biomedicine, 21:*61, 1974.
352. McKee, C., Jr., and Collins, R. D.: Intracellular leukocyte thrombi and aggregates as a cause of morbidity and mortality in leukemia. *Medicine, 53:*463, 1974.
353. Beard, M. F., Pitney, R. W., and Sanneman, E. H.: Serum concentrations of vitamin B12 in patients suffering from leukemia. *Blood, 9:*789, 1954.
354. Beard, M. F., Pitney, R. W., Sanneman, E. H., Kakol, M. J., and Moorhead, H. H.: Serum concentrations of vitamin B12 in acute leukemia. *Ann Intern Med, 41:*323, 1954.
355. Hall, C. A.: The plasma disappearance of radioactive Vitamin B12 in myeloproliferative diseases and other blood disorders. *Blood, 18:*717, 1961.
356. Weinstein, I. B., and Watkin, D. M.: Co^{58} B12 absorption, plasma transport and excretion in patients with myeloproliferative disorders, solid tumors, and nonneoplastic diseases. *J Clin Invest, 39:*1667, 1960.
357. Burns, C. P.: Serum-muramidase in leukemic reticuloendotheliosis. *Lancet, 2:*964, 1974.
358. Catovsky, D., Galton, D. A. G., and Griffin, C.: The significance of lysozyme estimations in acute myeloid and chronic monocytic leukemia. *Br J Haematol, 21:*565, 1971.
359. Firkin, F. C.: Serum muramidase in haematological disorders: Diagnostic value in neoplasmic states. *Aust N Z J Med, 1:*28, 1972.
360. Malmquist, J.: Serum and urinary lysozyme in leukemia and polycythemia vera. *Scand J Haematol, 9:*258, 1972.
361. Perillie, P. E., and Finch, S. C.: Muramidase studies in Philadelphia-chromosome-positive and chromosome-negative chronic granulocytic leukemia. *N Engl J Med, 283:*456, 1970.
362. Youman, J. D., Saarni, M. I., and Linman, J. W.: Diagnostic value of muramidase (lysozyme) in acute leukemia and preleukemia. *Mayo Clin Pro, 45:*219, 1970.
363. Baty, J. M., and Vogt, E. C.: Bone changes of leukemia in children. *Am J Roentgenol, 34:*310, 1935.
364. Brunner, S., Gubjerg, C. E., and Iversen, T.: Skeletal lesions in leukaemia in children. *Acta Radiol Stockh, 49:*419, 1958.
365. Campbell, E., Jr., Maldonado, W., and Suhrland, G.: Painful lytic bone lesion in an adult with chronic myelogenous leukemia. *Cancer, 35:*1354, 1975.
366. Chabner, B. A., Haskell, C. M., and Canellos, G. P.: Destructive bone lesions in chronic granulocytic leukemia. *Medicine, 48:*401, 1969.

367. Craver, L. F., and Copeland, M. M.: Changes of the bones in the leukemias. *Arch Surg, 30:*639, 1935.
368. Dresner, E.: The bone and joint lesions in acute leukaemia and their response to folic acid antagonists. *Quart J Med, 19:*339, 1950.
369. Erb, I. H.: Bone changes in leukemia. Part II. Pathology. *Arch Dis Childhood, 9:*319, 1934.
370. Follis, R. H., Jr., and Park, E. H.: Some observations on the morphologic basis for the roentgenographic changes in childhood leukemia. *Bull Hosp Joint Dis, 12:*67, 1951.
371. Jaffe, H. L.: Skeletal manifestations of leukemia and malignant lymphoma. *Bull Hosp Joint Dis, 13:*217, 1952.
372. Kalayjian, B. S., Herbut, P. A., and Erf, L. A.: The bone changes of leukemia in children. *Radiology, 47:*223, 1946.
373. Nixon, G. W., and Gwinn, J. L.: The roentgen manifestations of leukemia in infancy. *Radiology, 107:*603, 1973.
374. Pear, B. L.: Skeletal manifestations of the lymphomas and leukemias. *Semin Roentgenol, 9:*229-240, 1974.
375. Pettigrew, J. D., and Ward, H. P.: Correlation of radiologic, histiologic and clinical findings in agnogenic myeloid metaplasia. *Radiology, 93:*541, 1969.
376. Poynton, F. J., and Lightwood, R.: Lymphatic leukaemia, with infiltration of periosteum simulating acute rheumatism. *Lancet, 1:*1192, 1932.
377. Silberstein, M. J., Tangshewinsirikul, P., Chu, J. Y., and Graviss, E. R.: Bone changes in a neonate with congenital anemia. *Radiology, 131:*370, 1979.
378. Silverman, F. N.: The skeletal lesions in leukemia. *Am J Roentgenol, 59:*819, 1948.
379. Silverstein, M. N., and Kelly, P. J.: Leukemia with osteoarticular symptoms and signs. *Ann Int Med, 59:*637, 1963.
380. Simmons, C. R., Harle, T. S., and Singleton, E. B.: The osseous manifestations of leukemia in children. *Radiol Clin N A, 6:*115, 1968.
381. Snelling, C. E., and Brown, A.: Bone changes in leukemia. Part I. Clinical and roentgenological. *Arch Dis Childhood, 9:*315, 1934.
382. Sussman, M. L.: Myelosclerosis with leukoerythroblastic anemia. *Am J Roentgenol, 57:*313, 1947.
383. Thomas, L. B., Forkner, C. E., Jr., Feri, E., III, Besse, B. E., Jr., and Stabenau, J. R.: The skeletal lesions of acute leukemia. *Cancer, 14:*608, 1961.
384. Willson, J. K. V.: The bone lesions of childhood leukemia. *Radiology, 72:*672, 1959.
385. Hayhoe, F. G. J., and Cawley, J. C.: Acute leukemia: Cellular morphology, cytochemistry and fine structure. *Clin Haematol, 1:*49, 1972.
386. Hayhoe, F. G. J., Quagliano, D., and Doll, R.: *The Cytology and Cytochemistry of Acute Leukemias.* London, H. M. Stationery Office, 1964.
387. Kaplow, L. S.: Simplified myeloperoxidase stain using benzidine dihydrochloride *Blood, 26:*215, 1965.
388. Kaplow, L. S.: Substitute for benzidine in myeloperoxidase stains. *Am J Clin Pathol 63:*451, 1975.
389. Kaplow, L. S.: Cytochemistry of leukocyte alkaline phosphatase: Use of complex naphthol as phosphates in azo dye-coupling technics. *Am J Clin Pathol, 39:*439 1963.
390. Kaplow, L. S., and Burstone, M. S.: Acid-buffered acetone as a fixative for enzyme cytochemistry. *Nature, 200:*690, 1963.
391. Lillie, R. D., and Burtner, H. J.: Stable sudanophilia of human neutrophil leukocytes in relation to peroxidase and oxidase. *J Histochem Cytochem, 1:*8, 1953.

2. Sheehan, H. L., and Storey, G. W.: An improved method of staining leukocyte granules with Sudan black B. *J Pathol Bact, 59:*336, 1947.
3. Astaldi, G., Ronahelli, E. G., Birnardelli, E., and Strosselli, E.: An abnormal substance present in the erythroblasts of thalassemia major: Cytochemical investigations. *Acta Haematol, 12:*145, 1954.
4. Astaldi, G., and Verga, L.: The glycogen content of the cells of lymphatic leukaemia. *Acta Haematol, 17:*129, 1957.
5. Catovsky, D., Galetto, J., Okos, A., Miliani, E., and Galton, D. A. G.: Cytochemical profile of B and T leukemic lymphocytes with special reference to acute lymphoblastic leukemia. *J Clin Pathol, 27:*767, 1974.
6. Humphrey, G. B., Nesbit, M. E., and Brunning, R. D.: Prognostic value of the Periodic-Acid-Schiff (PAS) reaction in acute lymphoblastic leukemia. *Am J Clin Pathol, 61:*393, 1974.
7. Quagliano, D., and Hayhoe, F. G. J.: Observations on the Periodic Acid Schiff reaction in lymphoproliferative diseases. *J Pathol Bact, 78:*521, 1959.
8. Schmalzl, F., Hohn, D., Abbrederis, K., and Braunsteiner, H.: Acute lymphocytic leukemia: Cytochemistry and ultrastructure. *Blut, 29:*87, 1974.
9. Burstone, M. S.: Histochemical demonstration of acid phosphatase with naphthol AS-phosphate. *J Natl Cancer Inst, 21:*523, 1958.
0. Kaplow, L. S., and Burstone, M. S.: Cytochemical demonstration of acid phosphatase in hematopoietic cells in health and in various hematological disorders using Azo dye techniques. *J Histochem Cytochem, 12:*805, 1964.
1. Katayama, I., Li, C. Y., and Yam, L. T.: Histochemical study of acid phosphatase isoenzyme in leukemic reticuloendotheliosis. *Cancer, 29:*157, 1972.
2. Yam, L. T., Li, C. Y., and Finkel, H. T.: Leukemic reticuloendotheliosis: The role of tartrate-resistant acid phosphatase in diagnosis and splenectomy in treatment. *Arch Intern Med, 130:*248, 1972.
3. Li, C. Y., Lam, K. W., and Yam, L. T.: Esterases in human leukocytes. *J Histochem Cytochem, 21:*1, 1973.
4. Moloney, W. C., McPherson, K., and Fliegelman, L.: Esterase activity in leukocytes demonstrated by the use of naphthol AS-D chloroacetate substrate. *J Histochem Cytochem, 8:*200, 1960.
5. Rosenszajn, L., Leibovich, M., Shoham, D., and Epstein, J.: The esterase activity in megaloblasts, leukemic and normal hematopoietic cells. *Br J Haematol, 14:*605, 1962.
6. Schmalzl, F., and Braunsteiner, H.: The application of cytochemical methods to the study of acute leukemia. *Acta Haematol, 45:*209, 1971.
7. Yam, L. T., Li, C. Y., and Crosby, W. H.: Cytochemical identification of monocytes and granulocytes. *Am J Clin Pathol, 55:*283, 1971.
8. Prockop, D. J., and Davidson, W. D.: A study of urinary and serum lysozyme in patients with renal disease. *N Engl J Med, 240:*269, 1964.
9. Pruzanski, W., and Platts, M. E.: Serum and urinary proteins, lysozyme (muramidase), and renal dysfunction in mono- and myelomonocytic leukemia. *J Clin Invest, 49:*1694, 1970.
0. Silberstein, E. B.: Radionuclide therapy of hematologic disorders. *Semin Nucl Med, 9:*100-107, 1979.
1. Wallner, P.: Radiation therapy of malignant disease. *JAOA, 77:*606-621, 1978.
2. Gale, R. P., Opelz, G., Mickey, M. R., Graze, P. R., Saxon, A.: Immunodeficiency following allogenic bone marrow transplantation. *Transplant Proc, 10:*223-227, 1978.

413. Glasser, L.: Phagocytosis in acute leukemia. *Cancer, 45:*1365-1369, 1980.
414. Henon, P., Gerota, I., and Palacios, S.: Functional abnormalities of neutrophils i cancer patients: Inefficient phagocytosis and reverse endocytosis. *Biomedicir Express, 27:*261-266, 1977.
415. Louie, S., and Schwartz, R. S.: Immunodeficiency and the pathogenesis of lymphom and leukemia. *Semin Hematol, 15:*117-138, 1978.
416. Nachman, J. B., and Honig, G. R.: Fever and neutropenia in children with neoplast disease: An analysis of 158 episodes. *Cancer, 45:*407-412, 1980.
417. Aisner, J., Murillo, J., Schimpff, S. C., and Steere, A. C.: Invasive aspergillosis in acut leukemia: Correlation with nose cultures and antibiotic use. *Ann Intern Me 90:*4-9, 1979.
418. Atkinson, K., Storb, R., Prentice, R. L., Weiden, P. L., Witherspoon, R. P., Sullivar K., Noel, D., and Thomas, E. D.: Analysis of late infections in 89 long-terr survivors of bone marrow transplantation. *Blood, 53:*720-731, 1979.
419. Bodey, G. P.: Fungal infections complicating acute leukemia. *J Chron Dis, 19:*66 1966.
420. Bodey, G. P., Nies, B. A., and Freireich, E. J.: Multiple organism septicemia and acut leukemia. *Arch Intern Med, 116:*266, 1965.
421. Bodey, G. P., Rodriguez, V., Valdivieso, M., and Keating, M.: Gram-negative baci lary infections in cancer patients. *S Afr Med J, 52:*1049-1055, 1977.
422. Burgess, M. A., and DeGruchy, G. C.: Septicemia in acute leukemia. *Med J Aust 1:*1113, 1969.
423. Callen, P. W., Filly, R. A., and Marcus, F. S.: Ultrasonography and compute tomography in the evaluation of hepatic microabscesses in the immunosu pressed patient. *Radiology, 136:*433-434, 1980.
424. Cesario, T. C., Slater, L. M., Armentrout, S. A., Thrupp, L. D., and Tilles, J. G Septicemia in acute leukemia. *Med Pediatr Oncol, 5:*193-203, 1978.
425. Declerck, Y., Declerck, D., Rivard, G. E., and Benoit, P.: Septicemia in children wit leukemia. *Can Med Assoc J, 118:*1523-1526, 1978.
426. Favor, L. F., Tarpay, M., and Blackstock, R.: Septicemia in children with cancer. *Sout Med J, 72:*132-135, 1979.
427. Hoecker, J. L., Pickering, L. K., Groschel, D., and Kohl, S.: Streptococcus salivariu sepsis in children with malignancies. *J Pediatr, 92:*1145-1150, 1977.
428. Hoecker, J. L., Pickering, L. K., Groschel, D., Kohl, S., and Vaneys, J.: Curren concepts of bacteremia in children with malignancies. *Cancer, 44:*1939-194 1979.
429. King, K.: Septicemia in patients with haematological malignant disease. *Med J Aus 1:*603-606, 1980.
430. Koransky, J. R., Stargel, M. D., and Dowell, V. R., Jr.: Clostridium septicum ba teremia. Its clinical significance. *Am J Med, 66:*63-66, 1979.
431. Kosmidis, H. V., Lusher, J. M., Shope, T. C., Ravindranath, Y., and Dajani, A. S Infections in leukemic children: A prospective analysis. *J Pediatr, 96:*814-81 1980.
432. Ladisch, S. and Pizzo, P. A.: Staphylococcus aureus sepsis in children with cance *Pediatrics, 61:*231-234, 1978.
433. Mackie, P. H., Crockson, R. A., and Stuart, J.: C-reactive protein for rapid diagnos of infection in leukaemia. *J Clin Pathol, 32:*1253-1256, 1979.
434. Masur, H., Rosen, P. P., Armstrong, D.: Pulmonary disease caused by Candid species. *Am J Med, 63:*914-925, 1977.
435. Milligan, D. W., Kelly, J. K.: Pseudomembranous colitis in a leukaemic unit: A repo of five fatal cases. *J Clin Pathol, 32:*1237-1243, 1979.

436. Mirsky, H. S., and Cuttner, J.: Fungal infections in acute leukemia. *Cancer, 30:*348-352, 1972.
437. Neiman, P. E., Reeves, W., Ray, G., Flournoy, N., Lerner, K. G., Sale, G. E., and Thomas, E. D.: A prospective analysis — interstitial pneumonia and opportunistic viral infection among recipients of allogenic bone marrow grafts. *J Infect Dis, 136:*754-767, 1977.
438. Novak, R., and Feldman, S.: Salmonellosis in children with cancer: Review of 42 cases. *Am J Dis Child, 133:*298-300, 1979.
439. Rosen, P. P.: Cytomegalovirus infection in cancer patients. *Pathol Annu, 13:*175-208, 1978.
440. Singer, M. I., and House, J. L.: Invasive mycotic infections in the immunocompromised child. *Otolaryngol Head Neck Surg, 87:*32-34, 1979.
441. Watanabe, A., Higashi, T., Endo, H., and Nagashima, H.: Fulminant hepatic failure during remission from leukemia: Three cases associated with massive liver cell necrosis and hepatitis B virus. *Acta Med Okayama, 33:*245-257, 1979.
442. Wingard, J. R., Merz, W. G., and Saral, R.: Candida tropicalis: A major pathogen in immunocompromised patients. *Ann Intern Med, 91:*539-543, 1979.
443. Frei, E., Levin, R. H., Bodey, G. P., Morse, E. E., and Freireich, E. J.: The nature and control of infections in patients with acute leukemia. *Cancer Res, 25:*1511, 1965.
444. Lantz, B., and Reizenstein, P.: Management of septicemia and early death in acute leukemia. *Acta Med Scand, 202:*523-528, 1977.
445. Levine, A. S., Schimpff, S. C., Graw, R. G., Jr., and Young, R. C.: Haematologic malignancies and other marrow failure states: Progress in the management of complicating infections. *Semin Haemat, 11:*141, 1974.
446. Keating, M. J., and Penington, D. G.: Prophylaxis against septicemia in acute leukemia: The use of oral Framycetin. *Med J Austr, 2:*213, 1973.
447. Meyers, B. R., Wormser, G., Hirschman, S. Z., and Blitzer, A.: Rhinocerebral mucomycosis: Premortem diagnosis and therapy. *Arch Intern Med, 139:*557-560, 1979.
448. Mortensen, B. T., Mortensen, N., and Nissen, N. I.: Clinical experience with bacteraemia in patients with leukaemia and allied neoplastic diseases. *Chemotherapy, 24:*179-186, 1978.
449. Ortbals, D. W., Liebhaber, H., Presant, C. A., Van Amburg, A. D., and Lee, J. Y.: Influenza immunization of adult patients with malignant diseases. *Ann Intern Med, 87:*552-557, 1977.
450. Rodriguez, V., Bodey, G. P., Freireich, E. J., McCredie, K. B., Gutterman, J. U., Keating, M. J., Smith, T. L., and Gehan, E. A.: Randomized trial of protected environment-prophylactic antibiotics in 145 adults with acute leukemia. *Medicine, 57:*253-266, 1978.
451. Sinclair, A. J., Rossof, A. H., Coltman, C. A., Jr.: Recognition and successful management in pulmonary aspergillosis in leukemia. *Cancer, 42:*2019-2024, 1978.
452. Steinherz, P. G., Brown, A. E., Gross, P. A., Braun, D., Ghavimi, F., Wollner, N., Rosen, G., Armstrong, D., and Miller, D. R.: Influenza immunization of children with neoplastic diseases. *Cancer, 45:*750-756, 1980.
453. Sumaya, C. V., Williams, T. E., and Brunell, P. A.: Bivalent influenza vaccine in children with cancer. *J Infect Dis, 136:*656-660, 1977.
454. Winsnes, R.: Efficacy of zoster immunoglobulin in prophylaxis of varicella in high-risk patients. *Acta Paediatr Scand, 67:*77-82, 1978.
455. Buckner, C. D., Clift, R. A., Sanders, J. E., Meyers, J. D., Count, G. W., Farewell, V. T., and Thomas, E. D.: Protective environment for marrow transplant recipients: A prospective study. *Ann Intern Med, 89:*893-901, 1978.

456. Gaus, W., Wendt, F., and Wolf, G.: Protective isolation and antimicrobial decontamination in patients with high susceptibility to infection. A prospective cooperative study of gnotobiotic care in acute leukemia patients. II. Organizational and statistical concept. *Infection, 5:*248-254, 1977.

457. Kurrle, E., Bhaduri, S., Heipel, H., Hoelzer, D., Krieger, D., Vanek, E., and Kubanek, B.: The efficiency of strict reverse isolation and antimicrobial decontamination in remission induction therapy of acute leukemia. *Blut, 40:*187-195, 1980.

458. Levine, A. S., Siegel, S. E., Schreiber, A. D., Hauser, J., Preisler, H. D., Goldstein, I. M., Seidler, F., Simon, R., Perry, S., Bennett, J. E., and Henderson, E. S.: Protected environments and prophylactic antibiotics: A prospective controlled study of their utility in the treatment of acute leukemia. *N Engl J Med, 288:*477, 1973.

459. Pizzo, P. A., and Levine, A. S.: The utility of protected-environment regimens for the compromised host: A critical assessment. *Prog Hematol, 10:*311-332, 1977.

460. Schimpff, S. C., Greene, W. H., Young, V. M., Fortner, C. L., Jepsen, L., Lusback, N., Block, J. B., and Wiernick, P. H.: Infection prevention in acute non-lymphocytic leukemia: Laminar air flow room reverse isolation with oral nonabsorbable antibiotic prophylaxis. *Ann Intern Med, 82:*351, 1975.

461. Yates, J., and Holland, J. F.: A controlled study of isolation and endogenous microbial suppression in acute myelocytic leukemia patients. *Cancer, 32:*1490, 1973.

462. European Group of Bone Marrow Transplant: Symposium on Total Body Irradiation for Bone Marrow Transplantation. *Pathol Biol, 27:*317-318, 1979.

463. Peters, L. J., Withers, H. R., Cundiff, J. H., and Dicke, K. A.: Radiobiological considerations in the use of total-body irradiation for bone-marrow transplantation. *Radiology, 131:*243-247, 1979.

464. Schmitt, G., Schaeffer, U. W., Nowrousian, M. R., and Ohl, S.: Total body irradiation in conditioning patients for bone marrow transplantation. Irradiation technique and preliminary results at the West German Tumour Center, Universitatsklinikum Essen. *Pathol Biol, 27:*363-364, 1979.

465. Zwaan, F. E.: The role of total body irradiation in preparation for bone marrow transplantation in acute leukaemia. A review. *Pathol Biol, 27:*345-347, 1979.

466. Armitage, J. D., and Burns, C. P.: Treatment of refractory adult acute nonlymphoblastic leukemia with subcutaneous 5-Azacytidine. *Cancer Treat Rep, 61:*1721-1723, 1977.

467. Benjamin, R. S.: Adriamycin and other anthracycline antibiotics under study in the United States. *Recent Results Cancer Res, 63:*230-240, 1978.

468. Case, D. C., Jr.: Treatment of acute leukemia in adults. *J Maine Med Assoc, 69:*109-110, 1978.

469. Charron, D. L., Schmitt, T., and Degos, L.: Clinical investigation of lithium therapy in acute leukemia. *Adv Exp Med Biol, 127:*175-186, 1980.

470. Coltman, C. A., Jr., Bodey, G. P., Hewlett, J. S., Haut, A., Bickers, J., Balcerzak, S. P. Costani, J. J., Freireich, E. J., McCredie, K. B., Groppe, C., Smith, T. L., and Gehan, E. A.: Chemotherapy of acute leukemia: A comparison of vincristine cytarabine, and prednisone alone and in combination with cyclophosphamide or daunorubicin. *Arch Intern Med, 138:*1342-1348, 1978.

471. Davis, H. L., Jr., Von Hoff, D. D., Henny, J. E. and Rozencweig, M.: Role of antitumor antibiotics in current oncologic practice. *Recent Results Cancer Res 63:*21-29, 1978.

472. Ferrant, A., Hulhoven,R., Bosley, A., Cornu, G., Michaux, J. L., and Sokal, G.

Clinical trials with daunorubicin-DNA and adriamycin-DNA in acute lymphoblastic leukemia of childhood, acute nonlymphoblastic leukemia and bronchogenic carcinoma. *Cancer Chemother Pharmacol, 2:*67-71, 1979.

473. Griffin, T. W., Lister, T. A., Rybak, M. E., Rosenthal, D. S., Canellos, G. P., Woodruff, R., and Oliver, K. T.: Treatment of acute nonlymphocytic leukemia with neocarcinostatin. *Cancer Treat Rep, 63:*1853-1856, 1979.

474. Hewlett, J. S., Bodey, G. P., Wilson, H. E., and Stuckey, W. J.: Combination 6-Mercaptopurine and 6-Methylmercaptopurine Riboside in the treatment of adult acute leukemia: A southwest oncology group study. *Cancer Treat Rep, 63:*156-158, 1979.

475. Howell, S. B., Taetle, R., and Mendelsohn, J.: Thymidine as a chemotherapeutic agent: Sensitivity of normal human marrow, peripheral blood T cells, and acute nonlymphocytic leukemia. *Blood, 55:*505-510, 1980.

476. Lewis, B. J., Devita, V. T., Jr.: Combination chemotherapy of acute leukemia and lymphoma. *Pharmacol Ther, 7:*91-121, 1979.

477. Lippman, M. E.: Glucocorticoid receptors and effects in human lymphoid and leukemic cells. *Monogr Endocrinol, 12:*377-397, 1979.

478. Mandelli, F., Amadori, S., Fabiani, F., Grignani, F., Liso, V., Martelli, M., Neri, A., Petti, M. C., and Tonato, M.: Treatment of acute nonlymphocytic leukemia (ANLL) in elderly patients. Results of a multicentric study. *Haematologica* (Pavia), *64:*331-338, 1979.

479. Mandelli, F., Amadori, S., Pacilli, L., Tribalto, M.: Preliminary results of the combination methotrexate-asparaginase in patients with acute nonlymphoid leukemia. *Biomedicine Express, 29:*116-117, 1978.

480. Mathe, G., Misset, J. L., DeVassal, F., Gouveia, J., Hayat, M., Machover, D., Belpomme, D., Pico, J. L., Schwarzenberg, L., Ribaud, P., Musset, M., Jasmin, C., and DeLuca, L.: Phase II clinical trial with Vindesine for remission induction in acute leukemia, blastic crisis of chronic myeloid leukemia, lymphosarcoma, and Hodgkin's disease: Absence of cross-resistance with vincristine. *Cancer Treat Rep, 62:*800-809, 1978.

481. McKelvey, E. M., Burgess, M. A., McCredie, K. B., Murphy, W. K., and Bodey, G. P.: Neocarzinostatin: A phase I clinical trial with five-day intermittent and continuous infusions. *Cancer, 441:*1182-1188, 1979.

482. Peterson, B. A., Bloomfield, C. D., Bosl, G. J., Gibbs, G., and Malloy, M.: Intensive five drug combination chemotherapy for adult acute non-lymphocytic leukemia. *Cancer, 46:*663-668, 1980.

483. Prakash, U. B., Divertie, M. B., and Banks, P. M.: Aggressive therapy in acute respiratory failure from leukemic pulmonary infiltrates. *Chest, 75:*345-350, 1979.

484. Preisler, H. D., and Higby, D. J.: Therapy of acute nonlymphocytic leukemia: I. Clinical aspects. *N Y State J Med, 79:*879-884, 1979.

485. Richert-Boe, K. E., and Bagby, G. C., Jr.: Treating acute nonlymphocytic leukemia. *Geriatrics, 33:*50-55, 1978.

486. Rudnick, S. A., Cadman, E. C., Capizzi, R. L., Skeel, R. T., Bertino, Jr., and McIntosh, S.: High dose cytosine arabinoside (HDAEAC) in refractory acute leukemia. *Cancer, 44:*1189-1193, 1979.

487. Thompson, E. B., Norman, M. R., and Lippman, M. E.: Steroid hormone actions in tissue culture cells and cell hybrids — their relation to human malignancies. *Recent Prog Horm Res, 33:*571-615, 1976.

488. Von Hoff, D. D., Rozencweig, M. and Slavik, M.: Daunomycin: An anthracycline antibiotic effective in acute leukemia. *Adv Pharmacol Chemother, 15:*1-50, 1978.

489. Yap, B. S., McCredie, K. B., Benjamin, R. S., Bodey, G. P., Freireich, E. J.: Refractory acute leukemia in adults treated with sequential Colaspase and high-dose Methotrexate. *Br Med J, 2:*791-793, 1978.
490. Baldwin, R. W., Pimm, M. V.: BCG in tumor immunotherapy. *Adv Cancer Res, 28:*91-147, 1978.
491. Goodnight, J. E., and Morton, D. L.: Immunochemotherapy of cancer: Current status. *Prog Exp Tumor Res, 25:*61-88, 1980.
492. Leventhal, B. G., Mirro, J., Jr., and Yarbro, G. S.: Immune reactivity to tumor antigens in leukemia and lymphoma. *Semin Hematol, 15:*157-179, 1978.
493. Metzgar, R. S., and Mohanakumar, T.: Tumor-associated antigens of human leukemia cells. *Semin Hematol, 15:*139-156, 1978.
494. Minden, P., Odom, L. F., Tubergen, D. G., Hardtke, M. A., Sharpton, T. R., Rose, B., Zlotnick, A., and Carr, R. I.: Immune complexes in children with leukemia: Relationship to disease characteristics and to antibody response to mycobacterium bovis (BCG) in patients receiving BCG immunotherapy. *Cancer, 45:*60-68, 1980.
495. Morton, D. L., and Goodnight, J. E., Jr.: Clinical trials of immunotherapy: Present status. *Cancer, 42:*2224-2233, 1978.
496. Murphy, S., and Hersh, E.: Immunotherapy of leukemia and lymphoma. *Semin Hematol, 15:*181-203, 1978.
497. Beard, M. E.: Bone marrow transplantation: Technique and current indications. *N Z Med J, 91:*99-103, 1980.
498. Beatty, P. G., Oldham, R. K., and Greco, F. A.: Bone marrow transplantation — 1979. *J Tenn Med Assoc, 72:*361-364, 1979.
499. Beutler, E., Blume, K. G., Bross, K. J., Chillar, R. K., Ellington, O. B., Fahey, J. L., Farbstein, M. J., Schmidt, G. M., Spruce, W. E., and Turner, M. A.: Bone marrow transplantation as the treatment of choice for "good risk" adult patients with acute leukemia. *Trans Assoc Am Physicians, 92:*189-195, 1979.
500. Blume, K. G., Beutler, E., Bross, K. J., Chillar, R. K., Ellington, O. B., Fahey, J. L., Farbstein, M. J., Forman, S. L., Schmidt, G. M., Scott, E. P., Spruce, W. E., Turner, M. A., and Wolf, J. L.: Bone-marrow ablation and allogenic marrow transplantation in acute leukemia. *N Engl J Med, 302:*1041-1046, 1980.
501. Gale, R. P.: Autologous bone marrow transplantation in patients with cancer. *JAMA, 243:*540- 542, 1980.
502. Gorin, N. C., Najman, A., Salmon, C., Muller, J. Y., Petit, J. C., David, R., Stachowiak, J., Marie, F. H., Parlier, Y., and Duhamel, G.: High dose combination chemotherapy (TACC) with and without autologous bone marrow transplantation for the treatment of acute leukaemia and other malignant diseases: Kinetics of recovery of haemopoiesis. A preliminary study of 12 cases. *Eur J Cancer, 15:*1113-1119, 1979.
503. Hansen, J. A., Clift, R. A., Thomas, E. D., Buckner, C. D., Mickelson, E. M., and Storb, R.: Histocompatibility and marrow transplantation. *Transplant Proc, 11:*1924-1929, 1979.
504. Krein, B. M.: Allogenic bone marrow transplantation in the treatment of human leukemia. *JAOA, 77:*637-740, 1978.
505. Mathe, G., and Schwarzenberg, L.: Bone marrow transplantation (1958-1979): Conditioning and graft-versus-host disease, indications in aplasias and leukemias *Pathol Biol, 27:*337-343, 1979.
506. Thomas, E. D.: Current status of marrow transplantation for aplastic anemia and acute leukemia: The Philip Levine award lecture. *Am J Clin Pathol, 72:*887-892 1979.

507. Aisner, J., Schiffer, C. A., and Wiernik, P. H.: Granulocyte transfusions: Evaluation of factors influencing results and a comparison of filtration and intermittent centrifugation leukapheresis. *Br J Haematol, 38:*121-129, 1978.
508. Clift, R. A., Sanders, J. E., Thomas, E. D., Williams, B., and Buckner, C. D.: Granulocyte transfusions for the prevention of infection in patients receiving bone-marrow transplants. *N Engl J Med, 298:*1052-1057, 1978.
509. Mannoni, P., Rodet, M., Vernant, J. P., Brun, B., Coquin-Radeau, E. I., Bracq, C., Rochant, H., and Dreyfus, B.: Efficiency of prophylactic granulocyte transfusions in preventing infections in acute leukemia. *Rev Fr Transfus Immunohematol, 22:*503-518, 1979.
510. Schiffer, C. A., Aisner, J., and Wiernik, P. H.: Platelet transfusion therapy for patients with leukemia. *Prog Clin Biol Res, 28:*267-279, 1978.
511. Steinherz, P. G., and Reich, L. M.: Granulocyte transfusions in infected neutropenic children with malignancies. *Med Pediatr Oncol, 6:*65-76, 1979.
512. Brandt, L., Mitelman, F., and Panani, A.: Cytogenetic differences between bone marrow and spleen in a case of agnogenic myeloid metaplasia developing blast crisis. *Scand J Haematol, 15:*187, 1975.
513. Canellos, G. P., Nordland, J., and Carbone, P. P.: Splenectomy for thrombocytopenia in chronic granulocytic leukemia. *Ann Intern Med, 76:*447, 1972.
514. Gomez, G., Hossfeld, D. K., and Sokal, J. E.: Removal of abnormal clone of leukemic cells by splenectomy. *Br J Haematol, 2:*421, 1975.
515. Green, T. W., Conley, C. L., Ashburn, L. I., and Peters, H. R.: Splenectomy for myeloid metaplasia of the spleen. *N Engl J Med, 248:*211, 1953.
516. Ihde, D. C., Canellos, G. P., Schwartz, J. H., and Devita, V. T.: Splenectomy in the chronic phase of chronic granulocytic leukemia: Effects in 32 patients. *Ann Intern Med, 84:*17, 1976.
517. Mitelman, F., Brandt, L., and Nisson, P. G.: Cytogenetic evidence for splenic origin of blastic transformation in chronic myeloid leukaemia. *Scand J Haematol, 13:*87, 1974.
518. Mitelman, F., Nilsson, P. G., and Brandt, L.: Brief communication: Abnormal clones resembling those seen in blast crisis arising in the spleen in chronic myelocytic leukemia. *J Natl Cancer Inst, 54:*1319, 1975.
519. Spiers, A. S. D., Baikie, A. G., Galton, D. A. G., Richards, H. G. H., Wiltshaw, E., Goldman, J. M., Catovsky, D., Spencer, J., and Peto, R.: Chronic granulocytic leukemia: Effect of elective splenectomy on the course of disease. *Br Med J, 1:*175, 1975.
520. Spiers, A. S. D., Galton, D. A. G., Catovsky, D., Wiltshaw, E., Baikie, A. G., Kaur, J., Goldman, J. M., Lowenthal, R. M., and Buskard, N. A.: Splenectomy for complications of chronic granulocytic leukaemia. *Lancet, 1:*627, 1975.
521. Aur, R. J. A., Simone, J., Hustu, H. O., Walters, T., Burella, L., Pratt, C., and Pinkel, D.: Central nervous system therapy and combination chemotherapy of childhood lymphocytic leukemia. *Blood, 37:*272, 1971.
522. Belmusto, L., Regelson, W., Owens, G., Hananian, J., and Nigogosyan, G.: Intracranial extracerebral hemorrhages in acute lymphocytic leukemia. *Cancer, 17:*1079, 1964.
523. Bleyer, W. A.: Current status of intrathecal chemotherapy for human meningeal neoplasms. *Natl Cancer Inst Monogr, 46:*171-178, 1977.
524. Campbell, R. H., Marshall, W. C., and Chessells, J. M.: Neurological complications of childhood leukaemia. *Arch Dis Child, 52:*850-858, 1977.
525. Dereuck, J. L., Sieben, G. J., Sieben-Praet, M. R., Ngendahayo, P., DeCoster, W. J.,

and Vandereecken, H. M.: Wernicke's encephalopathy in patients with tumors of the lymphoid-hemopoietic systems. *Arch Neurol, 37:*338-341, 1980.

526. Evans, A. E., Gilbert, E. S., and Zandstra, R.: The increase incidence of central nervous system leukemia in children. *Cancer, 26:*404, 1970.
527. Fritz, R. D., Forkner, C. E., Jr., Freireich, E. J., Frei, E. III, and Thomas, L. B.: The association of fatal intracranial hemorrhage and "blastic crises" in patients with acute leukemia. *N Engl J Med, 261:*59, 1959.
528. Humphrey, G. B., Krous, H. F., Filler, J., Maxwell, J. D., and VanHoutte, J. J.: Treatment of overt CNS leukemia. *Am J Pediatr Hematol Oncol, 1:*37-47, 1979.
529. Hyman, C. B., Bogle, J. M., Brubaker, C. A., Williams, K., and Hammond, D.: Central nervous system involvement by leukemia in children. I. Relationship to systemic leukemia and description of clinical and laboratory manifestations. II. Therapy with intrathecal methotrexate. *Blood, 25:*1-13, 1965.
530. Jenkin, R. D.: Radiation in the treatment of meningeal leukemia. *Am J Pediatr Hematol Oncol, 1:*49-58, 1979.
531. Komp, D. M.: Diagnosis of CNS leukemia. *Am J Pediatr Hematol Oncol, 1:*31-35, 1975.
532. Law, I. P., and Blom, J.: Adult acute leukemia: Frequency of central nervous involvement in long term survivors. *Cancer, 40:*1304-1306, 1977.
533. Lukin, R., Tomsick, T. A., and Chambers, A. A.: Lymphoma and leukemia of the central nervous system. *Semin Roentgenol, 15:*246-250, 1980.
534. Havlight, G. M., Stuckey, S. E., Cabanillas, F. F., Keating, M. J., Tourtellotte, W. W., Schold, S. C., and Freireich, E. J.: Diagnosis of leukemia or lymphoma in the central nervous system by Beta 2-microglobulin determination. *N Engl J Med, 303:*718-722, 1980.
535. Nies, B. A., Thomas, L. B., and Freireich, E.: Meningeal leukemia: A follow-up study. *Cancer, 18:*546, 1965.
536. Nishimura, K., Hosoya, R., and Nakajima, K.: Sedimentation cytology in central nervous system leukemia with a new simple apparatus. *Br J Haematol, 40:*583-586, 1978.
537. Pochedly, C.: Prophylactic CNS therapy in childhood acute leukemia: Review of methods used. *Am J Pediatr Hematol Oncol, 1:*119-126, 1979.
538. Price, R. A., and Johnson, W. W.: The central nervous system in childhood leukemia. I. The arachnoid. *Cancer, 31:*520, 1973.
539. Sembiring, R.: Central nervous system leukemia in childhood. *Paediatr Indones, 17:*274-280, 1977.
540. Shankar, S. K., and Verma, K.: Cerebrospinal fluid cytology in patients with leukemias and lymphomas. *Indian J Med Res, 71:*90-95, 1980.
541. Spiers, A. S. D., and Clubb, J. S.: Meningeal involvement in acute leukemia of adults with a report on a patient treated by methotrexate intrathecally administered. *Med J Austr, 1:*930, 1966.
542. Thomas, L. B.: Pathology of leukemia in the brain and meninges: Postmortem studies of patients with acute leukemia and of mice given innoculation of L 1210 leukemia. *Cancer Res, 25:*1555, 1965.
543. Weizsaecker, M., and Koelmel, H. W.: Meningeal involvement in leukemias and malignant lymphomas of adults: Incidence, course of disease, and treatment for prevention. *Acta Neurol Scand, 60:*363-370, 1979.
544. Wold, R. N., Masse, S. R., Conklin, R., and Freireich, E. J.: Incidence of central nervous leukemia in adults. *Cancer, 33:*863, 1974.
545. Woodruff, R. K., Malpas, J. S., Wrigley, P. F., Lister, T. A., Paxton, A. M., and Janossy, G.: Meningeal leukemia in lymphoid blast crisis of chronic myeloid leukaemia. *Br Med J., 2:*1325-1326, 1977.

546. Belpomme, D., Dantchev, D., DuRusquec, D., Grandjon, D., Huchet, R., Pouillart, P., Schwarzenberg, L., Amiel, J. L., and Mathe, G.: T and B lymphocyte markers on the neoplastic cells of 20 patients with acute and 10 with chronic lymphocytic leukemia. *Biomedicine, 20:*109, 1974.
547. Bernard, J., Weil, M., and Jacquillat, C.: Prognostic factors in human acute leukemias. *Adv Biosci, 14:*97, 1975.
548. George, S. L., Fernbach, D. J., Vietti, T. J., Sullivan, M. P., Lane, D. M., Haggard, M. E., Berry, D. H., Lonsdale, D., and Komp, D.: Factors influencing survival in pediatric acute leukemia. *Cancer, 32:*1542, 1973.
549. Frei, E., III, Yankee, R., Krisham, A., Leavit, P., and Hart, J.: Cytokinetic evaluation of the effectiveness of remission induction treatment in patients with acute leukemia. *Adv Biosci, 14:*15, 1975.
550. Freireich, E. J., Gehan, E. A., and Spier, J. F.: The usefulness of multiple pretreatment patient characteristics for prediction of response and survival in patients with adult acute leukemia. *Adv Biosci, 14:*131, 1975.
551. Kersey, J. H., Sabad, A., Gajl-Peczalska, K., Hallgren, H. M., Yonis, E. J., and Nesbit, M.: Acute lymphoblastic cells with T (thymus derived) lymphocyte markets. *Science, 182:*1355, 1973.
552. Pierce, M. I., Borges, N. H., Heyn, R., Wolff, J. A., and Gilbert, E. S.: Epidermiological factors and survival experience in 1770 children with acute leukemia treated by members of Children's Cancer Group A. *Cancer, 23:*1296, 1969.
553. Sakurai, M., and Sandberg, A. A.: Prognosis of acute myeloblastic leukemia: Chromosomal correlations. *Blood, 41:*93, 1973.
554. Seligman, M., Preudhomme, J. L., and Brouet, J. C.: B and T cell markers in human proliferative blood diseases and primary immunodeficiencies. *Transplant Rev, 16:*83, 1973.
555. Sen, L., and Borella, L.: Clinical importance of lymphoblasts with T markers in childhood acute leukemia. *N Engl J Med, 292:*828, 1975.
556. Simone, J.: Prognostic factors in childhood acute lymphocytic leukemia. *Adv Biosci, 14:*27, 1975.
557. Tsukimoto, I., Wong, K. Y., and Lampkin, B. C.: Surface markers and prognostic factors in acute lymphoblastic leukemia. *N Engl J Med, 294:*245, 1976.
558. Walters, T. R., Bushne, M., and Simone, J.: Poor prognosis in negro children with acute lymphocytic leukemia. *Cancer, 29:*210, 1972.
559. Zippin, C., Cutler, S. J., Reeves, W. J., Jr., and Lum, D.: Variation in survival among patients with acute lymphocytic leukemia. *Blood, 37:*59, 1971.
560. Zippin, C., Cutler, S. J., and Lum, D.: Time trends in survival in acute lymphocytic leukemia. *J Natl Cancer Inst, 54:*581, 1975.

Chapter 5

Chordoma

ETIOLOGY

CHORDOMA IS A MALIGNANT primary bone tumor most likely caused by uncontrolled proliferation of cell remnants of primitive notochord. In addition, trauma has also been implicated in the pathogenesis of chordoma. The hypothesis is that trauma causes escape of notochordal tissue from its connective tissue capsule, which then gradually grows to tumorous proportion to cause symptoms. This trauma theory gains some support from Ribbert's experiment (1895)[1] of physaliphorous cells from punctured intervertebral discs of rabbits and from the report by Utne and Pugh (1955)[2] that twenty of their forty patients (50%) with sacrococcygeal chordoma had a positive history of injury. However, it can be argued that trauma merely aggravates the pre-existing chordomas and makes their victims more aware of the symptoms referable to these chordoma sites, which subsequently bring them to seek medical attention.

INCIDENCE

The axial skeleton from the skull to the coccyx is the exclusive primary tumor site for chordoma. The following is a list of chordoma's frequency of occurrence in decreasing order: sacrococcygeal region,[3-65] spheno-occipital synchondrosis region (cranial region),[66-93] cervical spine, [94-100] lumbar spine,[101-109] and thoracic spine.[110-115] Utne and Pugh (1955)[2] analyzed 505 cases of chordoma collected from world medical literature and found that sacrococcygeal chordoma comprised 45 percent; cranial chordoma, 39 percent; and vertebral chordoma, 16 percent. However, according to Jaffe (1958)[116] and Dahlin (1978),[117] the percentage of chordoma distribution is somewhat different: sacrococcygeal chordoma 55 percent, cranial chordoma 35 percent, and vertebral chordoma 10 percent. In spite of the fact that chordoma is an uncommon bone tumor, Cohen and his associates (1964)[118] found that it was the leading solitary primary bone tumor of the vertebral column.

It is interesting to note that the author and his colleagues (Wu et al., 1979)[119] reported an extremely rare case of chordoma in a sixty-three-year-old female patient that has caused destruction of the anterior arch of atlas and the odontoid process of axis (Figures 5-1A and 5-1B). A transoral approach was employed to biopsy the tumor and the unstable upper cervical region was stabilized by a posterior occipito-cervical fusion with iliac bone graft from the external occipital protuberance to the fourth cervical vertebra with satisfactory results for five years.

Similarly, Anderson and Meyer (1968)[120] reported occurrence of multicentric chordomas that can be brought about by either a simultaneous proliferation of the primitive nortochord remnants in the different parts of the axial skeleton or by metastasis from a solitary primary site, neither of which can be unequivocally and scientifically proven.

Generally speaking, chordomas affect males twice as frequently as females. The sacrococcygeal chordomas usually affect patients between forty to seventy years of age, whereas victims of spheno-occipital chordomas tend to be about a decade younger (age thirty to sixty years). Occasionally, chordomas also occur in children and even neonates.[6, 50, 56, 66, 85, 87, 89, 121]

CLINICAL SYMPTOMS AND SIGNS

The clinical complaints and findings of chordoma vary tremendously, depending on the sites of its involvement. For instance, sacrococcygeal chordoma, by virtue of its proximity to the cauda equina, sigmoid colon, rectum, and genito-urinary system, can cause low back pain; sciatica; saddle anesthesia; hypesthesia, paresthesia, paresis, and even paralysis of lower extremities; difficulty in urination, urinary retention and incontinence; and constipation, difficulty in defecation, fecal incontinence, and rectal bleeding. Sometimes, sacrococcygeal chordoma can present itself as a firm buttock mass (Figures 5-2A and 5-2B) and the large presacral chordomas are usually palpable by rectal or pelvic examination.

In contrast, chordoma in the spheno-occipital region is likely to produce early neurological symptoms because it can easily involve the sella, the brain stem, and the adjacent cranial nerves. Occasionally, spheno-occipital chordoma can erode through the base of the skull and extend into oropharynx,[69] nasopharynx,[72, 75] paranasal sinuses,[67, 71, 93] frontal sinus,[86] and the orbit.[68] The wide spectrum of symptoms produced by

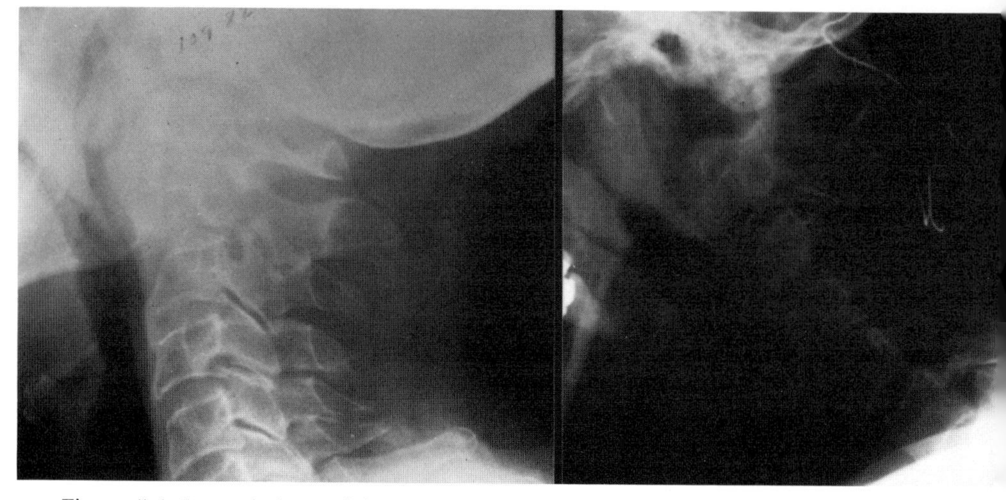

Figure 5-1. Lateral views of the upper cervical spine showing destruction of the anterior arch of the atlas and the odontoid process of the axis by a chordoma in a sixty-three-year-old white female patient who was treated with an occiput to C4 fusion with an iliac graft. The wire loop was used to hold the graft in proper position. From K. K. Wu, D. C. Mitchell, and E. R. Guise, Chordoma of the atlas, *The Journal of Bone and Joint Surgery, 61-A:*140-141, 1979.

spheno-occipital chordoma brings the sufferers to the attention of neurosurgeons, otolaryngologists, and ophthalmologists who usually confirm the diagnosis of cranial chordoma by biopsy of the offending tumor. Likewise, spinal chordoma can cause spinal cord and nerve symptoms by means of compression or direct invasion by the tumor tissue. Consequently, in addition to the pain in the spine, neurological signs such as sensory and motor deficits, changes in reflexes, muscle atrophy, etc., are likely to be found in the upper or lower extremities.

ROENTGENOGRAPHIC MANIFESTATIONS

Roentgenographically, sacro-coccygeal chordoma frequently causes expansion and destruction of the sacrum or sacrococcygeal region (Figures 5-3 and 5-4), which is often associated with an extraosseous tumor mass of varying size in which some degrees of radiopacities caused by calcification of the tumor tissue are commonly present. Intravenous pyelogram may show obstruction or displacement of the ureter or filling defect of the urinary bladder by the extraosseous portion of the chordoma. In addition, barium enema may demonstrate anterior displacement of the rectum or sigmoid colon and angiography may also show displacement of major pelvic blood vessels.

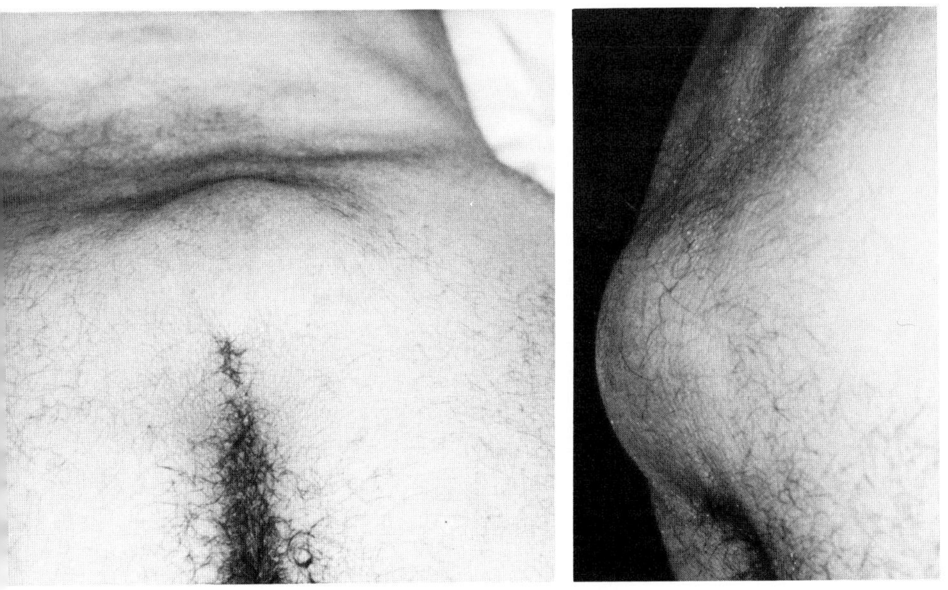

Figure 5-2A. Figure 5-2B.

Figures 5-2. This fifty-seven-year-old white male sought medical attention because of a one year history of a painless soft tissue mass over the dorsal and lower portion of his sacrum caused by a sacrococcygeal chordoma.

The cranial chordoma tends to be limited to the midline area initially, but can gradually expand in all directions. Spheno-occipital chordoma often causes osteolytic changes of the sphenoid and can also involve the sella turcica; petrous bone; sphenoid, paranasal and frontal sinuses, etc., in which scattered radiopacities can usually be seen in the invading soft tissue mass (Figure 5-5). Cerebral angiography may also reveal displacement of the major cerebral blood vessels by the chordoma tumor mass (Figures 5-6 and 5-7).

Spinal chordoma typically shows bone destruction of two or more adjacent vertebrae (Figures 5-8A and 5-8B) that may also contain foci of radiopacity and associated extraosseous tumor mass with similar calcification. The intervertebral disc between the involved vertebrae may or may not show significant destruction. It should be mentioned that computer assisted tomography is exceedingly helpful in delineating the exact extent of intraosseous and extraosseous involvement by chordomas in all locations.[122-125]

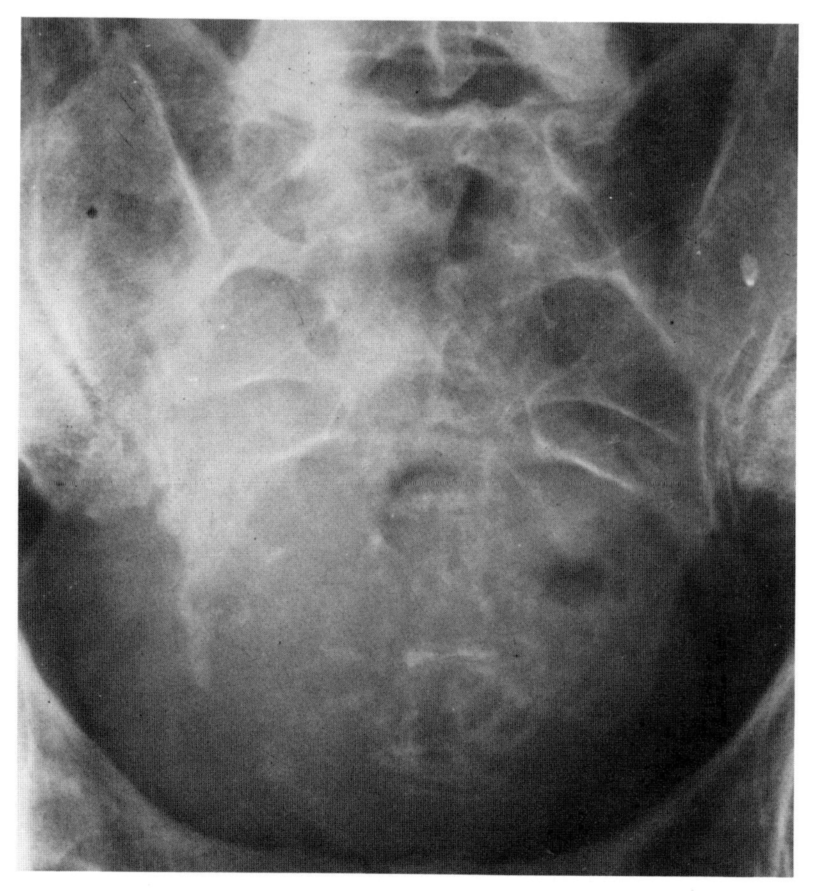

Figure 5-3. This fifty-two-year-old man with chronic low back pain had a sacrococcygeal chordoma that had produced destruction of the lower portion of his right sacrum.

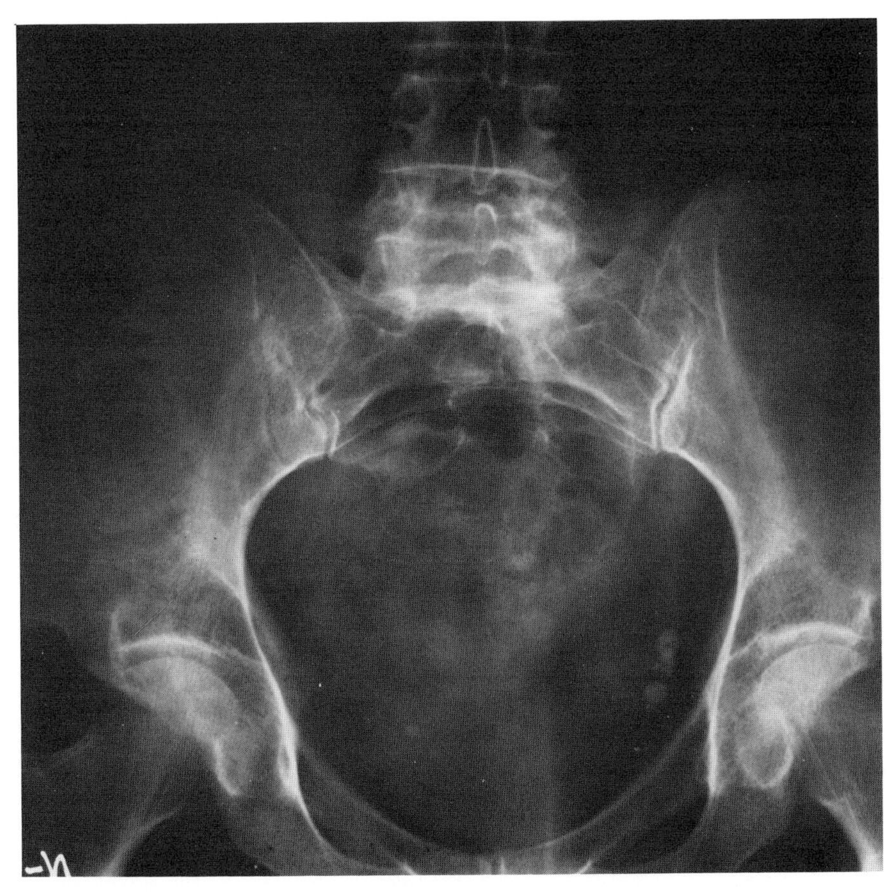

Figure 5-4. This fifty-eight-year-old female had a sacrococcygeal chordoma that had destroyed the right half of her sacrococcygeal junction.

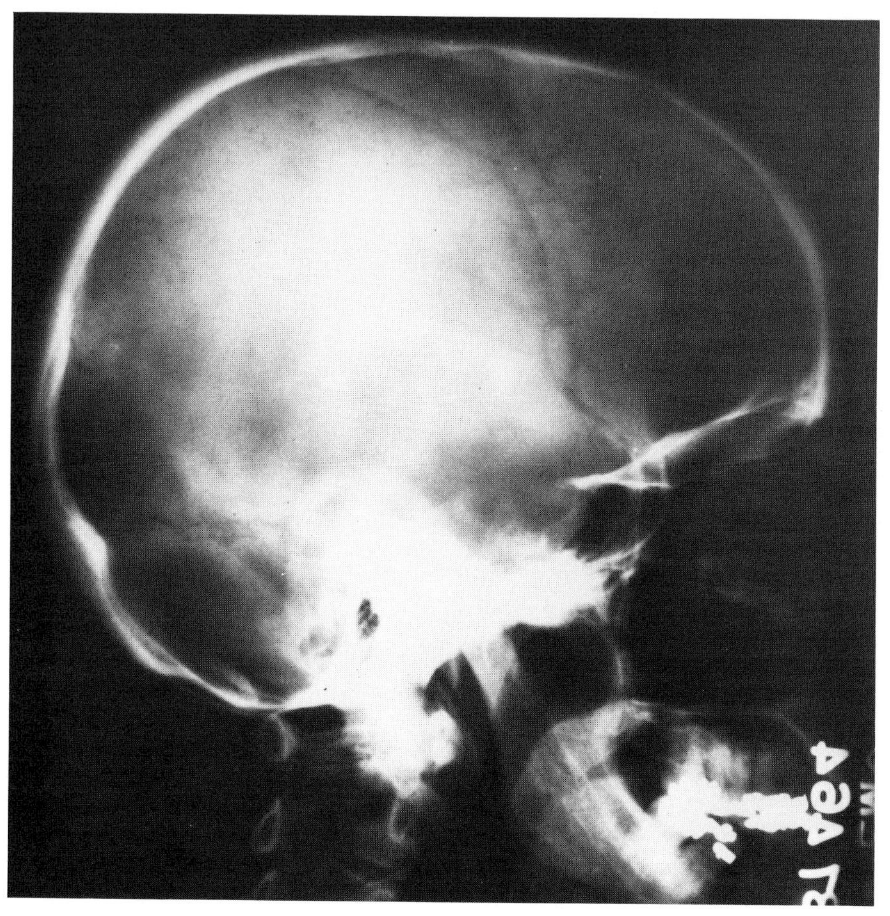

Figure 5-5. Lateral view of the skull showing destruction of the clinoids, clivus and dorsum sellae, and suprasellar calcification caused by a cranial chordoma.

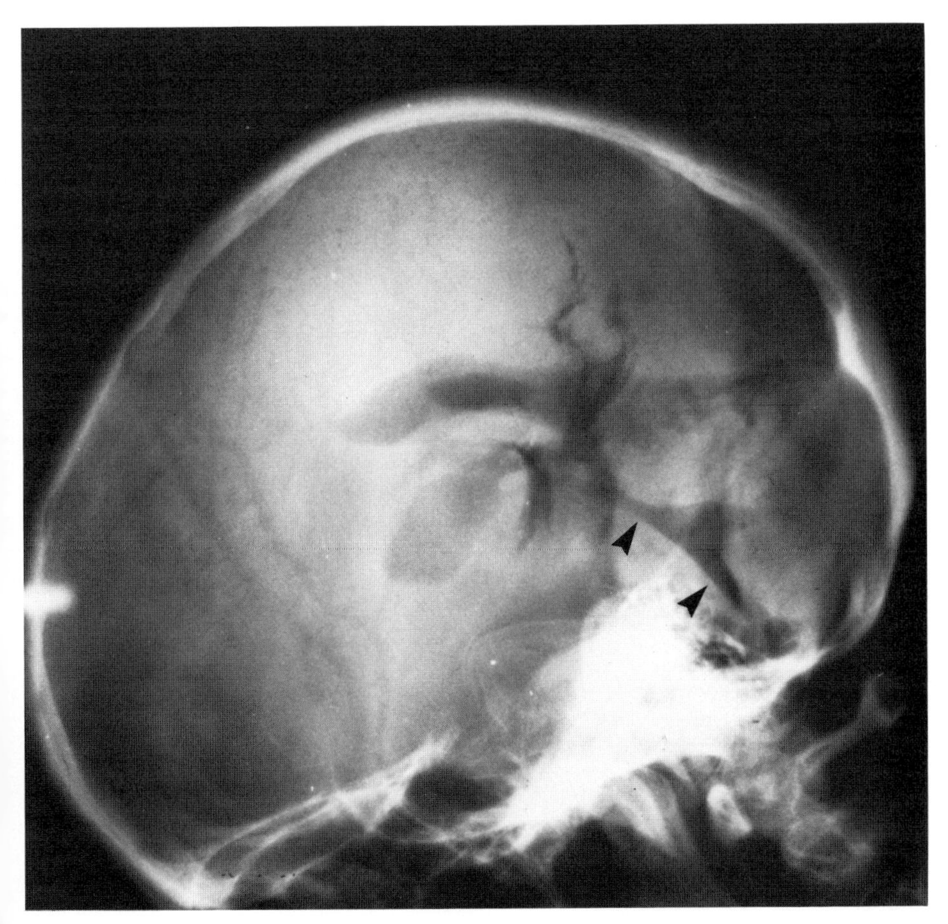

Figure 5-6. Pneumoencephalogram shows posterior displacement of the cerebral aqueduct and the fourth ventricle caused by an expanding intracranial chordoma.

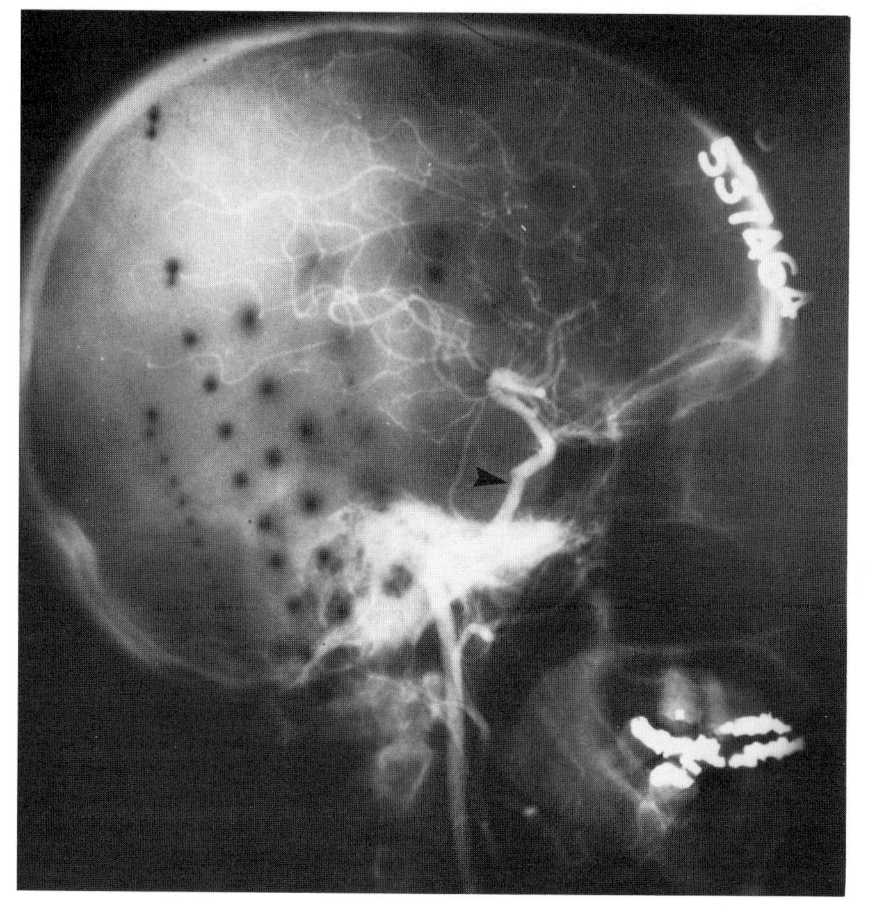

Figure 5-7. Cerebral arteriogram shows forward displacement of precavernous portion o the internal carotid artery.

Figure 5-8A. Routine lateral and oblique views of the cervical spine x-rays of this sixty-two year-old female patient with a constant neck pain shows mild deformity of the fifth an sixth cervical vertebral bodies.

Figure 5-8B. Laminograms of the same patient shown in Figure 5-8A show osteolytic an osteosclerotic changes in the fifth and sixth vertebral bodies caused by a cervical chordoma

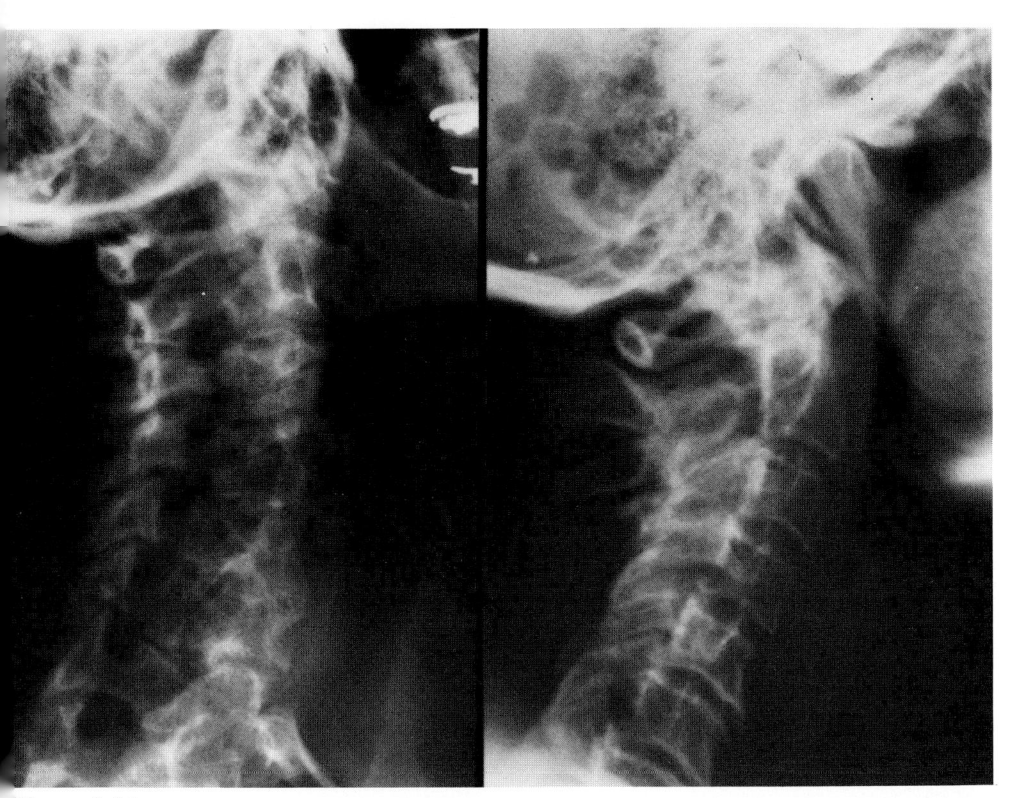

Figure 5-8A.

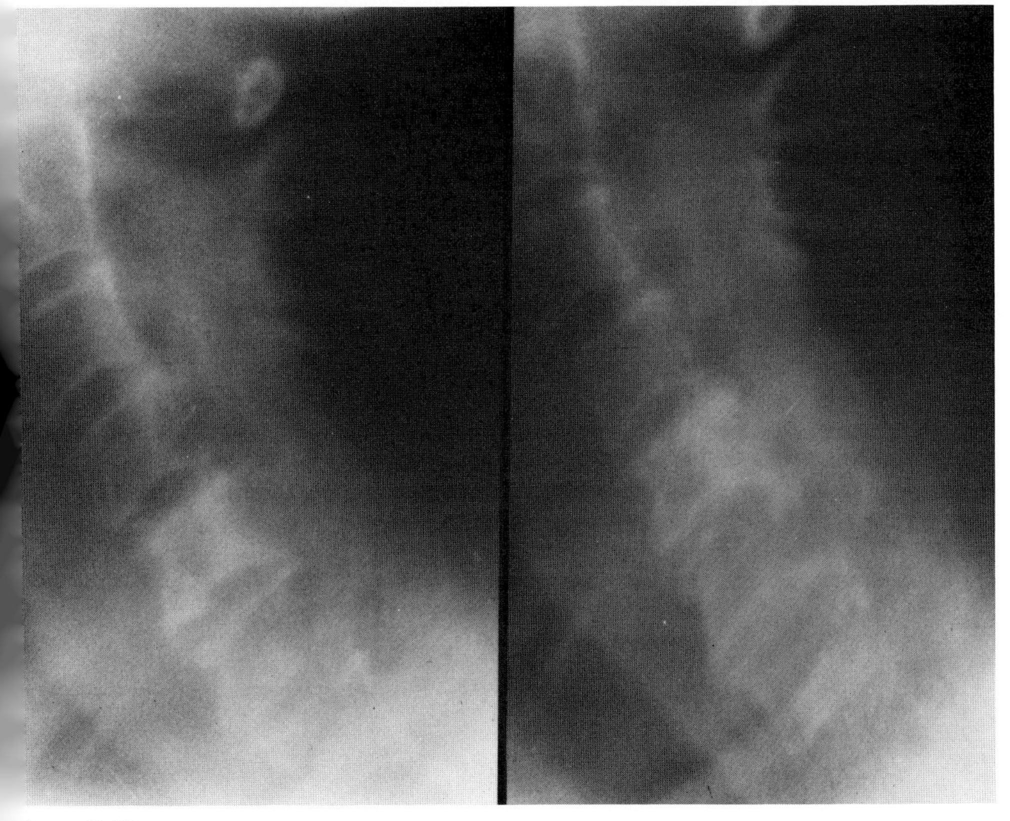

igure 5-8B.

PATHOLOGIC FEATURES

Gross Pathology

Sectioned surfaces of chordomas are glistening, semitranslucen grayish, yellowish, or reddish in color, with lobules separated by fibrou septa and enclosed by a thin connective tissue pseudo capsule (Figure 5-9) Foci of gelatinous cystic degeneration, hemorrhage, and occasional calci fication can also be seen. Sacrococcygeal chordomas are usually muc larger than the spinal or cranial chordomas. As a matter of fact, Faust et al (1944)[126] described a sacrococcygeal chordoma that was so large it fille the entire lower abdomen. Sacrococcygeal destruction is frequentl accompanied by a presacral extraosseous tumor mass that can encase o displace the sigmoid colon, rectum, ureter, urinary bladder, uterus, an adnexa from their normal locations. Spheno-occipital chordomas ofte show destruction of base of skull and involvement of the adjacent brai tissue and cranial nerves (Figure 5-10A and 5-10B), and a few of them ma

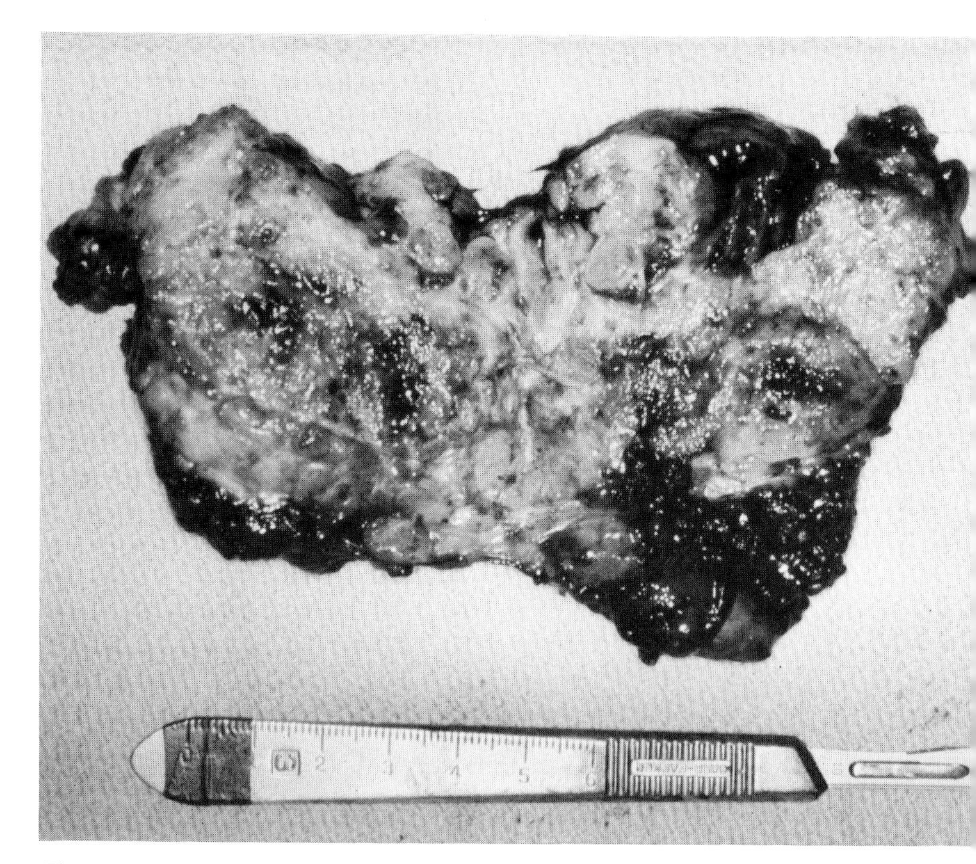

Figure 5-9. Cross section of a sacrococcygeal chordoma showing the soft, grayish, lobulated, semitranslucent, and hemorrhagic appearance of a typical chordoma.

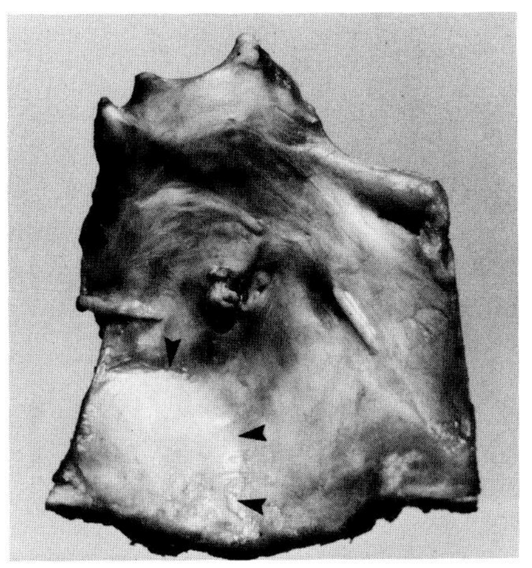

Figure 5-10A. Resected base of the skull showing a bulging spheno-occipital chordoma arising from the spheno-occipital synchondrosis region.

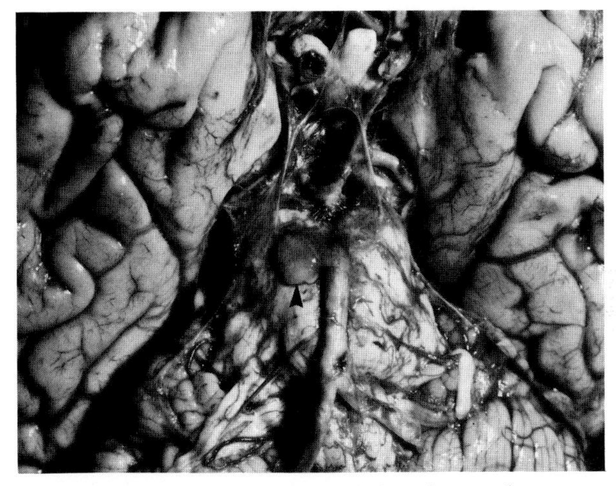

Figure 5-10B. The inferior surface of the brain belonging to the same patient shown in Figure 5-10A showing invasion of the pons and encasement of the basilar artery by a cranial chordoma.

even show extension into the nasopharynx, nasal sinus, sphenoid sinus, and the orbits. Vertebral chordomas commonly show destruction of more than one vertebral body, and the intervening intervertebral disk may or may not be destroyed. Compression of spinal cord and nerves and invasion of the prevertebral muscles and fascia by the chordoma tumor tissue are the common autopsy findings.

Microscopic Pathology

There is considerable variation in the histologic appearance of a chordoma (Figures 5-11, 5-12, and 5-13). In the highly cellular, peripheral area, the immature chordoma cells have a small, roundish nucleus with well-defined cytoplasmic border and show no or very little intracytoplasmic vacuoles. The more central portion of the tumor is less cellular and contains more mature cells that are characterized by the presence of many intracytoplasmic vacuoles. The vacuoles can coalesce into a single large vacuole to form the so-called signet-ring physaliphorous chordoma cells. In places where physaliphorous cells predominate, a mucinous substance is usually present in the extracellular space, and the cytoplasmic borders of these mature chordoma cells become indistinct.

In other areas, the histologic feature is dominated by pools of mucin of different sizes and only a few vacuolated chordoma cells can be seen. Occasionally, some tumor fields may show many immature and anaplastic cells with many mitotic figures, suggesting the appearance of a sarcomatous metaplasia.[127] The vacuolated chordoma cells and their associated

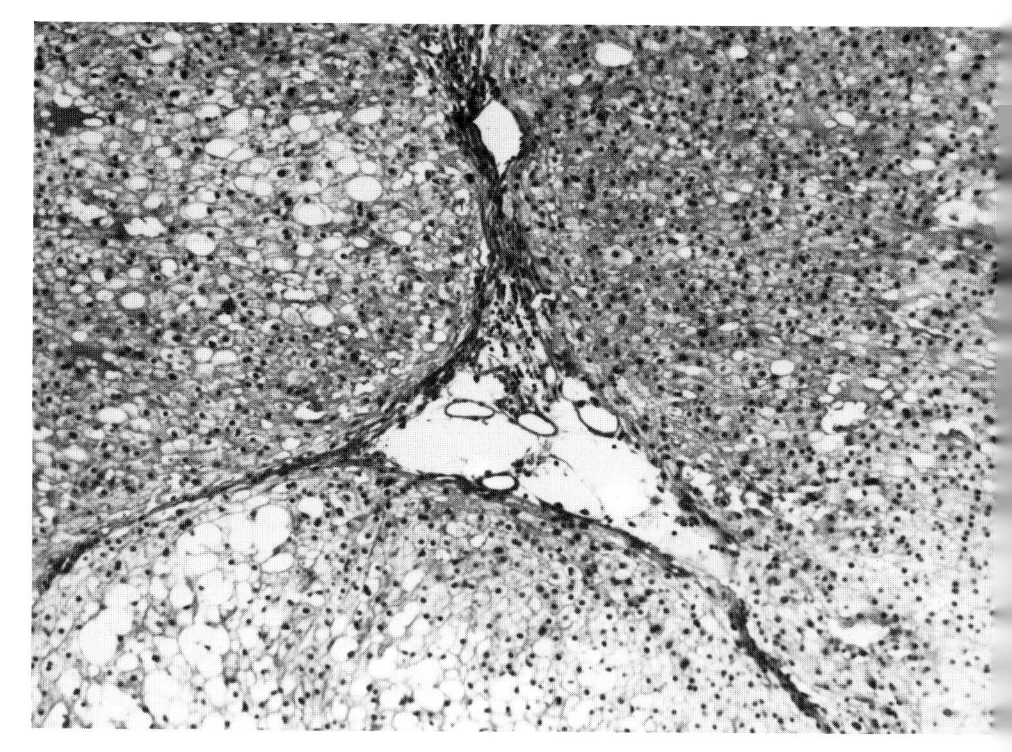

Figure 5-11. This photomicrograph (reduced 17% from 150×, H. & E.) shows the lobulated pattern of a chordoma that contains many round and hyperchromatic nuclei in association with a pale cytoplasm and a well defined cytoplasmic border. Note the presence of many oval empty spaces and their eccentrically located nuclei.

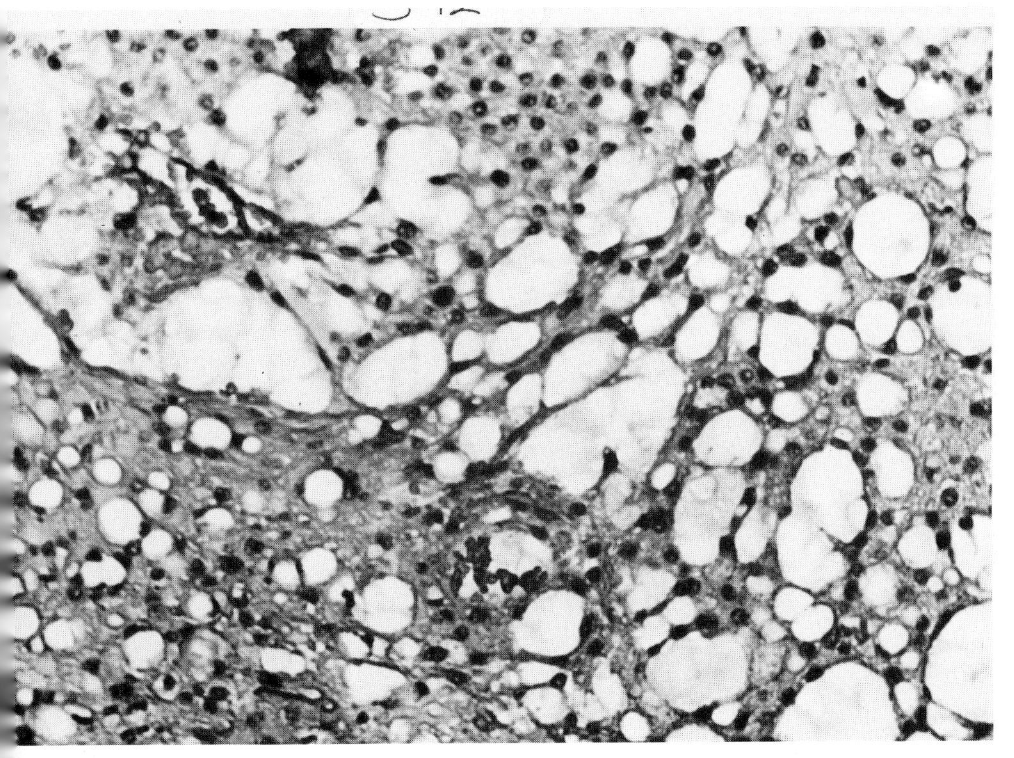

Figure 5-12. This photomicrograph (reduced 17% from 250×, H. & E.) shows chordoma cells in different stages of transformation. The less mature cells have a round nucleus with a vesicular cytoplasm and an indistinct cytoplasmic border whereas the mature chordoma cells have an eccentrically located, round, or pyknotic nucleus in close association with a large space in which mucinous material can be found.

intracellular and extracellular mucinous substance can sometimes be mistaken for myxoid chondrosarcoma. When this confusion arises, special histochemical staining procedures can be very helpful in differentiating chordoma from chondrosarcoma. The ground substance of chordoma remains unstained with phosphotungstic acid-hematoxylin and reticulin stains, whereas cartilage matrix is stained by both.[128]

By means of biochemical studies, Sweet et al. (1979)[91] found that the glycosaminoglycans of human chordoma and its metastasis were derived from the extracellular matrix and consisted of chondroitin 4- and 6-sulphate, keratin sulphate, and hyaluronate. The ratio of chondroitin sulphate to keratin sulphate was significantly lower in the metastasis than in the primary. Adams and Muir (1976)[129] and Hardingham and Adams (1976)[130] had also shown that the immature intervertebral disc contains relatively little hyaluronate and keratin sulphate, both of which rise proportionally with maturation and age, suggesting that the matrix of metastatic chordoma is less mature than that of its primary site.

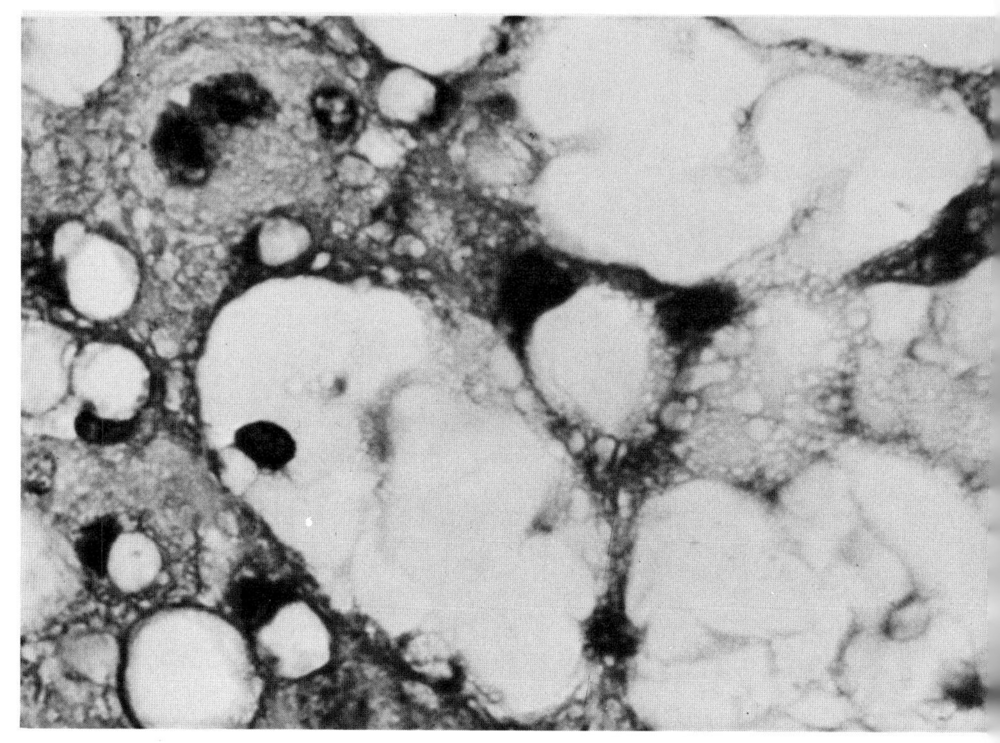

Figure 5-13. This photomicrograph (reduced 17% from 600×, H. & E.) shows the typica physaliphorous chordoma cells and the vacuolated cytoplasm of two less mature cells in the upper left corner with larger nuclei and indistinct cytoplasmic border. Note the presence o intracellular and extracellular mucinous substance.

The ultrastructure of human chordoma has been studied with electron microscope by several authors.[131-138] They found that the immature stel late cells, the mature physaliphorous cells, and transitional forms between the two are the same cells in different stages of maturation and differentia tion: the cells have the same intra- and extracellular glycogen containing vacuolar material. The electron microscope also shows that many of the vacuoles seen on the light microscopy are extracellular spaces enclosed b cytoplasmic processes. The true intracytoplasmic vacuoles appear to hav derived from both smooth and rough endoplasmic reticulum. In additio to the intra- and extracellular vacuoles, the presence of basal lamina desmosomes, and abundant microfilaments are the other characteristi features of chordomas.

Fu et al. (1975)[138] studied tissue culture of a sacrococcygeal chordom and found that the cells that proliferated in the early phase were mainl nonvacuolated stellate cells which gradually changed into vacuolated stel late cells. This finding further supports the conclusion that various ce types seen in chordoma merely represent variants of the same cell type an ifferent stages of maturity and differentiation. These *in vitro* chordoma ells also show that their golgi apparatus and endoplasmic reticulum are esponsible for producing their intracytoplasmic vacuoles, and they also ave the ability to produce collagen fibrils.

METASTASIS

Although chordomas do not frequently metastasize, their overall inciience of metastasis is about 10 percent.[36, 46, 56] Most metastatic chordonas have their origin in sacrococcygeal region.[5-6, 8-9, 11-14, 16-17, 23-24, 27-8, 31-33, 35, 42-45, 49-50, 52-54, 56-57, 61-63, 65] A few metastases originate in spiial chordomas[42, 78, 102-106] and very few metastases come from cranial hordomas.[42, 81, 85, 87, 90-92] Several factors are responsible for the relative revalence of metastasis by sacrococcygeal chordoma and the remarkable aucity of metastasis by cranial chordoma. In the first place, sacrococygeal chordomas are the most common type of chordoma and the law of robability naturally favors its incidence of metastasis. Secondly, chordonas are slowly growing tumors and usually take several years to metastaize. Sacrococcygeal chordomas have a lot of time and room to grow and nay attend great size before producing severe disturbances of the funcions of the cauda equina and the lower portion of the gastrointestinal and enito-urinary systems, which can eventually lead to death.

In contrast, cranial chordoma has relatively little time and room to grow efore the appearance of serious neurological symptoms that may quickly ause the patient's demise if aggressive measures are not taken to prevent r alleviate them. Consequently, patients with cranial chordomas may not urvive long enough to allow their tumors to develop metastases. To gain a etter understanding of the different clinical parameters of chordomas, Chambers and Schwinn (1979)[139] collected seventy cases of metastatic hordomas from the English medical literature, and their findings are ummarized in Table 5-I.

Table 5-I shows that metastasis from the sacrococcygeal region is about hree-and-one-half times more frequent than from the vertebral column nd ten times more frequent than from the cranial region. The average ime from onset of symptoms to diagnosis of primary tumor and from liagnosis of primary tumor to metastasis is three years, a significantly rolonged period of time for the chordoma to evolve. The following are he major sites of metastasis, listed in descending order: lung, lymphnode, iver, and bone. These account for 67.67 percent (or approximately twohirds) of the total metastatic sites.

Although chordomas do sometimes metastasize to bones, they usually o to the axial skeleton and rarely involve the upper or lower xtremities.[9, 14, 28, 39, 48-49, 56, 104-105] However, two cases of metastatic hordomas to the extremities were seen and treated at our medical center.

TABLE 5-I
CLINICAL DATA OF SEVENTY CASES OF METASTATIC CHORDOMAS

Age range	1 to 69 years (average age 44 years)
Primary site	
Sacrococcygeal	51 (or 72.86%)
Vertebral	14 (or 20%)
Cranial	5 (or 7.14%)
Average time from onset of symptoms to diagnosis of primary tumor	3 years
Average time from diagnosis of primary tumor to metastasis	3 years
Sites of metastasis	
Lung	40 (30.08%)
Lymphnode	23 (17.29%)
Liver	15 (11.28%)
Bone	12 (9.02%)
Skin and subcutaneous tissue	8 (6.02%)
Skeletal muscle	6 (4.51%)
Pleura, brain, and heart	5 each (3.76%, each)
Adrenal gland	3 (2.26%)
Peritoneum	2 (1.50%)
Omentum, urinary bladder, spleen, thyroid, kidney, pancreas, mesentery, pericardium, and cerebral leptomeninges	1 each (0.75%, each)
Total number of metastatic sites	133

One was a metastatic sacrococcygeal chordoma to the humeral head and neck (Figure 5-14) in a sixty-five-year-old man and the other a metastatic sacrococcygeal chordoma to the distal femoral region (Figure 5-15) in a fifty-nine-year-old man.

When a soft tissue or bone lesion in the extremities is diagnosed as a metastatic chordoma by means of ordinary light microscopy, the possibility of a chordoid sarcoma[140-142] should also be entertained. Chordoid sarcoma, also known as chordoid tumor,[143] chordoma periphericum [144-145] and parachordoma,[146] is an uncommon, slowly growing, and locally invasive malignant tumor that usually arises adjacent to tendon, synovium, and even bone of the extremities. It has a lobular and pseudoencapsulated gross appearance and microscopic features of cords of stellate cells with long cytoplasmic filopodia that interdigitate with each other to form many extracellular spaces containing loose ground substance and nests of vesicular cells embedded in a chondroid-like or myxoid matrix. Its appearance makes it look very much like metastatic chordoma. However, by means of electron microscopy, Robertson and Hogg (1980)[141] found a

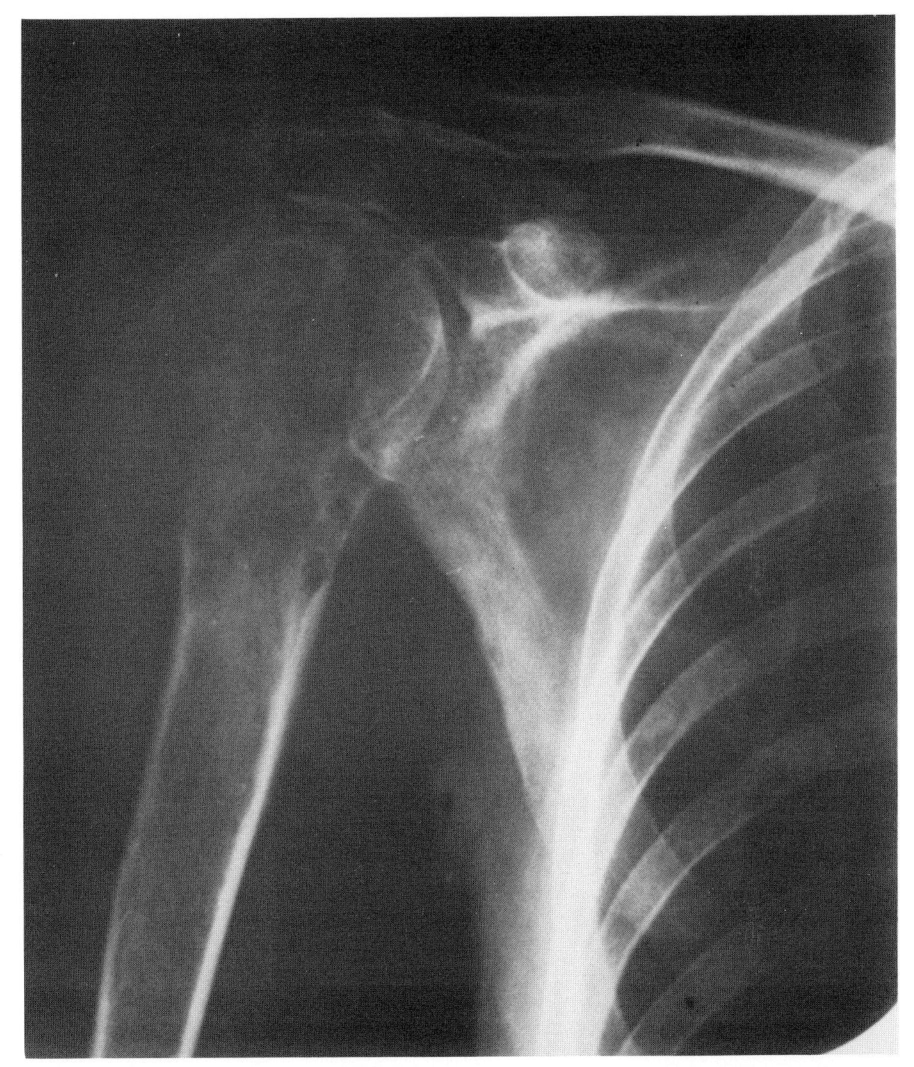

Figure 5-14. This shoulder x-ray shows an osteolytic lesion involving the whole humeral head and neck caused by a metastatic sacrococcygeal chordoma of a sixty-five-year-old man.

biphasic pattern containing epitheloid cells and stellate or spindle stromal cells with an incomplete basal lamina separating the two, suggesting a synovial origin of chordoid sarcoma. On the other hand, the typical intracellular vacuoles and intracytoplasmic complex in the form of alternating endoplasmic reticulum and flattened mitochondria separated by a constant interval of chordoma are completely absent in chordoid sarcoma. These basic ultrastructural differences clearly indicate that chordoma and chordoid sarcoma are two distinctive and fundamentally different tumor entities.

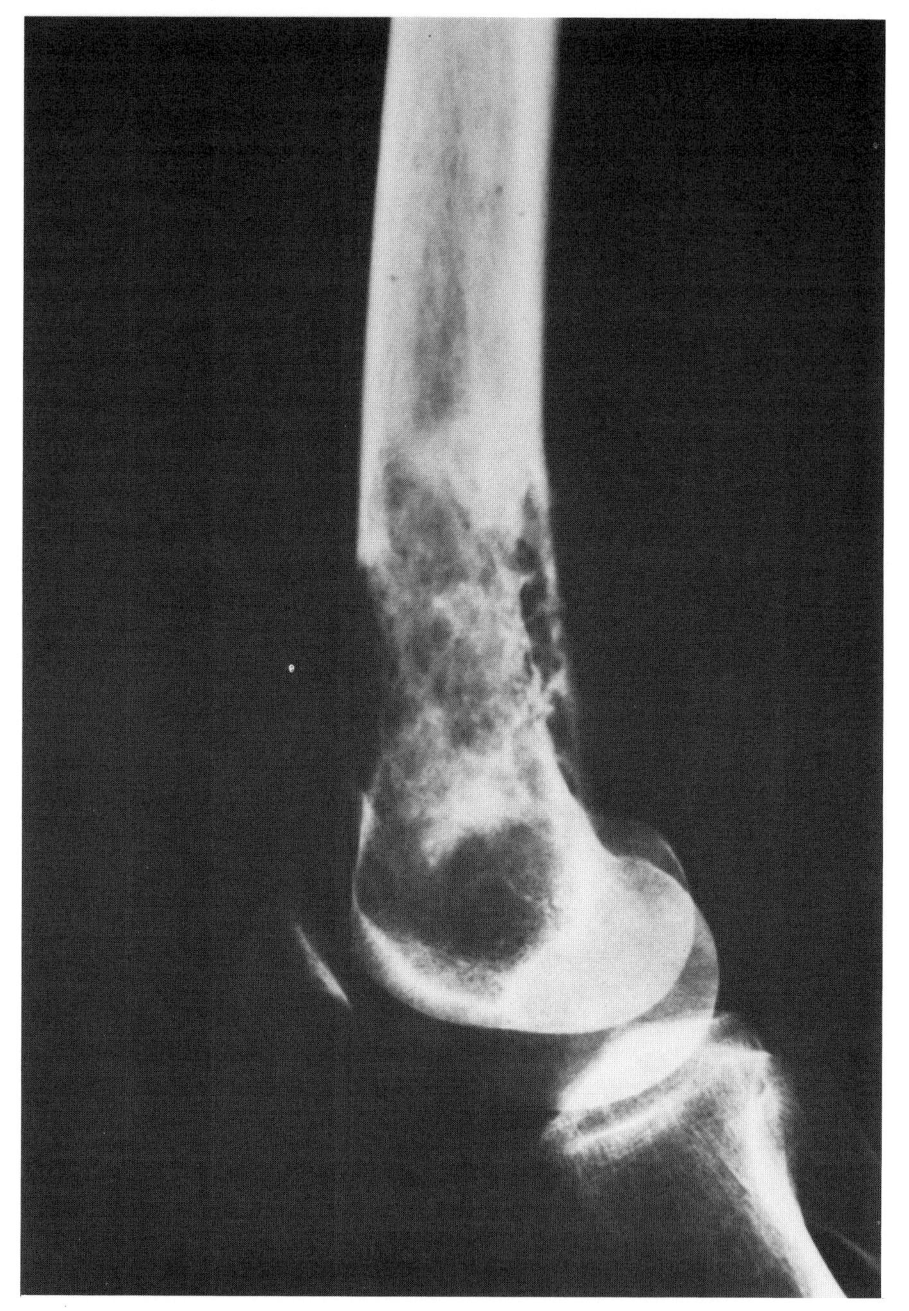

Figure 5-15. Lateral view of the knee shows an osteolytic lesion extending from the subchondral bone of the distal femur all the way to the metaphyseal-diaphyseal junction caused by a metastasizing sacrococcygeal chordoma of a fifty-nine-year-old man.

TREATMENT

Since chordoma is a slowly growing and late metastasizing malignant tumor, it naturally follows that total excision should be the treatment of choice. However, in practice, complete extirpation of chordoma is rarely achieved. For examples, in its cranial site, chordoma often involves the base of skull, brain, cranial nerves, intracranial blood vessels, and other less vital structures and a complete eradication of the primary cranial chordoma and the invaded surrounding tissues will surely cause disastrous neurological deficits and even immediate death. By the same token, an attempt to eliminate a large sacrococcygeal chordoma completely will most likely have to remove a large portion of the sacrum and the associated neural elements and the involved portions of the genitourinary and lower gastrointestinal systems. Needless to say, the resulting spinopelvic instability, bladder and bowel dysfunctions, and the neurologic deficits of the lower extremities are usually not medically acceptable.

In contrast, spinal chordomas offer some hopes for a complete surgical "cure," provided the spinal cord and nerves are not invaded. The author had participated in the removal of a chordoma from the lower cervical region of a sixty-two-year-old white female patient by excising the two diseased adjoining vertebral bodies and their intervertebral disk and bridging the resulting gap with an autogenous fibular graft. Although the patient has done very well so far, complete eradication of the disease can be claimed only after many years of complete absence of her initial disease.

In spite of the short-comings of surgical treatment of chordomas, incomplete surgical removal of chordoma has definite palliative value regardless of the site of the tumor and is usually the initial treatment of choice.[42, 56, 99, 147-159] The aim of surgical treatment of chordomas is to achieve as complete a removal of the tumor as possible without producing unacceptable impairments of vital bodily functions. The resulting unstable segment of the spine should be stabilized by appropriate surgical procedures. Since incomplete removal of chordoma is inevitably followed by local recurrence, repeated partial excisions can give patients dramatic symptomatic relief and can maintain the patients in reasonably good condition for many years, especially when the tumor is in the sacrococcygeal region where there is plenty of room for the tumor to grow. Surgery in this area has a definite lower mortality rate than the same type of operation in the spheno-occipital region.

Although chordomas are relatively radio-resistant, several authors have demonstrated the palliative effects from properly administered radiotherapy.[160-162] In addition, it is of interest to note that Razis et al. (1974)[97] were able to give a patient with an inoperable chordoma of the cervical spine, which was previously treated with tumor dose of radiation, significantly symptomatic relief with intravenous vincristine sulfate

(Oncovin). This suggests that chemotherapy may have a place in treating selected cases of chordoma. Furthermore, since chordoma is a slowly growing tumor and the lungs and liver are the favorite sites for its metastasis, removal of localized pulmonary and hepatic metastasis should be quite surgically feasible and will very likely improve its victims' long-term survival rate.

REFERENCES

1. Ribbert, H.: Uber die experimentelle erzeugung einer ecchondrosis physaliphora. *Verh D Congresses F Inn Med, 13:*455, 1895.
2. Utne, J. R., and Pugh, D. G.: The roentgenologic aspects of chordoma. *Am J Roentgenol Radium Ther Nucl Med, 74:*593, 1955.
3. Albert, H.: Chordoma with the report of a malignant case from sacrococcygeal region. *Surg Gynecol Obstet, 21:*766, 1915.
4. Alexander, W. A., and Struthers, J. W.: Sacrococcygeal chordoma. *J Pathol, 29:*61, 1926.
5. Anderson, W. B., and Meyers, H. J.: Multicentric chordoma: Report of a case. *Cancer, 21:*126-128, 1968.
6. Argaud, M. R., and Lestrade, A.: Sur la précocité de certains chordomes sacrococcygiens. *Bull Acad Med* (Paris), *95:*375-377, 1926.
7. Ariel, I. M., Verdu, C.: Chordoma: An analysis of twenty cases treated over a twenty year span. *J Surg Oncol, 7:*27-44, 1975.
8. Beaugie, J. M., Mann, C. V., and Butler, E. C.: Sacrococcygeal chordoma. *Br J Surg, 56:*588, 1969.
9. Bouvet, J. P., Leparc, J. M., and Auquier, L.: Metastasizing chordoma with extensive cutaneous sclerosis. *Ann Med Int* (Paris), *128:*877-881, 1977.
10. Brindley, G. V.: Sacral and presacral tumors. *Ann Surg, 121:*721, 1945.
11. Capelli, A., Jasonni, V., and Pizzoferrato, A.: Profilo morfologico ed istochimico dei chordomi. Considerazioni a proposito di un caso di chordoma maligno con metastasi. *Arch Ital Anat Istol Path, 42:*46-92, 1968.
12. Cato, E. T.: Chordoma. *Aust N Z J Surg, 1:*425-430, 1932.
13. Chalmers, J., and Heard, B. E.: A metastasizing chordoma—a further note. *J Bone & Joint Surg, 54:*526-529, 1972.
14. Combes, P. F., Naja, A., Lucot, H., and Sancerni, M.: Métastases multiples dun chordome sacro-coccygien. *J Radiol Electrol, 46:*692-695, 1965.
15. Congdon, C. C.: Benign and malignant chordomas. A clinico-anatomical study of twenty-two cases. *Am J Path, 28:*793, 1952.
16. Conway, C. A. G.: Case of sacrococcygeal chordoma with extensive metastases. *Mag London (Roy Free Hosp) School Med for Women, 24:*7-9, 1929.
17. Crawford, T.: The staining reactions of chordoma. *J Clin Path, 11:*110-113, 1958.
18. Dahlin, D. C., and MacCarty, C. S.: Chordoma: A study of fifty-nine cases. *Cancer, 5:*1170, 1952.
19. Debenham, G. P.: Chordoma of the gluteus maximus muscle. *Can Med Assoc J, 93:*558, 1965.
20. Dickson, J. A., and Lamb, C. A.: Sacral Chordoma. *Ann Surg, 93:*857, 1931.
21. Drukker, B. H., Lee, C. Y., and Kim, T. W.: Sacral chordoma. A rare cause of chronic pelvic and low back pain. *Obstet Gynecol, 49:*64-66, 1977.
22. Elem, B., Purohit, R., and Assanah, F. Y.: Sacrococcygeal chordoma. *Med J Zambia, 12:*25-26, 1978.

23. Faust, D. B., Gilmore, H. R., Jr., and Mudgett, C. S.: Chordomata: A review of the literature with report of a sacrococcygeal case. *Ann Int Med, 21:*678-698, 1944.
24. Fichardt, T., Villiers, P. C. de.: Chordoma. *S Afr Med J, 48:*383-391, 1974.
25. Firooznia, H., Pinto, R., Lin, J., Baruch, H. H., and Zausner, J.: Chordoma: Radiologic evaluation of 20 cases. *Am J Roentgenol, 127:*797, 1976.
26. Fletcher, E. M., Woltman, H. W., and Adson, A. W.: Sacrococcygeal chordoma: A clinical and pathological study. *Arch Neurol Psychiat, 33:*283-299, 1935.
27. Foote, R. F., Ablin, G., and Hall, W. W.: Chordoma in siblings. *Calif Med, 88:*383-386, 1958.
28. Fox, J. E., Batsakis, J. G., Dwano, L. R., and Arbor, A.: Unusual manifestation of a chordoma. *J Bone & Joint Surg, 50-A:*1618-1628, 1968.
29. Freeth, A., and Mair, J.: Chordoma as a cause of obstetric disproportion. *Br Med J, 1:*512, 1951.
30. Freier, D. T., Stanley, J. C., and Thompson, N. W.: Retrorectal tumors in adults. *Surg Gynecol Obstet, 132:*681, 1971.
31. Gartman, H.: Skin metastasis of a chordoma. *Z Hautkr, 51:*907-912, 1976.
32. Garusi, G., Donati, E., and Trinchi, E.: Metastasis from sacrococcygeal chordoma (frequency, diffusion and radiosensitivity). *Cancer, 22:*547-562, 1969.
33. Gentil, F., and Cooley, B. L.: Sacrococcygeal chordoma. *Ann Surg, 127:*432-433, 1948.
34. Goodnight, J. E., and Steckel, R. J.: Diagnostic oncology case study: Chronic low back pain and recent incontinence. *A J R, 133:*299-301, 1979.
35. Graf, L.: Sacrococcygeal chordoma with metastases. *Arch Path, 37:*136-139, 1944.
36. Gray, S. W., Singhabhandhu, B., Smith, R. A., and Skandalakis, J. E.: Sacrococcygeal chordoma: Report of a case and review of the literature. *Surgery, 78:*573-582, 1975.
37. Hale, J. E.: Sacrococcygeal chordoma. *Proc R Soc Med, 70:*276-8, 1977.
38. Harto-Garofalidis, G., Kambouroglu, G., and Fragiadakis, E. G.: Sacrococcygeal chordoma. *Br Med J, 56:*661, 1969.
39. Higginbotham, N. L., Phillips, R. F., Farr, H. W., and Hustu, H. O.: Chordoma. Thirty-five-year study at Memorial Hospital. *Cancer, 20:*1841, 1967.
40. Hsieh, C. K., and Hsieh, H. H.: Roentgenologic study of sacrococcygeal chordoma. *Radiology, 27:*101, 1936.
41. Johnson, W. R.: Post rectal neoplasms and cysts. *Aust N Z J Surg, 50:*163-166, 1980.
42. Kamrin, R. P., Potanos, J. N., and Pool, J. L.: An evaluation of the diagnosis and treatment of chordoma. *J Neurol Neurosurg Psychiat, 27:*157-165, 1964.
43. Kishikawa, H., and Tanaka, K.: Chordoma. Report of an autopsy case with fibrosarcoma. *Acta Pathol Jpn, 24:*299-308, 1974.
44. Knechtges, T. C.: Sacrococcygeal chordoma with sarcomatous feature (spindle cell anaplasia). *Am J Clin Pathol, 53:*612-616, 1970.
45. Lewis, N. D. C.: A contribution to the study of tumors from the primitive notochord. *Arch Int Med, 28:*434-452, 1921.
46. Littman, L.: Sacro-coccygeal chordoma. Review of 168 cases. *Ann Surg, 137:*80-90, 1953.
47. Mabrey, R. E.: Chordoma. A study of 150 cases. *Am J Cancer, 25:*501, 1935.
48. MacCarty, C. S., Vaugh, J. M., Coventry, M. D., and O'Sullivan, D. C.: Sacrococcygeal chordomas. *Surg Gynec & Obstet, 113:*551-554, 1961.
49. MacSweeney, A. J., and Sholl, P. R.: Metastatic chordoma. Use of mechlorethamine in chordoma therapy. *Arch Surg, 79:*152-155, 1959.
50. Montgomery, A. H., and Wolman, I. J.: Sacrococcygeal chordomas in children. *Am J Dis Child, 46:*1263-1281, 1933.

51. Paavolainen, P., and Teppo, L.: Chordoma in Finland. *Acta Orthop Scand, 47:*46-51, 1976.
52. Peters, W.: Ein Rezidivierendes, Boesartiges Chordom der Sacrococcygealen gegend mit metastasen. *Deutsche Zeitschr Chir, 151:*191-199, 1919.
53. Potoschnig, G.: Ein Fall von Malignem Chordom mit Metastasen. *Beitr Path Anat, 65:*356-362, 1919.
54. Pringle, S.: Sacrococcygeal teratoid tumor with formation of metastases in the groin. *Lancet, 1:*1643-1645, 1907.
55. Reich, W. J., and Nechtwo, M. J.: Similating an ovarian cyst. *Am J Obst & Gynec, 49:*265, 1945.
56. Rosenquist, H., and Saltzman, G. F.: Sacrococcygeal and vertebral chordoma and their treatment. *Acta Radiol, 52:*177-193, 1959.
57. Scevola, G.: On a case of metastasized chordoma. *Minerva Chir, 21:*789-794, 1966.
58. Shaw, J. F., Hamilton, T., and Thomson, D.: Chordoma presenting as a scrotal swelling. *J R Coll Surg Eding, 23:*100-103, 1978.
59. Steckler, R. M., and Martin, R. G.: Sacrococcygeal chordoma. *Am Surg, 40:*579-581, 1974.
60. Voigt, J. C., and Kenefick, J. S.: Sacrococcygeal chordoma presenting with stress incontinence of urine. *S Afr Med J, 45:*557, 1971.
61. Wang, C. C., and James, A. E.: Chordoma: Brief review of the literature and report of a case with widespread metastases. *Cancer, 22:*162-167, 1968.
62. Whitaker, R. H., and Cast, I. P.: Prolonged survival in a case of sacrococcygeal chordoma with metastases. *Br J Surg, 56:*392-395, 1969.
63. Willis, R. A.: Sacral chordoma with widespread metastases. *J Path Bact, 33:*1035-1043, 1930.
64. Wood, E. H., Jr., and Himadi, G. M.: Chordoma: A roentgenologic study of sixteen cases previously unreported. *Radiology, 54:*706, 1950.
65. Yarom, R., and Horn, Y.: Sacrococcygeal chordoma with unusual metastases. *Cancer, 25:*659-662, 1970.
66. Becker, L. E., Yates, A. J., Hoffman, H. J., and Norman, M. G.: Intracranial chordoma in infancy. Case Report. *J Neurosurg, 42:*349-352, 1975.
67. Berdal, P., and Myhre, E.: Cranial chordomas involving the paranasal sinuses. *J Laryngol Otol, 78:*906-919, 1964.
68. Blodi, F. C.: Unusual orbital tumors and their treatment. *Mod Probl Ophthalmol, 14:*565-588, 1975.
69. Burge, A. J.: A case of oropharyngeal chordoma. *J Laryngol Otol, 89:*115-119, 1975.
70. Burrow, J. L. F., and Stewart, M. J.: Malignant spheno-occipital chordoma. *J Neurol Psychopath, 4:*205, 1923.
71. Campbell, W. M., McDonald, T. J., Unni, K. K., and Laws, E. R., Jr.: Nasal and paranasal presentations of chordomas. *Laryngoscope, 90:*612-618, 1980.
72. Carvalho, G., and Coelho, L. H.: Chordoma of rhinopharynx. Report of a case. *Acta Cytol, 18:*425-428, 1974.
73. Cloward, R. B., and Passarelli, P.: Removal of giant clival chordoma by anterior cervical approach. *Surg Neurol, 11:*129-134, 1979.
74. Danziger, J., Allen, K. L., and Bloch, S.: Intracranial chordomas. *Clin Radiol, 25:*309-316, 1974.
75. Eisemann, M. L.: Spheno-occipital chordoma presenting as a nasopharyngeal mass. A case report. *Ann Otol Rhinol Laryngol, 89:*271-275, 1979.
76. Givner, I.: Ophthalmologic features of intracranial chordoma and allied tumors of the clivus. *Arch Ophthalmol, 33:*397-401, 1945.

77. Greens, R. A., and Weber, A. L.: X-ray of the mouth, intracranial chordoma. *Ann Otol Rhinol Laryngol, 89:*100-101, 1980.
78. Greenwald, C. M., Meaney, T. F., and Hughes, C. R.: Chordoma — uncommon destructive lesion of cerebrospinal axis. *JAMA, 163:*1240, 1957.
79. Harwick, R. D., and Miller, A. S.: Craniocervical chordomas. *Am J Surg, 138:*512-516, 1979.
80. Hefflinger, M. J., Dahlin, D. C., MacCarty, C. S., and Beabout, J. W.: Chordomas and cartilaginous tumors at the skull base. *Cancer, 32:*410, 1973.
81. Holzner, H.: Ungewoehnliche metastasie rung eines Chordoms. *Zbl Allg Path, 92:*12-18, 1954.
82. Kendall, B. E.: Cranial chordomas. *Br J Radiol, 50:*687-698, 1977.
83. Lim, G. H.: Clivus chordoma with unusual bone sclerosis and brainstem invasion. A case report with review of the radiology of cranial chordomas. *Austral Radiol, 19:*242-250, 1975.
84. Marc, J. A., and Schechter, M. M.: Radiological diagnosis of mass lesions within and adjacent to the foramen magnum. *Radiology, 114:*351-365, 1975.
85. Plese, J. P., Borges, J. M., Nudelman, M., LeFevre, A. B., and Sallum, J.: Unusual subarachnoid metastasis of an intracranial chordoma in infancy. *Childs Brain, 4:*251-256, 1978.
86. Pusalkar, A. G., and Steinbach, E.: Chordoma of the frontal sinus. *J Laryngol Otol, 93:*923-926, 1979.
87. Sassin, J. F., and Chutorian, A. M.: Intracranial chordoma in children. *Arch Neurol, 17:*89-93, 1967.
88. Schechter, M. M., Liebeskind, A. L., and Azar-Kia, B.: Intracranial chordomas. *Neuroradiology, 8:*67-82, 1974.
89. Scuotto, A., Albanese, V., and Tomasello, F.: Clival chordomas in children. *Acta Neurol* (Napoli), *35:*121-127, 1980.
90. Stough, D. R., Hartzog, J. T., and Fisher, R. G.: Unusual intradural spinal metastasis of a cranial chordoma. *J Neurosurg, 34:*560-562, 1971.
91. Sweet, M. B., Thonar, E. J., Berson, S. D., Skikne, M. I., Immelman, A. R., and Kerr, W. A.: Biochemical studies of the matrix of craniovertebral chordoma and a metastasis. *Cancer, 44:*652-660, 1979.
92. Uhr, N., and Churg, J.: Hypertrophic osteoarthropathy, report of a case associated with a chordoma of the base of the skull and lymphangitic pulmonary metastases. *Ann Int Med, 31:*681-691, 1949.
93. Zizmor, J., and Noyek, A. M.: Calcifying and osteoblastic tumors of the paranasal sinuses. *J Otolaryngol, 6:*22-44, 1977.
94. Bach, S. T.: Cervical chordoma. Report of a case. *Acta Otolaryngol, 69:*450-456, 1970.
95. Conley, J. J., and Clairmont, A. A.: Some aspects of cervical chordoma. *J Am Acad Ophthal Otol, 84:*145-147, 1977.
96. Prete, P., and Thorne, R. P.: Low cervical chordoma: Report of two cases with documentation by computed tomography and review of the literature. *Orthop, 3:*643-648, 1980.
97. Razis, D. V., Tsatsaronis, A., Kyriazides, I., and Triantafyllou, D.: Chordoma of the cervical spine treated with Vincristine sulfate. *J Med* (Basel), *5:*274-277, 1974.
98. Samuel, K. C., Singh, K. N., and Garg, R. K.: Malignant chordoma of cervicothoracic region — A case report. *Indian J Pathol Bacteriol, 12:*122-125, 1969.
99. Windle-Taylor, P. C.: Cervical chordoma: Report of a case and the technique of transoral removal. *Br J Surg, 64:*438-441, 1977.

100. Wright, D.: Nasopharyngeal and cervical chordoma. Some aspects of their development and treatment. *J Laryng, 81:*1337-1355, 1967.
101. Baker, H. W., and Coley, B. L.: Chordoma of lumbar vertebrae. *J Bone & Joint Surg, 35-A:*403, 1953.
102. Clay, A., Dupont, A., and Gosselin, B.: Observation anatomo-clinique dun chordome lombaire avec metastases viscerales multiples. *Arch Anat Path* (Paris), *17:*111-114, 1969.
103. Guethert, H., and Henkel, H.: Ein Metastasie kendes Chordom der Lendenwirbelsaeule. *Zentrabl Allg Path, 77:*376-380, 1941.
104. Jenni, J., and Sulser, H.: Metastasierendes Chordom der Lumbosakralwierelsaeule. *Schweiz Med Wschr, 103:*697-701, 1973.
105. Markwalder, T. M., Markwalder, R. V., Robert, J. L., and Krneta, A.: Metastatic chordoma. *Surg Neurol, 12:*473-479, 1979.
106. Maynard, R. B.: A case of chordoma with pulmonary metastases. *Aust N Z J Surg, 22:*215-219, 1953.
107. McCormack, M. P.: Upper lumbar chordoma. *J Bone & Joint Surg, 42-B:*565, 1960.
108. Morris, A. A., and Rabinovitch, R.: Malignant chordoma of lumbar region. *Arch Neurol & Psychiat, 57:*547, 1947.
109. Richards, S. L.: Lumbar vertebra chordoma. *Arch Path, 40:*128, 1945.
110. Aleksic, S., Budzilovich, G. N., Nirmel, K., Ransohoff, J., and Feigin, I.: Subarachnoid dissemination of thoracic chordoma. *Arch Neurol, 36:*652-654, 1979.
111. Castellano, G. C., and Johnston, H. W.: Intrathoracic chordoma presenting as a posterior mediastinal tumor. *South Med J, 68:*109-112, 1975.
112. Gregorius, F. K., and Batzdorf, U.: Removal of thoracic chordoma by staged laminectomy and thoracotomy: A case report. *Am Surg, 43:*631-634, 1977.
113. Gregorius, F. K., and Batzdorf, U.: Removal of thoracic chordoma by staged laminectomy and thoracotomy: Case Report. *Am Surg, 45:*535-537, 1979.
114. Hansson, C. J.: Chordoma in a thoracic vertebra. *Acta Radiol, 22:*598, 1941.
115. Hutton, J., and Young, A.: Chordoma, a report of two cases, a malignant sacrococcygeal chordoma and a chordoma of the dorsal spine. *Surg Gynecol Obstet, 48:*333, 1929.
116. Jaffe, H. L.: *Tumors and Tumorous Conditions of the Bone and Joints.* Philadelphia, Lea & Febiger, 1958, pp. 451-462.
117. Dahlin, D. C.: *Bone Tumors,* 3rd ed. Springfield, Charles C Thomas, 1978, pp. 329-343.
118. Cohen, D. M., Dahlin, D. C., and MacCarthy, C. S.: Apparently solitary tumors of the vertebral column. *Mayo Clin Proc, 39:*509, 1964.
119. Wu, K. K., Mitchell, D. C., and Guise, E. R.: Chordoma of the atlas. *J Bone & Joint Surg, 61-A:*140-141, 1979.
120. Anderson, W. B., and Meyers, H. I.: Multicentric chordomas. *Cancer, 21:*126, 1968.
121. Nix, W. L., Steuber, C. P., Hawkins, E. P., Stenback, W. A., Pokorny, W. J., and Fernbach, D. J.: Sacrococcygeal chordoma in a neonate with multiple anomalies. *J Pediatr, 93:*995-998, 1978.
122. Byrd, S. E., Harwood-Nash, D. C., Barry, J. F., Fitz, C. R., and Boldt, D. W.: Coronal computed tomography of the skull and brain in infants and children. Part II. Clinical value. *Radiology, 124:*710-714, 1977.
123. Glydensted, C., and Karle, A.: Computed tomography of intra- and juxtasellar lesions. A radiological study of 108 cases. *Neuroradiology, 14:*5-13, 1977.
124. McLeod, R. A., Stephens, D. H., Beabout, J. W., Sheedy, P. F., and Hattery, R. R.: Computed tomography of the skeletal system. *Semin Roentgenol, 13:*235-247, 1978.

125. Nakagawa, H., Huang, Y. P., Malis, L. I., and Wolf, B. S.: Computed tomography of intraspinal and paraspinal neoplasms. *J Comput Assist Tomography, 1:*377-390, 1977.
126. Faust, D. B., Gilmore, H. R., Jr., and Mudgett, C. S.: Chordomata. *Ann Int Med, 21:*678, 1944.
127. Knechtges, T. C.: Sacrococcygeal chordoma with sarcomatous features (spindle cell metaplasia). *Am J Clin Pathol, 53:*612-616, 1970.
128. Crawford, T.: The staining reactions of chordoma. *J Clin Pathol, 11:*110, 1958.
129. Adams, P., and Muir, H.: Qualitative changes with age of proteoglycans of human lumbar disc. *Ann Rheum Dis, 35:*289-296, 1976.
130. Hardingham, T. E., and Adams, P.: A method for determination of hyaluronate in the presence of other glycosaminoglycans and its application to intervertebral disc. *Biochem J, 159:*143-147, 1976.
131. Cancilla, P., Morecki, R., and Hurwitt, E.: Fine structure of a recurrent chordoma. *Arch Neurol, 11:*289-295, 1964.
132. Erlandson, R. A., Tradler, B., Lieberman, P. H., and Higginbotham, N. L.: Ultrastructure of human chordoma. *Cancer Res, 28:*2115-2125, 1968.
133. Friedman, I., Harrison, D. F. N., and Bird, E. S.: The fine structures of chordoma with particular reference to the physaliphorous cells. *J Clin Path, 15:*116-125, 1962.
134. Kay, S., and Schatzki, P. F.: Ultrastructural observations of a chordoma arising in the clivus. *Human Path, 3:*403-413, 1972.
135. Murad, T. M., and Murthy, M. S. N.: Ultrastructure of a chordoma. *Cancer, 25:*1204-1215, 1970.
136. Pena, C. E., Horvat, B. L., and Fisher, E. R.: The ultrastructure of chordoma. *Am J Clin Path, 53:*544-551, 1970.
137. Spjut, H. J., and Luse, S. A.: Chordoma: An electron microscopic study. *Cancer, 17:*643-656, 1964.
138. Fu, Y. S., Prichett, P. S., and Young, H. F.: Tissue culture study of a sacrococcygeal chordoma with further ultrastructural study. *Acta Neuropath, 32:*225-233, 1975.
139. Chambers, P. W., and Schwinn, C. P.: A clinicopathologic study of metastases. *Am J Clin Pathol, 72:*765-776, 1979.
140. Martin, R. F., Melnick, F. J., Warner, N. E., Terry, R., Bullock, W. K., and Schwinn, C. P.: Chordoid sarcoma. *Am J Clin Pathol, 59:*623-635, 1972.
141. Robertson, D. I., and Hogg, G. R.: Chordoid sarcoma, ultrastructural evidence supporting a synovial origin. *Cancer, 45:*520-527, 1980.
142. Weiss, S. W.: Ultrastructure of the so-called "chordoid sarcoma." *Cancer, 37:*300-306, 1976.
143. Stewart, F. W.: *Case 211, Division of Laboratories and Research.* Albany, New York, 1948.
144. Laskowski, J.: Zarys onkologii. Pathology of tumors. In Kolodziejska, H. Pzwl, Warszawa, 1955, pp. 91, 99.
145. Laskowski, J.: *Abstracts of Papers, VIII International Cancer Congress.* Medgiz. Moscow, Publ. House, 1962, p. 262.
146. Dabska, M.: Parachordoma: A new clinicopathologic entity. *Cancer, 40:*1586-1592, 1977.
147. Bailey, R. W., and Badgley, C. E.: Stabilization of the cervical spine by anterior fusion. *J Bone & Joint Surg, 42-A:*565-594, 1960.
148. Cloward, R. B., and Passarelli, P.: Removal of giant clival chordoma by an anterior cervical approach. *Surg Neurol, 11:*129-134, 1979.
149. Coley, B. L.: Sacral chordoma: One year after radical excision. *Ann Surg, 105:*463, 1937.

150. Drobni, S., and Kudasz, J.: Abdominoperineal resection for enormous presacral cysts and tumors. *Am J Proctol, 26:*33-36, 1975.
151. Falconer, M. A., Bailey, I. C., and Duchen, L. W.: Surgical treatment of chordoma and chondroma of the skull base. *J Neurosurg, 29:*261-275, 1968.
152. Fielding, J. W., Pyle, R. N., and Fiett, V. G.: Anterior vertebral body resection and bone grafting for benign and malignant tumors. *J Bone and Joint Surg, 61-A:*251-253, 1979.
153. Gregorius, F. K., and Batzdorf, U.: Removal of thoracic chordoma by staged laminectomy and thoracotomy: A case report. *Am Surg, 43:*631-634, 1977.
154. Hardy, J., and Vezina, J. L.: Transsphenoidal neurosurgery of intracranial neoplasm. *Adv Neurol, 15:*261-273, 1976.
155. Laws, E. R., Jr., Trautmann, J. C., Hollenhorst, R. W., Jr.: Transsphenoidal decompression of the optic nerve and chiasm. Visual results in 62 patients. *J Neurosurg, 46:*717-722, 1977.
156. Localio, S. A., Eng, K., and Ransom, J. H.: Abdominosacral approach for retrorectal tumors. *Ann Surg, 191:*555-560, 1980.
157. McCune, W. S.: Management of sacrococcygeal tumors. *Ann Surg, 159:*911, 1964.
158. Mixter, C. G., and Mixter, W. J.: Surgical management of sacrococcygeal and vertebral chordoma. *Arch Surg, 41:*408, 1940.
159. Stener, B., and Gunterberg, B.: High amputation of the sacrum for extirpation of tumors. Principles and techniquc. *Spine, 3:*351-366, 1978.
160. Pearlman, A. W., and Friedman, M.: Radical radiation therapy of chordoma. *Am J Roentgenol Radium Ther Nucl Med, 108:*333, 1970.
161. Sennett, E. J.: Chordoma, its roentgen diagnostic aspects and its response to roentgen therapy. *Am J Roentgenol Radium Ther Nucl Med, 69:*613, 1953.
162. Tewfik, H. H., McGinnis, W. L., Nordstrom, D. G., and Latourette, H. B.: Chordoma: Evaluation of clinical behavior and treatment modalities. *Int J Radiat Oncol Biol Phys, 2:*959-962, 1977.

Chapter 6

Myeloma

INCIDENCE

MYELOMA, ALSO KNOWN as multiple myeloma, myelomatosis, plasma cell myeloma, or plasmacytoma, is the most common primary bone tumor.[1-4] It is usually caused by neoplastic proliferation of a single clone of plasma cells that have their origin in the primitive marrow reticulum of bones with hematopoietic red marrow such as spine, skull, ribs, and pelvis. By studying bone marrow kinetics in patients with multiple myeloma, Mellstedt et al. (1979)[5] found that both the plasma cell and lymphoid cell populations contributed to the proliferation of malignant cells in myeloma, and B-lymphocytes are part of the malignant cell clone in myelomatosis which can very well be the precursors to the myeloma plasma cells.

The most common skeletal site of myeloma is the spinal column, especially vertebral bodies of the thoracic and lumbar spine. Carson et al. (1955)[6] reported a 66 percent incidence of vertebral column involvement by myeloma in their series. Myeloma shows a stronger predilection for male than female patients, and the great majority of its victims are between 50 to 70 years of age. Occasionally, children can also become victims of multiple myeloma.[7-11] It has been estimated that the incidence of occurrence of myeloma is about 3 cases per 100,000 population per year.

Although myeloma is predominantly multicentric in origin, a number of solitary myeloma cases have been reported.[12-44] Like multiple myeloma, solitary myeloma is most commonly found in the spine and to a lesser extent in pelvic and femoral regions. It differs from multiple myeloma in its remarkable lack of abnormal blood and urinary findings, absence of constitutional symptoms, little cellular atypism, normal sternal marrow examination, predilection for younger patients (about half of the patients with solitary myeloma are under fifty years of age), and much better prognosis. Stewart and Taylor (1932)[45] and Wright (1961)[46] had reported surgical "cures" of solitary myeloma ranging from sixteen to thirty years. However, most authors agree that solitary myeloma is a precursor of multiple myeloma and the reported incidence of transformation of solitary myelomata to multiple myeloma varied from 33 percent to 75 percent.[47-50]

It should be mentioned that extramedullary plasmacytoma[51-77] involving the upper respiratory passage, nasal and oral pharynx, paranasal sinuses, conjunctiva, parotid gland, thyroid, spleen, vagina, vulva, testis, mucosal lining of various visceral organs, and soft tissues of the neck and other parts of the body is a distinctive clinical entity. Although extraskeletal myelomata normally lack systemic symptoms, abnormal sternal marrow examination and positive blood and urinary findings, some of them may develop into skeletal myelomatosis[78-81] whereas the others seem to run a relatively benign course. Excision, electrocoagulation, and irradiation have been shown to be quite effective in eradicating these localized extramedullary plasmacytomas. Consequently, the prognosis of extraskeletal myeloma is better than solitary intramedullary myeloma and is much better than multiple myeloma.

Occasionally, plasma cells can also invade the blood stream and cause plasma cell leukemia.[82-94] Approximately 10 percent to 25 percent of myeloma patients develop amyloidosis[95-113] that can involve the gastrointestinal tract, cardiovascular system, kidney, liver, spleen, lung, tongue, bone, adrenal gland, muscle and other viscerae, and soft tissues. Sometimes, myeloma can occur in Paget's disease of bone,[114-121] and, rarely, it can be induced by radiation.[122]

CLINICAL SYMPTOMS AND SIGNS

The most common complaint of myeloma patients is bone pain, especially in the back or chest region. Constitutional symptoms, such as generalized weakness, weight loss, anorexia, fever, malaise, etc., can also be present. Compression of spinal cord and nerve by vertebral compression fractures and intraspinal deposits of myelomatous tissue and infiltration of spinal and peripheral nerves by the myeloma paraproteins can produce a wide spectrum of neurological symptoms and signs:[123-138] pain, hypesthesia, paresthesia, paralysis, paresis, reflex changes, muscular atrophy, clonus, bladder and bowel disturbances, etc. In addition, pathologic fractures of the spine can produce severe kyphoscoliosis and significant shortening of stature.

Sternal and multiple rib fractures can create an unstable rib cage that moves paradoxically with respiration and causes respiratory difficulties.[139-141] Congestive heart failure secondary to cardiac amyloidosis and infection and thromboembolic and thrombocytopenic complications of the lungs can bring about chest pain, hemoptysis, coughs, and dyspnea. Hypercalcemia brought about by polyostotic osteolysis in response to 'osteoclast-activating factor"[142-144] secreted by lymphocytes and plasma cells can produce polyuria, polydypsia, muscular weakness, constipation, nausea, vomiting, mental confusion, coma, and even death.

Less than 10 percent of myeloma patients develop hyperviscosity syndrome,[145-152] which is caused by polymerization of myeloma globulins (usually IgG and sometimes IgA) with high intrinsic viscosity. The following are its manifestations: headache; disturbance of vision; dizziness; mental confusion; somnolence; coma; seizure; hearing loss; congestive heart failure; and spontaneous bleeding from nose, mucous membrane, and gastrointestinal, genitourinary, or respiratory tract. Sometimes, myeloma globulins are responsible for producing cold hypersensitivity from cryoglobulinemia[153-155] with the clinical manifestations of Raynaud-type phenomenon, circulation impairment, vascular occlusion, and gangrene upon exposure to cold due to the presence of cold precipitable myeloma globulins. It should be emphasized that bacterial, fungal, and viral infections of the respiratory, urinary, and other systems of the body and acute and chronic renal failure account for a significant portion of myeloma patients' clinical complaints. Occasionally, myopathies involving the proximal muscle groups can also be present in myelomatosis.

LABORATORY STUDIES

Abnormal laboratory studies in myeloma depend on the extent of skeletal myelomatosis and the degrees of renal and other visceral involvements. In a healthy person, different plasmacytic cells produce a balanced synthesis of different heavy chain immunoglobulins, which include IgG, IgA, IgD, IgE, and IgM, and two light chain globulins of either kappa or lambda variety. In myeloma, excessive proliferation of a single clone of plasma cells produces a large quantity of a single protein, which can be structurally normal with immunological activity, a distorted proportion of heavy and light chains, or an excessive amount of defective globulins and constituent polypeptide subunits.

Among the myeloma cases belonging to the heavy chain family, approximately 70 percent are of the IgG variety; 28 percent of IgA; and 2 percent of IgD, IgE, and IgM. In addition, about 50 percent of the myeloma patients can produce significant amount of light chain globulin (Bence-Jones proteins) with molecular weight in the 20,000 to 25,000 range, which is rapidly excreted by the kidney, resulting in a low serum concentration of Bence-Jones proteins. As a result, immunoelectrophoresis of both serum and urine from patients suspected of having myeloma will positively identify serologically distinct heavy and/or light chain types of myeloma.[156-188] It should be pointed out that the routine dipstick method for detecting urinary myeloma proteins and the classic Bence-Jones heat precipitation method,[189] which demonstrates precipitation of Bence-Jones proteins at 50 degrees to 60 degrees C. and dissolution of the same proteins at 90 degrees to 95 degrees C., are much less specific and sensitive than immunoelectrophoresis. Furthermore, isolated cases of Bence-Jones proteinuria have been found in patients with lymphoma, chronic lymphocytic leukemia, metastatic carcinoma, amyloidosis, macroglobulinemia, and even in an occasional individual with no clinically detectable disease.[190-191]

It is of interest to note that about 1 percent of the myeloma cases belongs to the so-called non-secretory myeloma[192-205] that does not have myeloma globulins in either the serum or urine because of impairment in either the synthesis or the release of the abnormal globulins into the systemic circulation from the myeloma cells. However, these intracellular immunoglobulins can be clearly demonstrated by the immunofluorescence or immunoperoxidase techniques.[206-212]

Other less specific laboratory findings of myeloma may include the following:[213-215] anemia; elevated erythrocytic sedimentation rate; leukopenia; thrombocytopenia; hyperglobulinemia; hypoalbuminemia; hyperuricemia; hypercalcemia; deficiency of blood coagulation factors;[216-223] elevated serum alkaline phosphatase, BUN, and creatinine; hypercalsuria; hyperuricosuria; hyperproteinuria (Bence-Jones proteins and albumen); hematuria; urinary casts, etc. These findings are merely reflections of skeletal destruction and impairment of the normal functions of various visceral organs caused by the myeloma cells and the abnormal proteinaceous substances produced by them.

It should be noted that sternal and iliac marrow puncture smears are of vital diagnostic importance.[224-226] About 75 percent of the myeloma patients show a greater than 30 percent of bone marrow plasmacytosis with large numbers of immature plasma cells containing basophilic cytoplasm, eccentric nucleus and clumped chromatin, and multinucleated cells with prominent nucleoli and intracytoplasmic deposits of myeloma proteins at time of diagnosis. As the disease progresses further, nearly 100 percent positive bone marrow smears will be the routine laboratory findings.

STAGING

The clinical staging of myeloma[227-234] is based on estimation of the total myeloma tumor cell mass in the whole body. The total mass can be calculated when the amount of immunoglobulins synthesized by myeloma cells in culture[235] and the turnover of radiolabeled immunoglobulins[236] in the same patient have been determined by employing the following formula:

$$\text{Total Number of Myeloma Cells in the Body} = \frac{\text{Total Body Myeloma Protein Synthetic Rate}}{\text{Cellular Myeloma Protein Synthetic Rate}}$$

Clinically, the total myeloma tumor mass bears a significant correlation to the extent of bone destruction and the degrees of hypercalcemia, anemia, and serum and urinary myeloma protein concentrations. On the basis of these simple laboratory and radiological findings, three clinical stages of multiple myeloma have been recognized.

STAGE I.
1. absence of anemia, hypercalcemia, and multiple skeletal lesion — may have solitary skeletal plasmacytoma
2. low serum and urinary myeloma immunoglobulins
3. low total body myeloma cell mass

STAGE II.
1. intermediate total body myeloma cell mass
2. the extent of abnormal laboratory findings falls between Stage I and Stage III

STAGE III.
1. high total body myeloma cell mass
2. one or more of the following abnormal laboratory findings
   a. anemia
   b. hypercalcemia
   c. multiple osteolytic lesions
   d. high serum and urinary myeloma immunoglobulins

ROENTGENOGRAPHIC MANIFESTATIONS

Roentgenographically, skeletal lesions of myeloma are usually polyostotic and purely osteolytic in nature with minimal or no periosteal bone formation. In the spine, although the vertebral bodies are the favorite sites of involvement, the pedicles and posterior neural arches can also be involved. Sometimes, myelomatous paraspinal soft tissue mass can also be present. The great majority of myeloma lesions of the spine usually falls under several different patterns:

- solitary lesions, resembling primary bone tumor (Figures 6-1 and 6-2)
- generalized osteoporosis, hard to be distinguished from many metabolic bone diseases such as senile and postmenopausal osteoporosis, osteomalacia, Cushing's syndrome, etc. (Figure 6-3)
- osteoporosis associated with one or more compression fractures (Figures 6-4, 6-5 and 6-6)

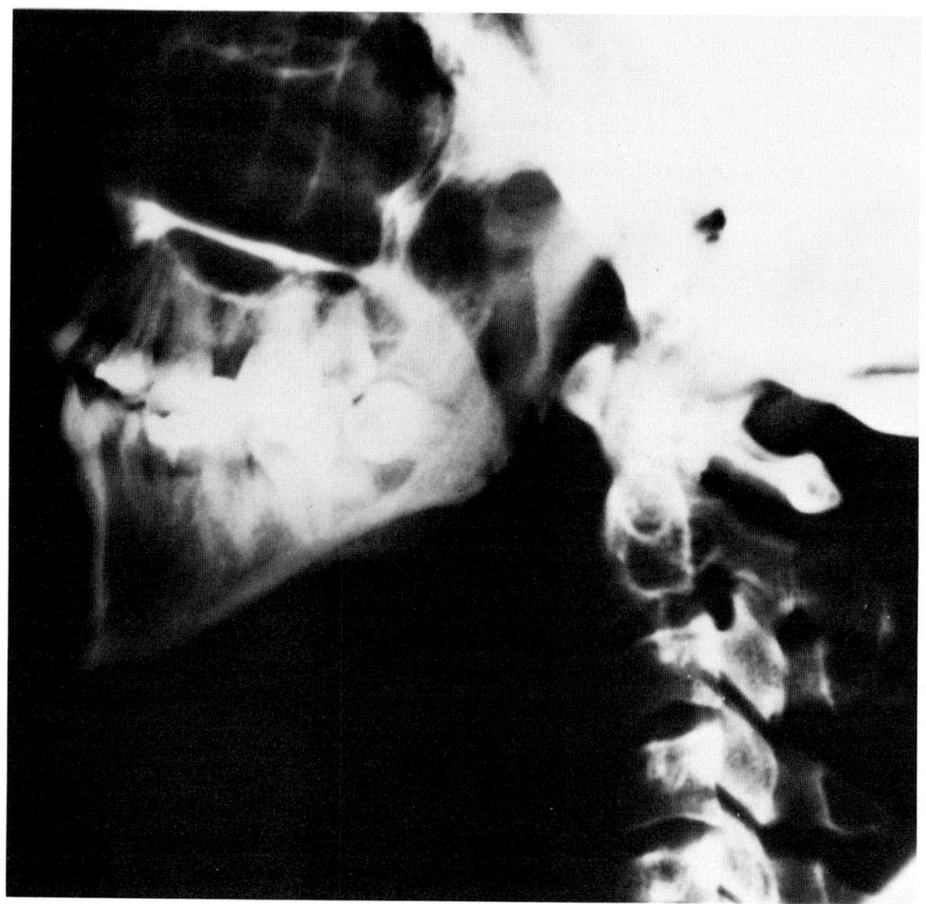

Figure 6-1. X-ray of cervical spine shows a solitary osteolytic lesion involving the body, pedicle, and lamina of the second cervical vertebra. The patient was a twenty-four-year-old female with severe neck pain. Subsequent biopsy revealed the presence of a solitary myeloma in C2. Note the reversal of the normal cervical lordosis in the upper cervical region due to paraspinal muscle spasm.

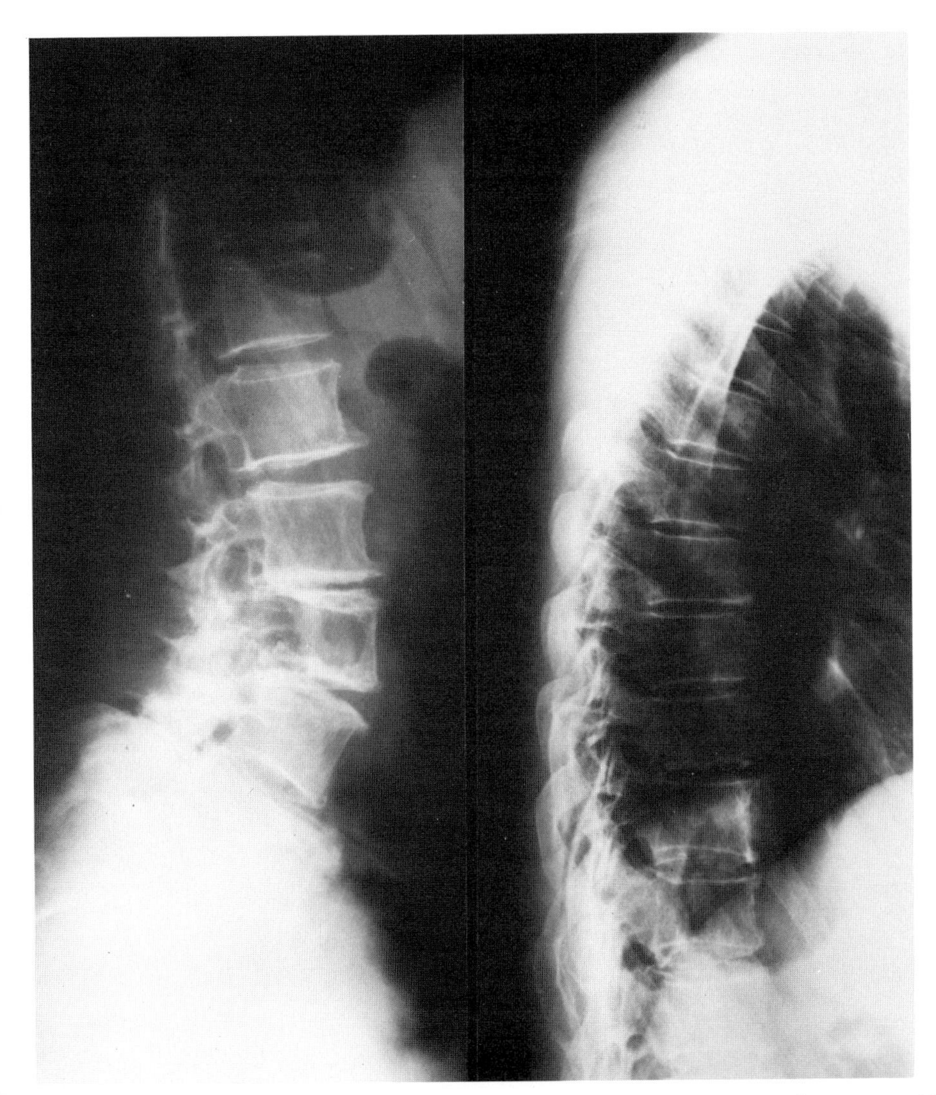

Figure 6-2. Roentgenographs of the thoracic and lumbar spine of a seventy-three-year-old male reveals a large osteolytic lesion involving almost the entire fourth lumbar vertebral body and suggesting the presence of a primary bone tumor. This is an uncommon roentgenographic manifestation of multiple myeloma.

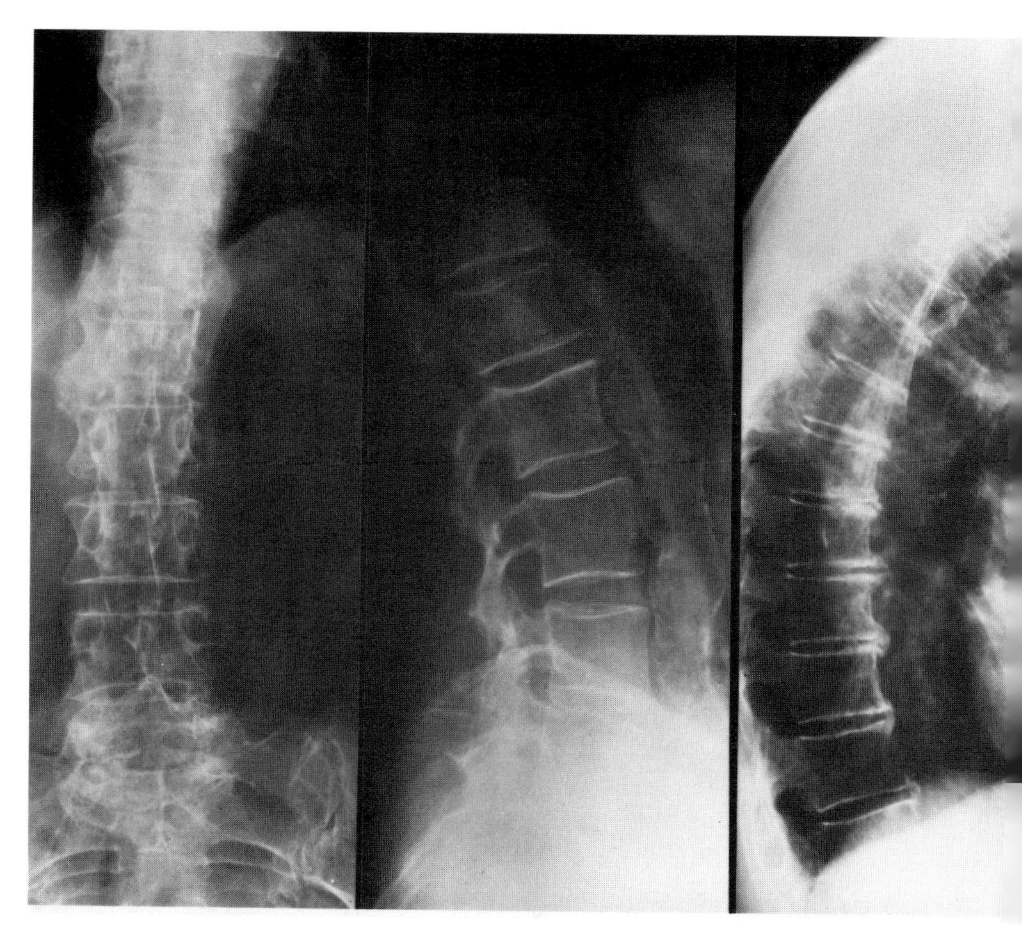

Figure 6-3. This set of spine x-rays belonged to a seventy-year-old man with multiple myeloma. Note the generalized osteoporosis throughout the entire thoracic and lumbar spine without any compression fracture or osteolytic lesions.

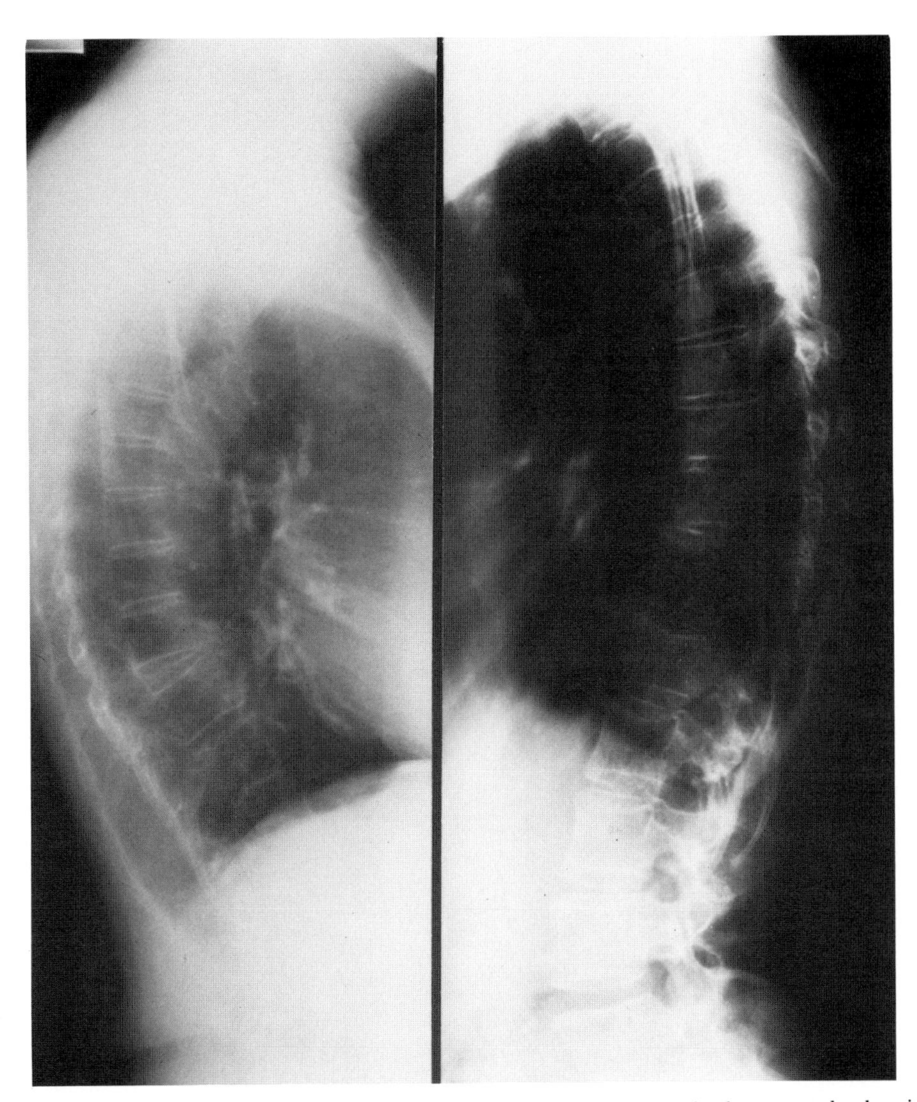

Figure 6-4. This fifty-eight-year-old female with multiple myeloma had constant back pain caused by a complete collapse of the ninth vertebral body, which appears as a merely white line.

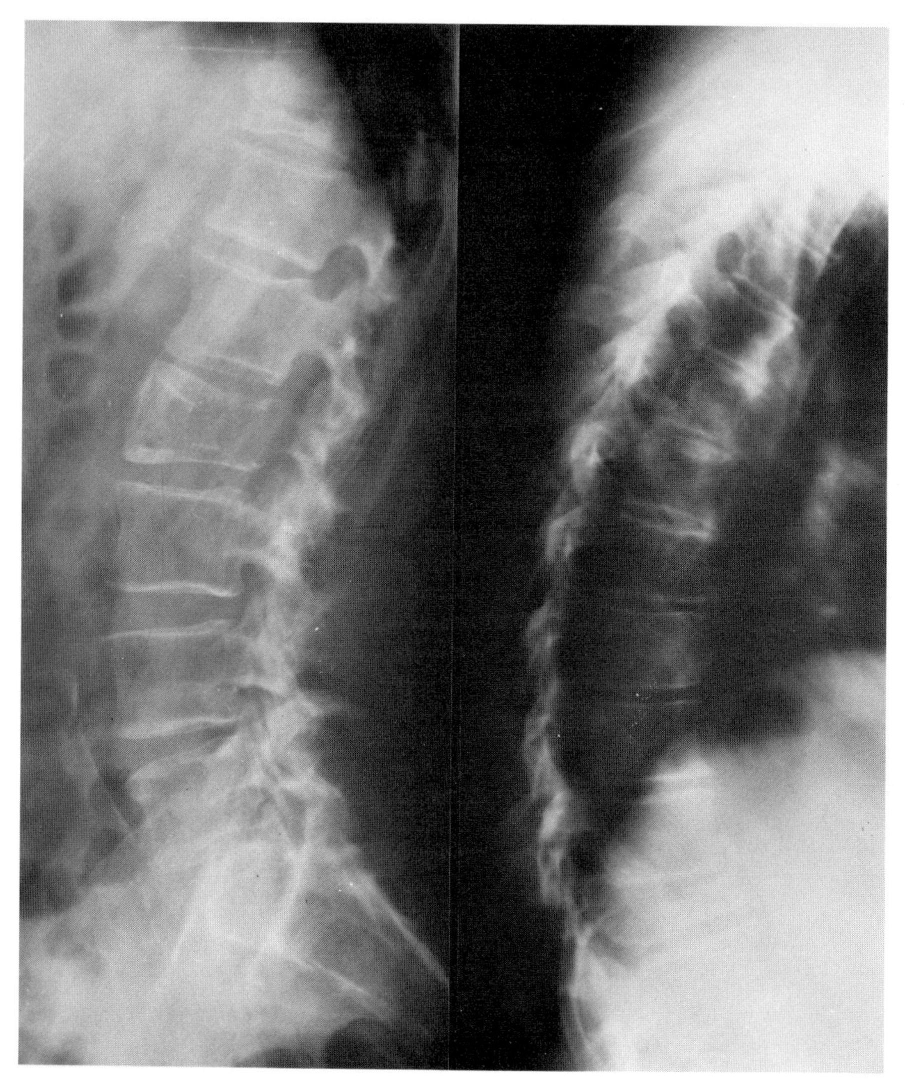

Figure 6-5. This seventy-seven-year-old woman with multiple myeloma had a compression fracture of her T11 and L2 vertebral bodies and a moderate degree of osteoporosis throughout her thoracic and lumbar spine.

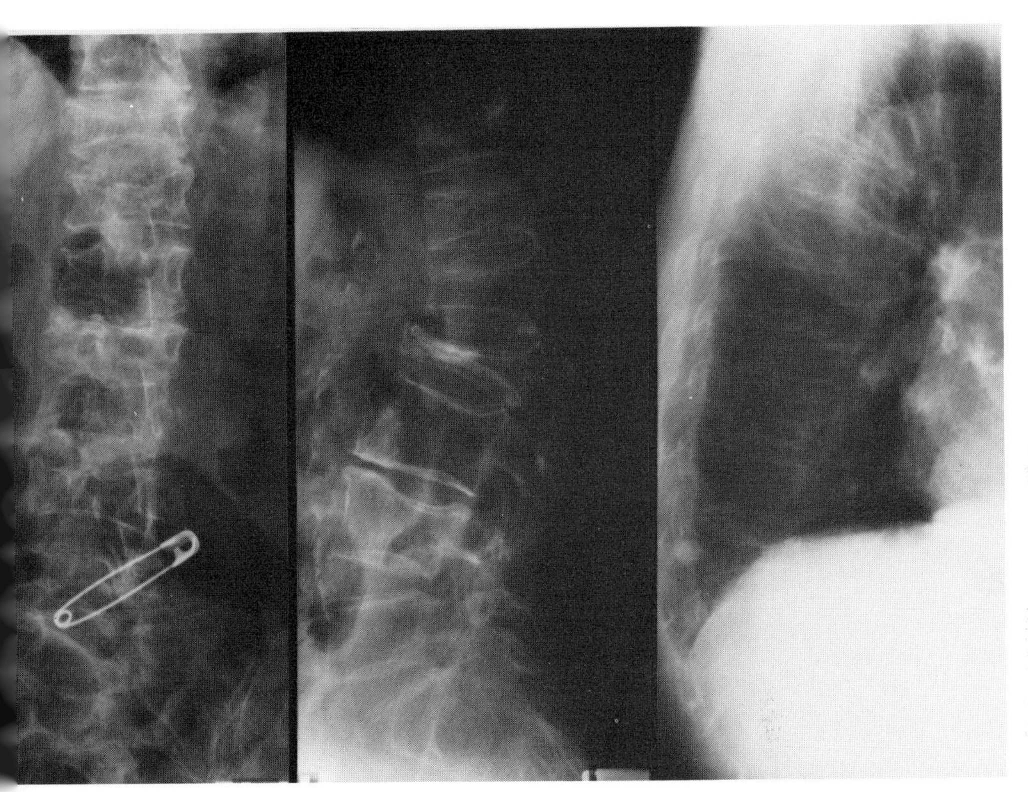

Figure 6-6. This set of spine x-rays belonged to a seventy-two-year-old female patient with multiple myeloma. Note the multiple vertebral compression fractures and the severe osteoporosis throughout the entire thoracic and lumbar spine.

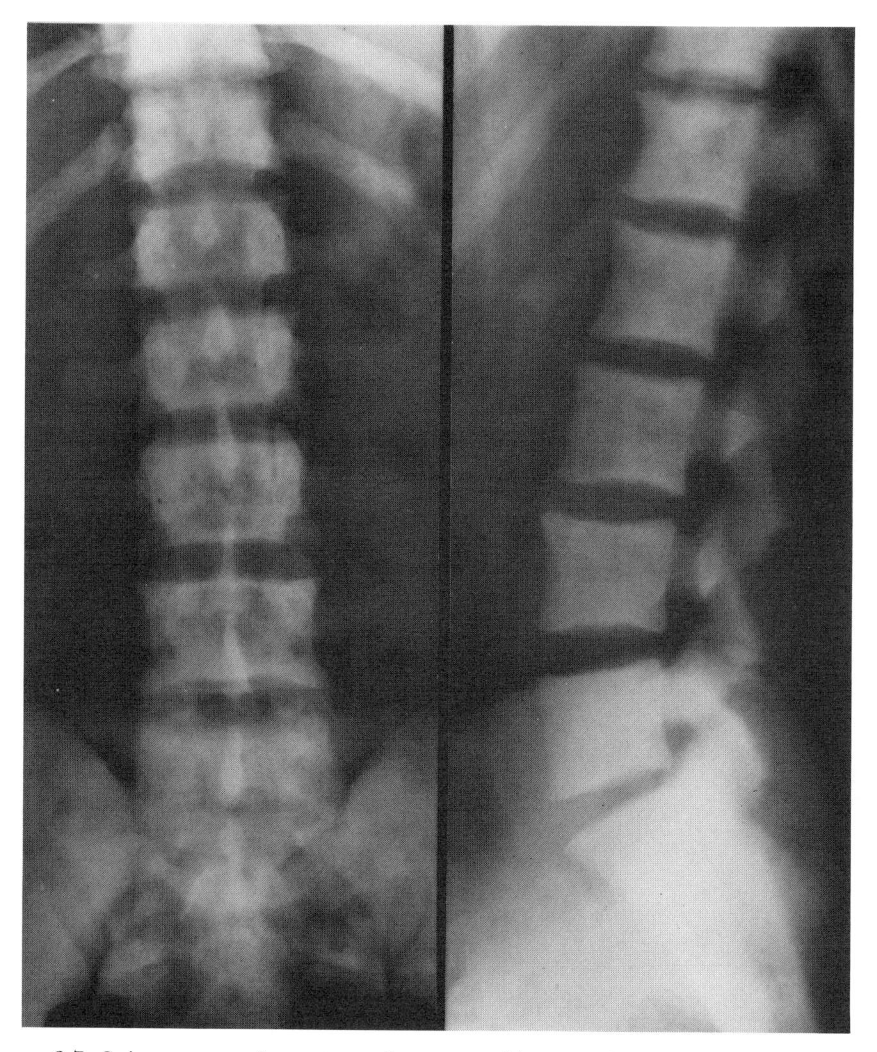

Figure 6-7. Spine x-rays of a seventy-four-year-old man with multiple myeloma show extensive osteosclerotic bone changes in association with small foci of osteolysis throughout the thoracolumbar spine. Bone sclerosis is a rare roentgenographic manifestation of multiple myeloma.

- generalized osteosclerosis or a mixture of osteosclerotic and osteolytic lesions throughout the spine (Figure 6-7), both of which are fairly uncommon radiological manifestations

Prolonged systemic administration of corticosteroids undoubtedly contributes to the generalized osteoporosis, and the osteoclast-activating factor secreted by lymphocytes and plasma cells from multiple myeloma patients may cause additional bone destruction. It is felt that calcitonin,[237-240] an inhibitor of bone resorption, may be partially responsible for producing osteosclerosis of myeloma,[241-254] which is sometimes associated with peripheral polyneuropathy.[255-261] Bone scans with radionuclides[262-266] such as radioactive gallium and technetium compounds can reveal lesions not demonstratable by routine radiography and are quite useful in distinguishing solitary myeloma from multiple meyloma.

PATHOLOGICAL FEATURES

Gross Pathology

The gross appearance of multiple myeloma varies from the hard, yellowish-white or grayish-white osteosclerotic lesions with myeloma-induced trabecular thickening and normal intervertebral disks (Figure 6-8) to the soft, gelatinous, reddish-gray or grayish-white osteolytic lesions in which punched-out lesions filled with myeloma tissue and foci of hemorrhage and cystic degeneration can usually be found (Figure 6-9). Reduction in number and thickness of the spongy trabeculae, occupation of the marrow space with reddish-gray and grayish-white tumor tissue, erosion or perforation of the cortex from the medullary side with or without extraosseous tumor extension, compression fracture of vertebral bodies, expansion of intervertebral disks, and evidence of spinal cord or nerve compression by the extruded bone, disk, or tumor tissue are the other autopsy findings (Figure 6-10).

Microscopic Pathology

Microscopically, typical myeloma cells have a rather uniform round or oval eccentric nucleus that has clumped chromatin, producing the so-called wheel-spoke or clock-face appearance, and a pinkish cytoplasm with well-defined cytoplasmic border (Figures 6-11 and 6-12). The less mature myeloma cells are significantly bigger and contain more nuclear and cytoplasmic materials and cellular pleomorphism (Figure 6-13). Occasionally, multinucleated plasma cells and mitoses can also be present. In osteosclerotic lesions, although the histology of myeloma cells is like that of osteolytic lesions, the involved bone usually shows tremendous trabecular thickening brought about by the myeloma-induced osteoblastic activity (Figures 6-14 and 6-15). However, in both the osteosclerotic and osteolytic

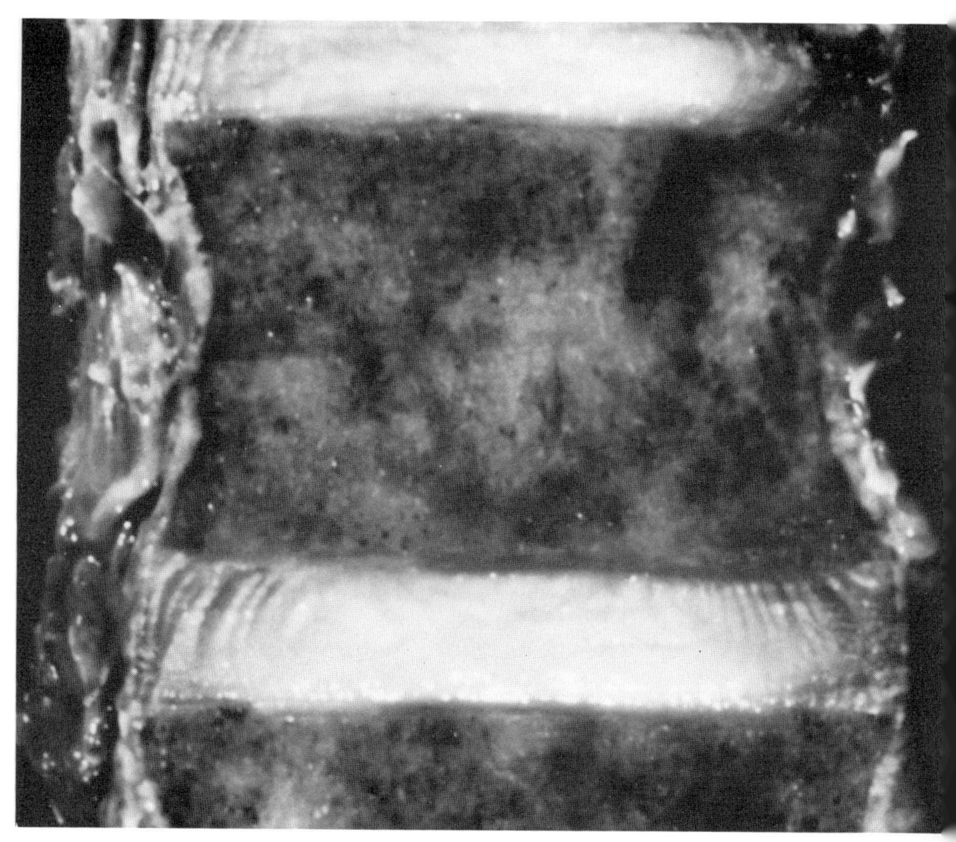

Figure 6-8. Longitudinal section of a lower thoracic vertebra from a sixty-seven-year-old man who died of osteosclerotic form of multiple myeloma shows extensive myeloma-induced new bone formation within the vertebral body that prevents the adjacent intervertebral disks from bulging into the myeloma-infiltrated vertebral body.

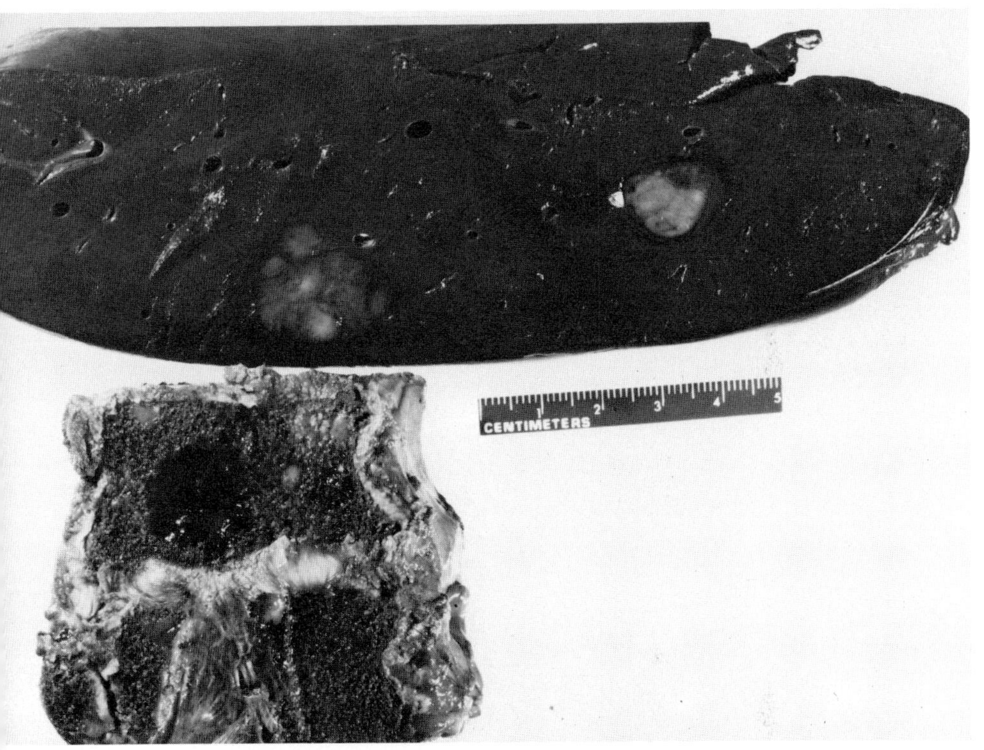

Figure 6-9. Longitudinal section of two lower thoracic vertebrae showing several round reddish-gray myeloma foci imbedded in the trabecular bone. Note the similarity in gross appearance between the intraosseous myeloma foci and the intrahepatic myeloma deposits and the punched-out hemorrhagic cyst in the upper vertebral body.

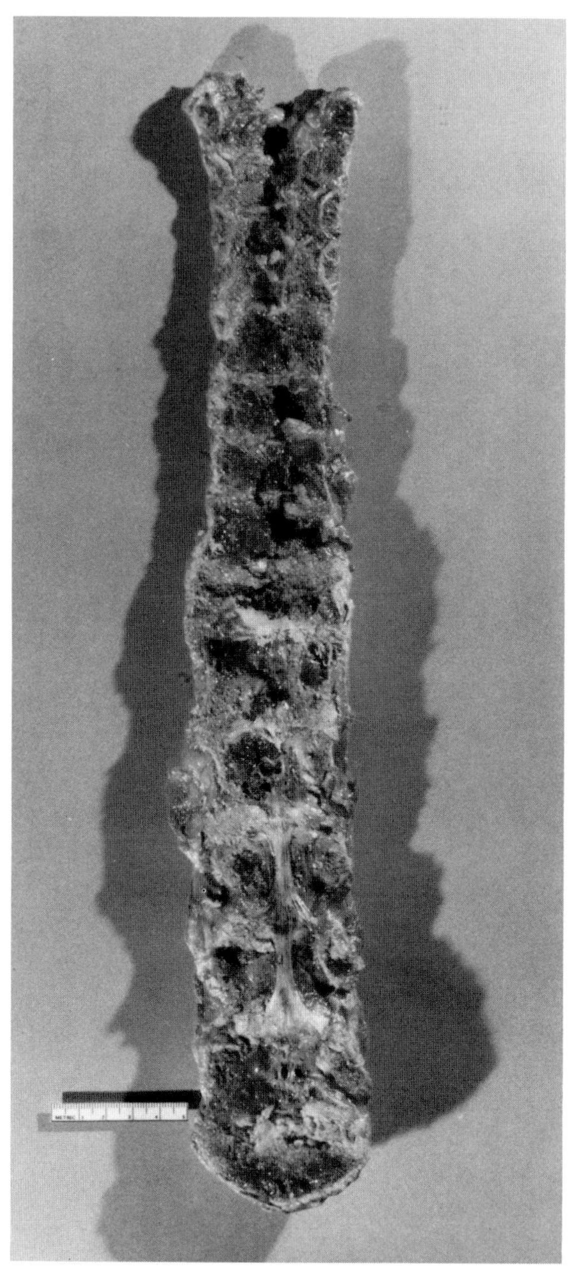

Figure 6-10. Longitudinal section of the entire thoracic and lumbar spine of a myeloma patient showing multiple compression fractures of the vertebral bodies and the corresponding expanded intervertebral disks.

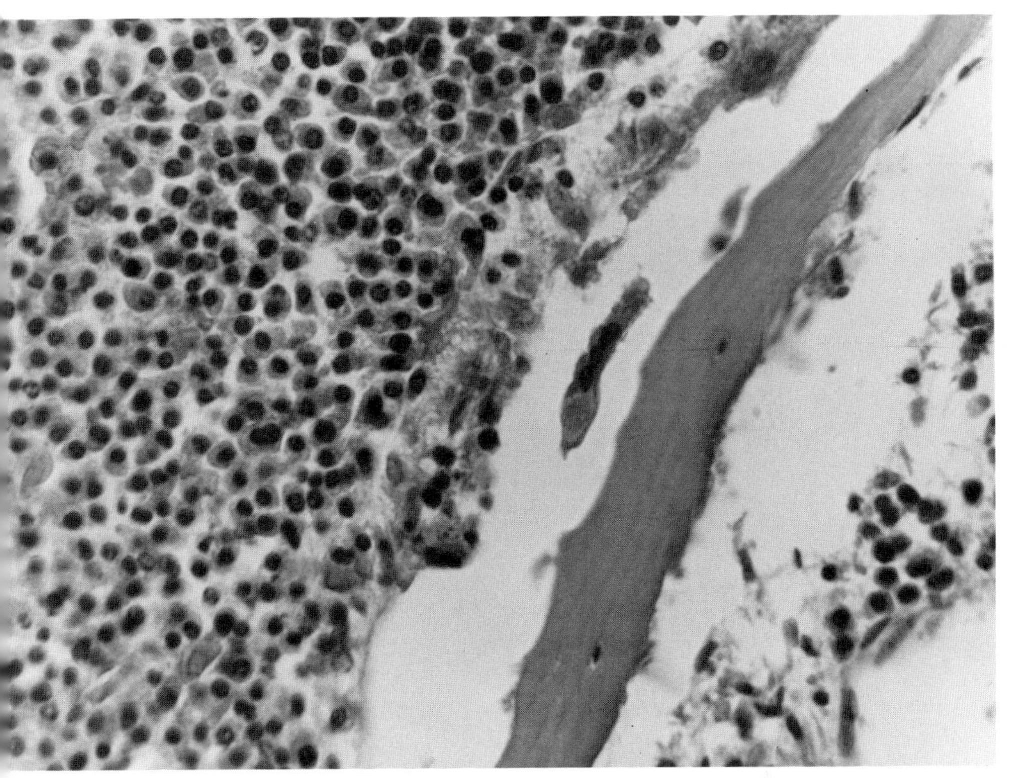

Figure 6-11. This photomicrograph (reduced 15% from 390 ×, H. & E.) shows trabecular erosion by many myeloma cells that all have a well-defined cytoplasmic border and show little cellular atypism.

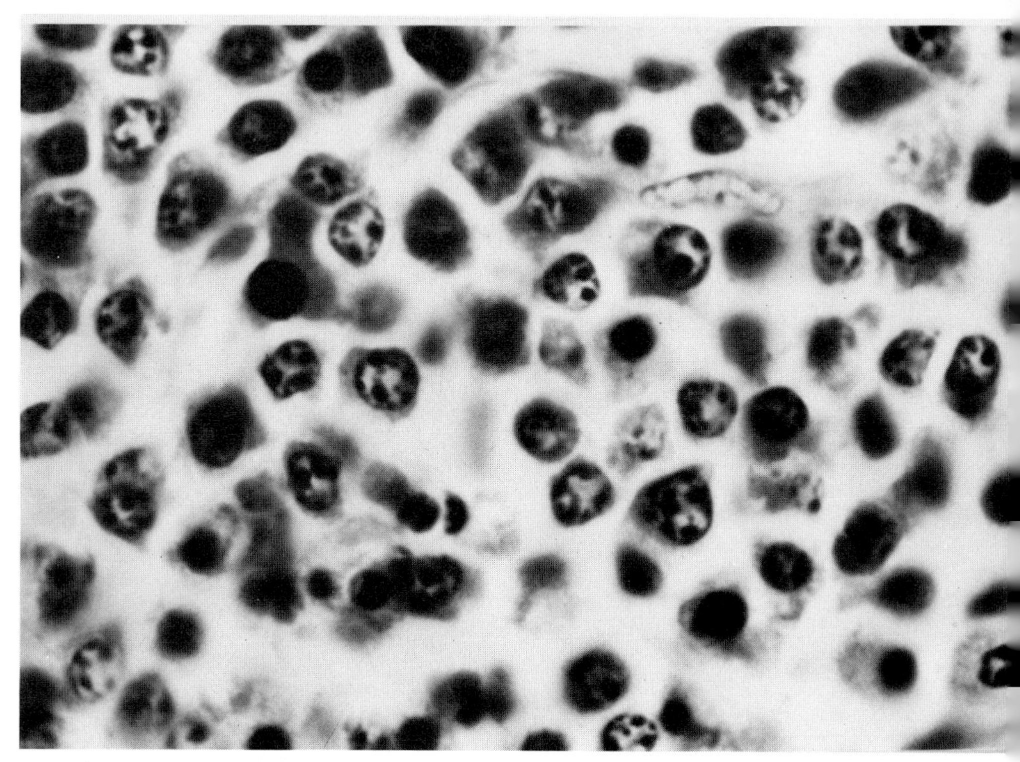

Figure 6-12. This photomicrograph (reduced 17% from 900×, H. & E.) shows many fairly uniform myeloma cells with round and eccentric nuclei, many of which have clumped chromatin, which produces the so-called clock face or wheel spoke appearance.

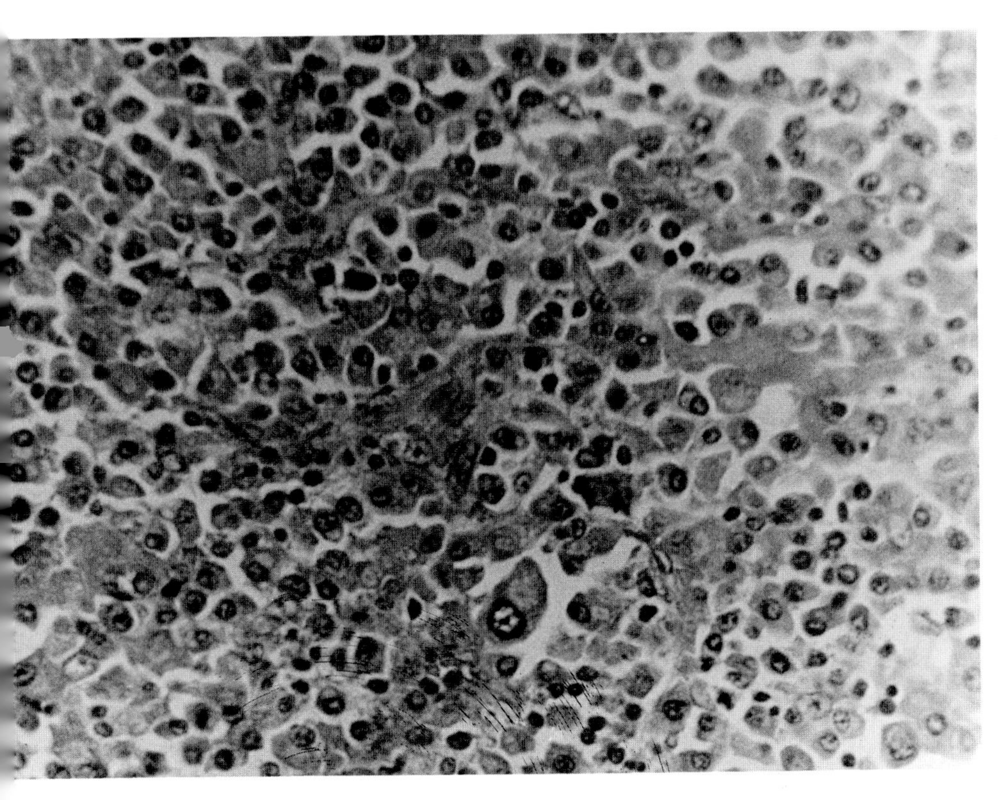

Figure 6-13. This photomicrograph (reduced 15% from 390×, H. & E.) shows a less mature form of myeloma characterized by the presence of more nuclear and cytoplasmic materials per cell and moderate degree of cellular pleomorphism. Note the giant myeloma cell in the lower central portion of this picture with a wheel-spokelike nucleus and abundant cytoplasm enclosed by a distinct cytoplasmic border.

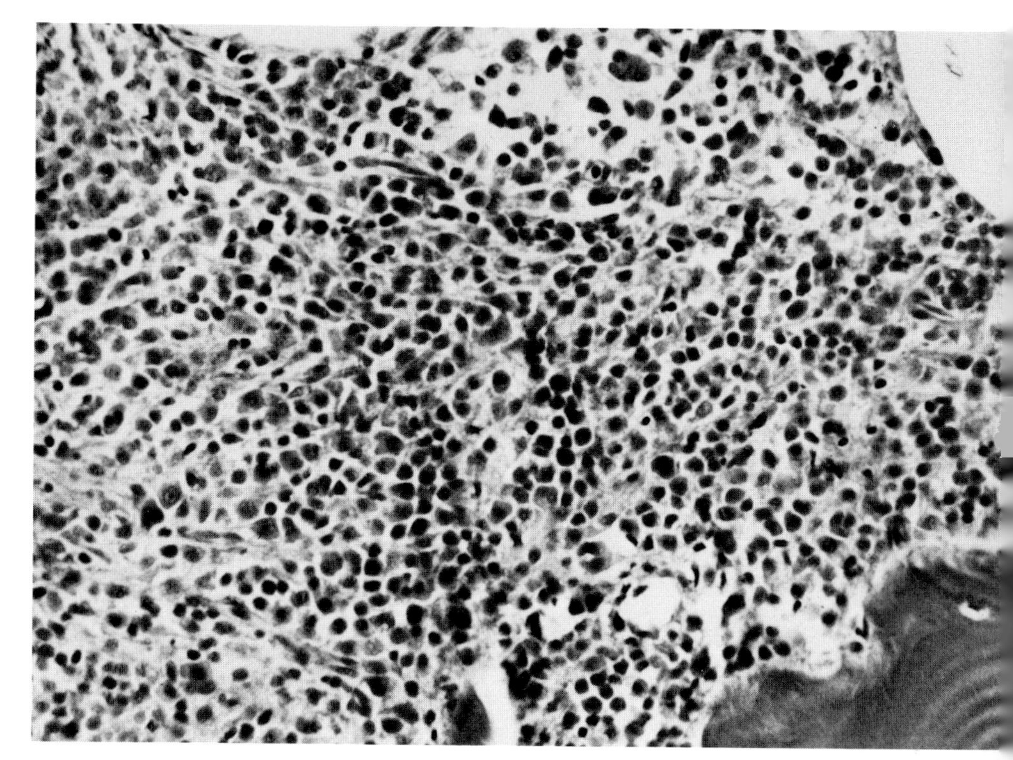

Figure 6-14. This photomicrograph (reduced 17% from 250×, H. & E.) belonging to a[n] osteosclerotic myeloma shows many typical myeloma cells with distinct cytoplasmic border[s] and a piece of thickened lamellar bone in the right lower corner of this picture.

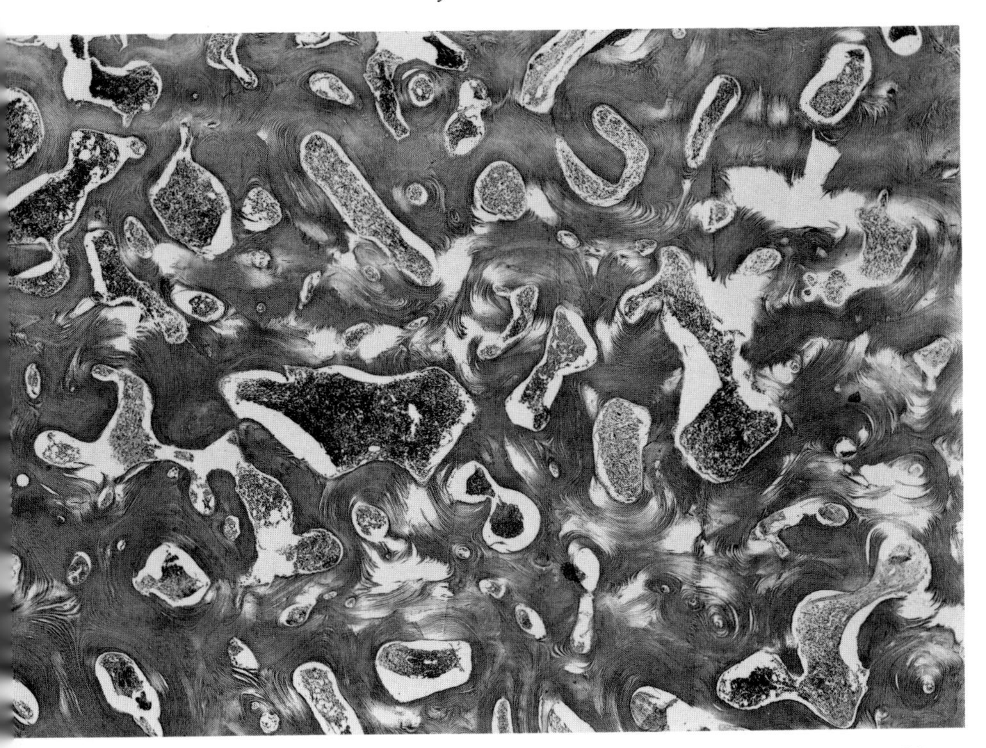

igure 6-15. This photomicrograph (reduced 17% from 25×, H. & E.) from a patient with steosclerotic myeloma shows tremendous thickening of the bony trabeculae caused by nyeloma-induced osteoblastic activity. Note the presence of numerous dense cement lines reating a mosaic pattern of the bone and resembling the histologic appearance of Paget's isease of bone.

esions of myeloma, the intramedullary proliferation of myeloma cells ften causes complete obliteration of the normal fatty septa of bone narrow. Electron microscopic examination of myeloma cells by several uthors had demonstrated the presence of intracytoplasmic myeloma roteins and abnormal pattern of the rough endoplasmic reticulum with nultiple concentric lamellar bodies and single sac loops.[267-269]

TREATMENT

Owing to the wide ramifications of systemic and local involvements and omplications of myeloma, treatment should be carefully tailored to suit ach myeloma patient's individual need.[270-275] Anemia and thrombocy-openia can be alleviated by proper nutrition and blood and platelet ransfusions.[276] Hypercalcemia from increased bone resorption possibly aused by an "osteoclast-activating factor" secreted by lymphocytes and lasma cells of multiple myeloma patients can be treated with adequate ydration; and systemic corticosteroids, calcitonin, and mithramycin, either singly or in various combinations.[277-278] Different diphosphonates[279-281] such as dichloromethylene diphosphonate, a pyrophosphate analogue, have been shown to inhibit osteoclastic activity and suppress both bone resorption and mineralization, resulting in decreased urinary excretion of calcium and hydroxyproline, skeletal lesions and pain. In addition, by treating myeloma patients with different combinations of sodium floride, calcium carbonate, and vitamin D, Kyle (1980)[282] was able to show increased bone formation demonstrated by microradiography and videodensitometry and increased compression strength of vertebral bodies. Similar observations were made by Cohen and Gardner (1964)[283] and Cohen (1966).[284] Hyperuricemia secondary to high turnover of myeloma cells and cytotoxic effects of chemotherapy can be properly managed with adequate hydration and hypouricemic agent such as allopurinal (Zyloprim®). Systemic administration of chemotherapeutic agents in various combinations,[285-293] e.g. alkylating agents and Prednisone®, is usually required in treating advanced and widely disseminated forms of myeloma cases. The important signs of improvement for chemotherapy include decreased serum myeloma immunoglobulins and urinary Bence-Jones proteins, hematologic improvement, cessation of further skeletal destruction or occasional reossification of osteolytic lesions, improved resistance to different infections, and diminution or total disappearance of clinical complaints. Recently, the feasibility of growing human myeloma cells in cell culture enabled investigators to test the sensitivity of myeloma cells to different chemotherapeutic agents prior to administrating the same agents to myeloma patients. Their preliminary findings showed a good correlation between *in vitro* and *in vivo* drug sensitivity of myeloma cells.[294] Needless to say, this new technique has to be fully perfected before coming into general use.

Since infection is still the most frequent specific cause of death in myeloma patients who often have neutropenia and significantly decreased concentration of normal immunoglobulins, respiratory and urinary tract infection, septicemia, and other infections[295-306] should be vigorously treated with appropriate antibiotics and other supportive treatments. Myeloma patients with flail chest caused by sternal and multiple rib fractures should be given ventilatory support with positive airway pressure in order to prevent fatal pulmonary complications. Pulmonary embolism, intrathoracic plasmacytoma, and pleural effusion associated with pleural plasmacytoma[307-314] should also receive special medical attention.

Renal failure is the second most common cause of death in myeloma patients. It is brought about by nephrocalcinosis, uric acid nephropathy, renal amyloidosis, renal tubular acidosis, toxicity of Bence-Jones proteins to the proximal tubular cells, blockage of the renal tubules by the precipitation of Bence-Jones proteins, recurrent pyelonephritis, glomerulonephropathy, myelomatous obstructive uropathy, etc.[315-337] It should be vigorously treated with peritoneal or hemodialysis, plasmapheresis, and, rarely, renal transplantation.[338-342] Hyperviscosity syndrome caused by excessive myeloma immunoglobulins with high intrinsic viscosity and cold sensitivity from cryoglobulinemia can be alleviated by means of plasmapheresis.[343] Plasmapheresis removes the offending myeloma paraproteins from the serum and can simultaneously reduce the chances of spontaneous bleeding from various organs because myeloma paraproteins can react with various coagulation factors to bring about hemorrhagic diasthesis.

It should be noted that solitary and extraskeletal myelomas should be treated with radiotherapy or surgical excision, and chemotherapy is usually contraindicated due to its long-term oncogenic effects. In addition, radiotherapy is effective in relieving bone pain and retarding or arresting further bone destruction caused by multiple myeloma due to the radiosensitivity of myeloma cells, and both the regional and whole body radiotherapy is in the general use.[344-351] In addition, local treatments of myeloma of the spine consist of surgical or irradiational treatment of a certain portion of the spine where the myeloma process has destroyed the bony elements to the extent that dangerous instability is present or pressure on the spinal cord or nerves has taken place. Radiotherapy can destroy the relatively radiosensitive myeloma cells, especially the less mature and actively proliferating variety, whereas surgical laminectomy, removal of the pressing tumor tissue, bone and disk fragments, and stabilization of the destroyed area can at least temporarily spare the myeloma patients of the tremendous morbidity and the impending potentially fatal outcome.

PROGNOSIS

The prognosis of myeloma[352-361] depends on the site and extent of its involvement and the cellular morphology of the predominant tumor cells:

- Extraskeletal myeloma has the best prognosis; solitary skeletal myeloma, less favorable prognosis; and multiple myeloma, the worst prognosis.
- The small-cell, mature, and well-differentiated type of myeloma has a definitely better prognosis than the large-cell, immature, and pleomorphic variety.
- The presence of severe infections or renal failure in myeloma patients makes them poor candidates for long-term survival.
- The higher the stage of myeloma the poorer the prognosis.
- When plasmacytoma, hyperviscosity syndrome, amyloidosis and flail chest are present and involve the vital organs, e.g. kidney, heart, lung, etc., the prognosis is unfavorable.

- Acute leukemia arising from a pre-existing myeloma case[362-364] can bring about the patient's demise in a short period of time.
- Elderly myeloma patients tend to fare significantly worse than younger patients with the same myelomatous skeletal and visceral involvements.
- Failure to show favorable response to chemotherapy, radiotherapy, and other modalities of therapy will allow the relentless myeloma process to progress in an uncontrolled manner and bring about its victim's early demise.

REFERENCES

1. Advani, S. H., Soman, C. S., Talwalkar, G. V., Iyer, Y. S., and Bhatia, H. M.: Multiple-myeloma: Review of 231 cases. *Indian J Cancer, 15:*55-61, 1978.
2. Kapadia, S. B.: Multiple myeloma: A clinicopathologic study of 62 consecutively autopsied cases. *Medicine* (Baltimore), *59:*380-392, 1980.
3. Kyle, R. A.: Multiple myeloma: Review of 869 cases. *Mayo Clin Proc, 50:*29-40, 1975.
4. Nordenson, N. G.: Myelomatosis. A clinical review of 310 cases. *Acta Med Scand, 179:*178, 1966.
5. Mellstedt, H., Killander, D., and Pettersson, D.: Bone marrow kinetic studies on three patients with myelomatosis. *Acta Med Scand, 202:*413-417, 1977.
6. Carson, C. P., Ackerman, L. V., and Maltby, J. D.: Plasma cell myeloma. *Am J Clin Path, 25:*849-888, 1955.
7. Gordon, H., and Schneider, B.: Plasma-cell myeloma in child: Report of case. *Int Clin, 4:*173-181, 1940.
8. Hewell, G. M., and Alexanian, R.: Multiple myeloma in young person. *Ann Intern Med, 84:*441-443, 1976.
9. Porter, F. S., Jr.: Multiple myeloma in a child. *J Pediatr, 62:*602, 1963.
10. Schmaus, K. A.: Multiples myelom (plasmacytom) bei einem Jugend Lichen. *Chirurg, 21:*48, 1950.
11. Slavens, J. J.: Multiple myeloma in a child. *Am J Dis Child, 47:*821-835, 1934.
12. Baitz, T., and Kyle, R. A.: Solitary myeloma in chronic osteomyelitis. Report of case *Arch Intern Med, 113:*872-876, 1964.
13. Carter, P. M., and Rushman, R. W.: Solitary plasmacytoma of the clavicle. *Proc R Soc Med, 67:*1097-1098, 1974.
14. Christopherson, W. M., and Miller, A. J.: A reevaluation of solitary plasma-cell myeloma of bone. *Cancer, 3:*240-252, 1950.
15. Cutler, M., Buschke, F., and Cantril, S. T.: Course of single myeloma of bone. *Surg Gynec and Obstet, 62:*918, 1936.
16. Dalgaard, E. B., and Dalgaard, J. B.: Solitary plasmacytoma with terminal dissemination. *Acta Radiol, 37:*231, 1952.
17. Fujiwara, S., Matsushima, T., Kitamura, K., Iwashita, H., Numaguchi, Y.: Solitary plasmacytoma in the cerebellopontine angle. *Surg Neurol, 13:*211-214, 1980.
18. Gupta, S. P., and Prabhakar, B. R.: Peripheral neuropathy and solitary myeloma. *Br Med J, 2:*1004, 1965.
19. Harding, W. G., II, and Kimball, T. S.: Solitary myeloma (plasmacytoma) of the femur: Report of one case. *Am J Cancer, 16:*1184-1192, 1932.
20. Hinds, E. C., Pleasants, J. E., and Bell, W. E.: Solitary plasma-cell myeloma of the mandible. *Oral Surg, 9:*193-202, 1956.

21. Jackson, H., Jr., Parker, F., Jr., and Bethea, J. M.: Studies of disease of the lymphoid and myeloid tissues. Plasmacytomata and their relation to multiple myelomata. *Am J M Sc, 181:*169, 1931.
22. Jacobson, R. J., Levy, J. K., Shulman, G., and DeMoor, N. G.: Solitary myeloma. *S Afr Med J, 49:*1347-1351, 1975.
23. Johnson, L. C., and Meador, G. E.: The nature of benign "solitary myeloma" of bone. *Bull Hosp Joint Dis, 12:*298-313, 1951.
24. Kaplan, G. A., and Bennett, J.: Solitary myeloma of lumbar spine successfully treated with radiation. Report of a case. *Radiol, 91:*1017-1018, 1968.
25. Lewin, H., and Stein, J. M.: Solitary plasma cell myeloma with new bone formation. *Am J Roentgenol Radium Ther Nucl Med, 79:*630-637, 1958.
26. Lumb, G.: Solitary plasmacytoma of bone with renal changes. *Br J Surg, 36:*16-22, 1948.
27. McLauchlan, J.: Solitary myeloma of the clavicle with long survival after total excision. Report of a case. *J Bone & Joint Surg, 55-B:*357-358, 1973.
28. Mendenhall, C. M., Thar, T. L., and Mellion, R. R.: Solitary plasmacytoma of bone and soft tissue. *Int J Radiat Oncol Biol Phys, 6:*1497-1501, 1980.
29. Pasternack, J. G., and Waugh, R. L.: Solitary myeloma of bone. *Ann Surg, 110:*427-436, 1939.
30. Paul, L. W., and Pohle, E. A.: Solitary myeloma of bone. *Radiology, 35:*651-667, 1940.
31. Raven, R. W., and Willis, R. A.: Solitary plasmocytoma of the spine. *J Bone & Joint Surg, 31-B:*369-375, 1949.
32. Read, D., and Warlow, C.: Peripheral neuropathy and solitary plasmacytoma. *J Neurol Neurosurg Psychiatry, 41:*177-184, 1978.
33. Ritz, N. D., and Meyer, L. M.: Solitary plasmacytoma of bone with subsequent multiple myeloma. *Acta Haematol, 8:*224-232, 1952.
34. Rushton, D. I.: Peripheral sensorimotor neuropathy associated with a localized myeloma. *Br Med J, 2:*203-205, 1965.
35. Spitzer, R., and Price, L. W.: Solitary myeloma of the mandible. *Br Med J, 1:*1027-1028, 1948.
36. Todd, I. D. H.: Treatment of solitary plasmacytoma. *Clin Radiol, 16:*395-399, 1965.
37. Toth, B. J., and Wintermantel, J. A.: Apparently solitary myeloma with subsequent generalization. *Radiology, 41:*472, 1943.
38. Udoji, W. C., and Frigy, A. F.: Cytoplasmic fibrils in plasma cells of a solitary myeloma. *Am J Clin Pathol, 70:*836-839, 1978.
39. Urbanski, S. J., Bilbao, J. M., Horvath, E., Kovacs, K., So, W., and Ward, J. V.: Intrasellar solitary plasmacytoma terminating in multiple myeloma: A report of a case including electron microscopical study. *Surg Neurol, 14:*233-236, 1980.
40. Valderrama, J. A. F., and Bullough, P. G.: Solitary myeloma of the spine. *J Bone & Joint Surg, 50-B:*82-90, 1968.
41. Willis, R. A.: Solitary plasmacytoma of bone. *J Pathol, 53:*77-85, 1941.
42. Woodruff, R. K., Malpas, J. S., and White, F. E.: Solitary plasmacytoma. II. Solitary plasmacytoma of bone. *Cancer, 43:*2344-2347, 1979.
43. Wright, C. J. E.: Long survival in solitary plasmacytoma of bone. *J Bone & Joint Surg, 43-B:*767-771, 1961.
44. Yentis, I.: The so-called solitary plasmacytoma of bone. *J Fac Radiol, 8:*132-144, 1957.
45. Stewart, M. J., and Taylor, A. L.: Observations on solitary plasmacytoma. *J Path & Bact, 35:*541, 1932.
46. Wright, C. J. E.: Long survival in solitary plasmacytoma of bone. *J Bone & Joint Surg, 43-B:*767, 1961.

47. Gootnick, L. T.: Solitary myeloma: Review of sixty-one cases. *Radiology, 45:*385-391, 1945.
48. Meyer, J. E., and Schulz, M. D.: "Solitary" myeloma of bone. *Cancer, 34:*438-440, 1974.
49. Mill, W. B., and Griffith, R.: The role of radiation therapy in the management of plasma cell tumors. *Cancer, 45:*647-652, 1980.
50. Tong, D., Griffin, T. W., Laramore, G. E., Kurtz, J. M., Russell, A. H., Groudine, M. T., Herron, T., Blasko, J. C., and Tesh, D. W.: Solitary plasmacytoma of bone and soft tissues. *Radiology, 135:*195-198, 1980.
51. Ahmed, N., Ramos, S., Sika, J., Leveen, H. H., and Piccone, V. A.: Primary extramedullary esophageal plasmacytoma. *Cancer, 38:*943-947, 1976.
52. Batsakis, J. G., Fries, G. T., Goldman, R. T., and Karlsberg, R. C.: Upper respiratory tract plasmacytoma. *Arch Otolaryngol, 29:*613-618, 1964.
53. Bjorn-Hansen, R.: Primary plasmocytoma of the spleen. *Am J Roentgenol, 117:*81, 1973.
54. Chang, S. C., Jing, B. S.: Solitary plasmacytoma in cranial cavity. *J Neurosurg, 33:*471, 1971.
55. Corwin, J., and Lindberg, R. D.: Solitary plasmacytoma of bone vs. extramedullary plasmacytoma and their relationship to multiple myeloma. *Cancer, 43:*1007-1013, 1979.
56. Dolin, S., and Dewar, J. P.: Extramedullary plasmacytoma. *Am J Pathol, 32:*83-103, 1956.
57. Doss, L. L.: Simultaneous extramedullary plasmacytomas of the vagina and vulva: A case report and review of the literature. *Cancer, 41:*2468-2474, 1978.
58. Douglass, H. O., Jr., Sika, J. V., and Leveen, H. H.: Plasmacytoma: A not so rare tumor of the small intestine. *Cancer, 28:*456-460, 1971.
59. Edwards, G. A., and Zawadski, Z. A.: Extraosseous lesions in plasma cell myeloma. A report of 6 cases. *Am J Med 43:*194-205, 1967.
60. Ewing, M. R., and Foote, F. W., Jr.: Plasma-cell tumor of the mouth and upper air passages. *Cancer, 5:*499-513, 1952.
61. Ferlito, A., Polidoro, F., and Recher, G.: Extramedullary plasmacytoma of the parotid gland. *Laryngoscope, 90:*486-493, 1980.
62. Fishkin, B. G., and Spiegelberg, H. L.: Cervical lymphnode metastasis as the first manifestation of localized extramedullary plasmacytoma. *Cancer, 38:*1641-1644, 1976.
63. Fruhling, L., and Chadli, A.: Le sarcome plasmocytaire extrasquelettique. *Ann Anat Pathol, 8:*317-376, 1963.
64. Gromer, R. C., and Duvall, A. J., III: Plasma cytoma of the head and neck. *J Laryngol Otol, 58:*861-872, 1973.
65. Halliday, D., Davey, F. R., Call, F., and Marucci, A. A.: Identification of intracellular immunoglobulin in extramedullary myeloma. *Arch Pathol Lab Med, 101:*522-525, 1977.
66. Hellwig, C.: Extramedullary plasma cell tumors as observed in various locations. *Arch Pathol, 36:*95-111, 1943.
67. Jaeger, E.: Das extramedullare plasmacytoma. *Itschr F Krebstorsch, 52:*349-383, 1941.
68. Levin, H. S., and Mostofi, F. K.: Symptomatic plasmacytoma of the testis. *Cancer, 25:*1193-1203, 1970.
69. Mancilla-Jimenez, R., and Tavassoli, F. A.: Solitary meningeal plasmacytoma. *Cancer, 38:*798-806, 1976.
70. McCall, J. W., and Bailey, C. H., Jr.: Extramedullary plasmacytoma of the upper air passages. *Trans Am Laryngol Assoc, 81:*235-246, 1960.

71. Moosy, J., and Wilson, C.: Solitary intracranial plasmacytoma. *Arch Neurol, 16:*212, 1967.
72. More, J. R. S., Dawson, D. W., Ralston, A. J., and Craig, I.: Plasmacytoma of the thyroid. *J Clin Pathol, 21:*661-667, 1968.
73. Nielsen, S. M., Schenken, J. R., and Cawley, L. P.: Primary colonic plasmacytoma. *Cancer, 30:*261-267, 1962.
74. Remigio, P. A., and Klaum, A.: Extramedullary plasmacytoma of the stomach. *Cancer, 27:*562-568, 1971.
75. Soumerai, S., and Gleason, E. A.: Asynchronous plasmacytoma of the stomach and testis. *Cancer, 45:*396-400, 1980.
76. Stout, A. P., and Kenney, F. R.: Primary plasma-cell tumors of upper air passages and oral cavity. *Cancer, 2:*261-278, 1949.
77. Woodruff, R. K., Whittle, J. M., and Malpas, J. S.: Solitary plasmacytoma. I. Extramedullary soft tissue plasmacytoma. *Cancer, 43:*2340-2343, 1979.
78. Kotner, L. M., and Wang, C. C.: Plasmacytoma of the upper air and food passages. *Cancer, 30:*414-418, 1972.
79. Poole, A. G., and Marchetta, F. C.: Extramedullary plasmacytoma of the head and neck. *Cancer, 22:*14-21, 1968.
80. Webb, H. E., Harrison, E. G., Masson, J. K., and Remine, W. H.: Solitary extramedullary myeloma (plasmacytoma) of the upper part of the respiratory tract and oropharynx. *Cancer, 15:*1142-1155, 1962.
81. Wiltshaw, E.: The natural history of extramedullary plasmacytoma and its relation to solitary myeloma of bone and myelomatosis. *Medicine, 55:*217-238, 1976.
82. Grammens, G. L., and Ellis, R. W.: Multiple myeloma terminating as plasma cell leukemia and coinciding with a change in light chain production. *Minn Med, 63:*179-180, 1980.
83. Kyle, R., Maldonado, J. E., and Bayrd, E. D.: Plasma cell leukemia: Report on 17 cases. *Arch Intern Med, 144:*813-818, 1974.
84. Moss, W. T., and Ackerman, L. V.: Plasma cell leukemia. *Blood, 1:*396-406, 1946.
85. Muller, G. L., and McNaughton, E.: Multiple myeloma (plasmacytomata) with blood picture of plasma cell leukemia. *Folia Haemat, 46:*17, 1931.
86. Nagaratnam, N., Talwaite, S. N., Fernando, D. J., Deen, M. F., and Kulasegaram, V.: Uncommon manifestations of myelomatosis and plasma cell leukaemia. *Ceylon Med J, 22:*167-171, 1977.
87. Newman, W., Diefenbach, W. C. L., Quinn, M., and Meyer, L. M.: A case of acute plasma-cell leukemia supporting the concept of unity of plasma cellular neoplasia. *Cancer, 5:*514-520, 1952.
88. Pater, A. J., Jr., and Castle, W. B.: Plasma cell leukemia. *Am J M Sc, 191:*788, 1936.
89. Pedraza, M. A.: Plasma-cell leukemia with unusual immunoglobulin abnormalities. *Am J Clin Pathol, 64:*410-415, 1975.
90. Piney, A., and Riach, J. S.: Multiple myeloma. Aleukaemic and leukaemic. *Folia Haemat, 46:*37, 1931.
91. Raha, P. K., and Basumullick, R. N.: Plasma cell leukemia with some uncommon features. *J Indian Med Assoc, 74:*174-175, 1980.
92. Rubinstein, M. A.: Multiple myeloma as a form of leukemia. *Blood, 4:*1049, 1949.
93. Sharnoff, J. G., Belsky, H., and Melton, J.: Plasma cell leukemia or multiple myeloma with osteosclerosis. *Am J Med, 17:*582, 1954.
94. Wetter, O., Linder, K. H., Hossfeld, D. K., Lunscken, C., Schmitt-Graff, A.: Plasma cell dyscrasias — a comparative study of cell surface properties in plasma cell leukemia and myeloma. *Leuk Res, 4:*249-259, 1980.

95. Akin, R. K., Barton, K., and Walters, P. J.: Amyloidosis, macroglossia, and carpal tunnel syndrome associated with myeloma. *J Oral Surg, 33:*690-692, 1975.
96. Bayrd, E. D., and Bennett, W. A.: Amyloidosis complicating myeloma. *Med Clin North Am, 34:*1151-1164, 1950.
97. Breathnach, S. M., and Wells, G. C.: Amyloid vascular disease: Cord-like thickening of mucocutaneous arteries, intermittent claudication and angina in a case with underlying myelomatosis. *Br J Dermatol, 102:*591-595, 1980.
98. Dahlin, D. C., and Dockerty, M. B.: Amyloid and myeloma. *Am J Pathol, 26:*581-593, 1950.
99. Fadell, E. J., and Morris, H. C.: Amyloidoma presenting as a primary sternal tumor. *Am J Surg, 108:*75-79, 1964.
100. Flick, W. G., and Lawrence, F. R.: Oral amyloidosis as initial symptom of multiple myeloma. A case report. *Oral Surg, 49:*18-20, 1980.
101. French, B. T.: Amyloid arthropathy in myelomatosis-intracytoplasmic synovial deposition. *Histopathology, 4:*21-28, 1980.
102. Glenner, C. G., Terry, W. D., and Isersky, C.: Amyloidosis: Its nature and pathogenesis. *Sem Hematol, 10:*65-86, 1973.
103. Grossman, R. E., and Hensley, G. T.: Bone lesion in primary amyloidosis. *Am J Roentgenol Radium Ther Nucl Med, 65:*585-589, 1951.
104. Isobe, T., and Osserman, E. F.: Patterns of amyloidosis and their association with plasma cell dyscrasia, monoclonal immunoglobulins and Bence-Jones proteins. *N Engl J Med, 290:*473-477, 1974.
105. Kavanaugh, J. H.: Multiple myeloma. Amyloid arthropathy and pathological fracture of the femur. A case report. *J Bone & Joint Surg, 60-A:*135-137, 1978.
106. Kyle, R. A.: Amyloidosis: Part 2. *Int J Dermatol, 20:*20-25, 1981.
107. Kyle, R. A., and Bayrd, E. D.: "Primary systemic amyloidosis and myeloma. Discussion of relationship and review of 81 cases. *Arch Intern Med, 107:*344-353, 1961.
108. Lowell, D. M.: Amyloid-producing plasmacytoma of the pelvis. Case report and review of the literature. *Arch Surg, 94:*899-903, 1967.
109. Melato, M., Falconieri, G., Pascali, E., and Pezzoli, A.: Amyloid casts within renal tubules: A singular finding in myelomatosis. *Virchows Arch Pathol Anat, 387:*133-145, 1980.
110. Druzanski, W., Hasselback, R., Katz, A., and Parr, D. M.: Multiple myeloma (light chain disease) with rheumatoid-like amyloid arthropathy and mu-heavy chain fragment in the serum. *Am J Med, 65:*334-341, 1978.
111. Pruzanski, W., and Katz, A.: Clinical and laboratory findings in primary generalized and multiple-myeloma-related amyloidosis. *Can Med Assoc J, 114:*906-909, 1976.
112. Roslund, J., Sundgerg, K., and Tovi, D.: Plasma cell myeloma of thoracic vertebra with amyloid deposits. *Acta Pathol Microbiol Scand, 49:*273-279, 1960.
113. Trump, D. L., Allen, H., Olson, J., Wright, J., and Humphrey, R. L.: Epidermolysis bullosa acquisita. Association with amyloidosis and multiple myeloma. *JAMA, 243:*1461-1462, 1980.
114. Grader, J., and Moynihan, J. W.: Multiple myeloma and osteogenic sarcoma in a patient with Paget's Disease. *JAMA, 176:*685-687, 1961.
115. Gross, R. J., and Yelin, G.: Multiple myeloma complicating Paget's Disease. *Am J Roentgenol Radium Ther Nucl Med, 65:*585-589, 1951.
116. Hanisch, C. M.: Paget's Disease complicated by multiple myeloma. *Bull Hosp Joint Dis, 11:*43-47, 1950.
117. Mehbod, H., and Sweeney, W. M.: Multiple myeloma in Paget's Disease. *JAMA, 177:*531, 1961.

118. Price, C. H. G.: Myeloma occurring with Paget's Disease of Bone. *Skeletal Radiol, 1:*15-19, 1976.
119. Reich, C., and Brodsky, A. E.: Coexisting multiple myeloma and Paget's Disease of bone treated with Stilbamidine. *J Bone & Joint Surg, 30-A:*642-646, 1948.
120. Rosenkrantz, J. A., and Gluckman, E. C.: Coexistence of Paget's Disease of bone and multiple myeloma. Case reports of 2 patients. *Am J Roentgenol Radium Ther Nucl Med, 78:*30-38, 1957.
121. Scurr, J. A.: Myeloma occurring in Paget's Disease. *Proc R Soc Med, 65:*725, 1972.
122. Cuzick, J.: Radiation-induced myelomatosis. *N Engl J Med, 304:*204-210, 1981.
123. Clarke, E.: Spinal cord involvement in multiple myelomatosis. *Brain, 79:*332, 1956.
124. Dahlstrom, U., Jarpe, S., and Lindstrom, F. D.: Paraplegia in myelomatosis — a study of 20 cases. *Acta Med Scand, 205:*173-178, 1979.
125. Driedger, H., and Pruzanski, W.: Plasma cell neoplasia with peripheral polyneuropathy. A study of five cases and a review of the literature. *Medicine* (Baltimore), *59:*301-310, 1980.
126. Garrett, M. J.: Spinal myeloma and cord compression. Diagnosis and management. *Clin Radiol, 20:*42, 1969.
127. Jacox, H. W., and Kahn, E. A.: Multiple myeloma with spinal cord involvement. *Am J Roentgenol Radium Ther Nucl Med, 30:*201-205, 1933.
128. Kelly, J. J., Jr., Kyle, R. A., Miles, J. M., O'Brien, P. C., and Dyck, P. J.: The spectrum of peripheral neuropathy in myeloma. *Neurology* (N.Y.), *31:*24-31, 1981.
129. McKissock, W., Bloom, W. H., and Chynn, K. Y.: Spinal cord compression caused by plasma cell tumors. *J Neurosurg, 18:*68, 1961.
130. Nelson, C. L., Jr., and Evarts, C. M.: Multiple myeloma with cord compression. Report of a case. *J Bone & Joint Surg, 50-A:*305-310, 1968.
131. Schulman, P., Sun, T., Sharer, L., Hyman, P., Vinciguerra, V., Feinstein, M., Blanck, R., Susin, M., and Degnan, T. J.: Meningeal involvement in IgD myeloma with cerebrospinal fluid paraprotein analysis. *Cancer, 46:*152-155, 1980.
132. Sen, S. K., Hunter, S. B., Dent, C. A., and Green, L. D.: Multiple myeloma: Presenting as a neurological disorder. *J Natl Med Assoc, 72:*135-139, 1980.
133. Silverstein, A., and Doniger, D. E.: Neurologic complications of myelomatosis. *Arch Neurol, 9:*534, 1963.
134. Snyder, L. J., and Cohen, C.: Multiple myeloma with spinal cord compression as initial finding. *Ann Int Med, 26:*1169, 1948.
135. Sod, L. M., and Wiener, L. M.: Intradural extramedullary plasmacytoma. *J Neurosurg, 16:*107, 1959.
136. Spiers, A. S., Halpern, R., Ross, S. C., Neiman, R. S., Harawi, S., and Zipoli, T. E.: Meningeal myelomatosis. *Arch Intern Med, 140:*256-259, 1980.
137. Svien, H. J., Price, R. D., and Bayrd, E. D.: Neurosurgical treatment of compression of the spinal cord caused by myeloma. *JAMA, 153:*784-786, 1953.
138. Victor, M., Banker, B. Q., and Adams, R. D.: The neuropathy of multiple myeloma. *J Neurol Neurosurg Psychiatry, 21:*73-88, 1958.
139. Fleegler, B., Fogarty, C., Owens, G., Cohen, E., and Cassileth, P. A.: Pathologic flail chest complicating multiple myeloma. *Arch Intern Med, 140:*414-415, 1980.
140. Mansouri, A.: Flail chest and multiple myeloma. *JAMA, 243:*1036, 1980.
141. Rammohan, G., and Karbowitz, S. R.: Spontaneous flail chest in multiple myeloma: Successful recovery. *N Y State J Med, 81:*235-236, 1981.
142. Durie, B. G., Salmon, S. E., and Mundy, G. R.: Relation of osteoclast activating factor production to extent of bone disease in multiple myeloma. *Br J Haematol, 47:*21-30, 1981.

143. Luben, R. A.: An assay for osteoclast activating factor (OAF) in biological fluids: Detection of OAF in the serum of myeloma patients. *Cell Immunol, 49:*74-80, 1980.
144. Mundy, G. R., Raisz, L. G., Cooper, R. A., Schechter, G. P., and Salmon, S. E.: Evidence for the secretion of an osteoclast stimulating factor in myeloma. *N Engl J Med, 291:*1041, 1974.
145. Benninger, G. W., and Kreps, S. I.: Aggregation phenomenon in an IgG multiple myeloma resulting in the hyperviscosity syndrome. *Am J Med, 51:*287-293, 1971.
146. Bloch, K. J., and Maki, D. G.: Hyperviscosity syndromes associated with immunoglobulin abnormalities. *Sem Hemat, 10:*113-124, 1973.
147. Capra, J. D., and Kunkel, M. G.: Aggregation of IgG 3 proteins. Relevance to the hyperviscosity syndrome. *J Clin Invest, 49:*610-621, 1970.
148. Fahey, J., Barth, W., and Solomon, A.: Serum hyperviscosity syndrome. *JAMA, 192:*120-123, 1965.
149. Pruzanski, W., Chu, R., Damji, N. F., Galler, S., and Norman, C. S.: Anemia splenomegaly and hyperviscosity syndrome. *Can Med Assoc J, 123:*731-737, 1980.
150. Pruzanski, W., and Watt, J. B.: Serum viscosity and hyperviscosity syndrome in IgG multiple myeloma. *Ann Intern Med, 77:*853-860, 1972.
151. Ray, P. K., Besa, E., Idiculla, A., Rhoads, J. E., Jr., Bassett, J. G., and Cooper, D. R.: Efficient removal of abnormal immunoglobulin G from plasma of a multiple myeloma patient. Description of a new method for treatment of the hyperviscosity syndrome. *Cancer, 45:*2633-2638, 1980.
152. Smith, E., Kochwa, S., and Wasserman, L. R.: Aggregation of IgG globulin in vivo. The hyperviscosity syndrome in multiple myeloma. *Am J Med, 39:*35-45, 1965.
153. Leonard, R. C.: Effect of temperature upon relative viscosity of normal and myeloma serum. *Br J Haematol, 47:*161, 1981.
154. Narita, H., Ogata, K., Kikuchi, I., and Inoue, S.: A case of cryoglobulinemic gangrene in myeloma with fatal outcome despite successful skin grafting. *Dermatologica, 160:*125-130, 1980.
155. Virella, G.: IgG subclasses in relation to viscosity and cryoglobulin syndromes. *Br Med J, 2:*322-327, 1971.
156. Adam, W. S., Alling, E. L., and Lawrence, J. S.: Multiple myeloma: Its clinical and laboratory diagnosis with emphysis on electrophoretic abnormalities. *Am J Med, 6:*141-161, 1961.
157. Azar, H. A., and Potter, M.: *Multiple Myeloma and Related Disorders.* Hagertown, Md. Harper & Row, 1973, Vol. I.
158. Bartoloni, C., Flamini, G., Gentiloni, N., Russo, M. A., Barone, C., Gambassi, G., and Terranova, T.: Immunochemical and ultrastructural study of multiple myeloma with a heavy chain protein in the serum. *J Clin Pathol, 33:*936-945, 1980.
159. Bloth, B., Christensson, T., and Mellstedt, H.: Extreme hyponatremia in patients with myelomatosis: An effect of cationic paraproteins. *Acta Med Scand, 203:*273-275, 1978.
160. Broder, S., Humphrey, R., Durm, M., Blackman, M., Meade, B., Golman, C., Strober W., and Waldmann, T.: Impaired synthesis of polyclonal (non-para-protein) immunoglobulins by circulating lymphocytes from patients with multiple myeloma. *N Engl J Med, 293:*887, 1975.
161. Canova, R., Casalino, C., Fischioni, P., Geissa, P., Marraffa, G., Montanaro, M., and Fabiani, F.: IgA kappa multiple myeloma in a young man. *Haematologica* (Pavia) *65:*244-249, 1980.
162. Dammacco, F., Miglietta, A., Tribalto, M., Mandelli, F., and Bonomo, L.: The expanding spectrum of clinical and laboratory features of IgE myeloma (report of a case and review of the literature). *Ric Clin Lab, 10:*583-590, 1980.

163. Dworsky, E., Sletten, K., Harboe, M., and Wetteland, P.: Structural studies of three IgG kappa proteins from a patient with multiple myeloma. *Scand J Immunol, 12:*281-287, 1980.
164. Ford, H. C., Casey, B. R., Walker, S., and Mason, A.: Multiple myeloma with an IgD kappa monoclonal protein. *Am J Clin Pathol, 74:*105-107, 1980.
165. Forsumann, O., and Nilsson, G.: A case of multiple myeloma with flaming plasma cells, but no significant M-compound in serum or urine. *Acta Med Scand, 181:*33, 1967.
166. Fritsche, H. A., and DeLeon, E.: The determination of serum immunoglobulins by automated nephelometric analysis. *Am J Med Tech, 41:*136-145, 1975.
167. Gach, J., Simon, L., and Salmon, J.: Multiple myeloma without M-type proteinemia. Report of a case with immunologic and ultrastructure studies. *Am J Med, 50:*835, 1971.
168. Gallango, M. L., Suinaga, R., and Ramirez, M.: Bence-Jones myeloma with a tetramer of kappa-type globulin in serum. *Clin Chem, 26:*1741-1744, 1980.
169. Ganeval, D., Noel, L. H., Droz, D., and Leibowitch, J.: Systemic lambda light-chain deposition in a patient with myeloma. *Br Med J Clin Res, 282:*681-683, 1981.
170. Heremans, E. P., and Waldenstrom, J.: Cytology and electrophoretic pattern in myeloma. *Acta Med Scand, 170:*575-589, 1961.
171. Hobbs, J. R.: Immunochemical class of myelomatosis. *Br J Haemat, 16:*899-906, 1969.
172. Jancelewicz, Z., Tokatski, K., Sugai, S., and Pruzanski, W.: IgD multiple myeloma. *Arch Intern Med, 135:*87-94, 1975.
173. Kim, I., Harley, J. B., and Weksler, B.: Multiple myeloma without initial paraprotein. *Am J Med Sci, 264:*267, 1972.
174. Kyle, R. A., and Bayrd, E. D.: *The Monoclonal Gammopathies: Multiple Myeloma and Related Plasma Cell Disorders.* Springfield, Ill., Charles C Thomas, 1976.
175. Kyle, R. A., Bayrd, E. D., McKenzie, B. R., and Heck, F. J.: Diagnostic criteria for electrophoretic patterns of serum and urinary proteins in multiple myeloma. *JAMA, 174:*245, 1960.
176. Kyle, R. A., and Greipp, P. R.: The laboratory investigation of monoclonal gammopathies. *Mayo Clin Proc, 53:*719-739, 1978.
177. Leb, L., Grimes, E. T., Balogh, K., and Merritt, J. A.: Monoclonal macroglobinemia with osteolytic lesions. *Cancer, 39:*227-231, 1977.
178. Nerenberg, S. T.: Gamma globulin studies of biopsy material and serum in solitary plasmacytoma of the spine. *Cancer, 24:*750-757, 1969.
179. Nicholls, M., Vincent, P. C., Repka, E., Saunders, J., and Gunz, F. W.: Isotypic discordance of paraproteins and lymphocyte surface immunoglobulins in myeloma. *Blood, 57:*192-195, 1981.
180. Osserman, E. F., and Lawlor, D. P.: Abnormal serum and urinary proteins in thirty-five cases of multiple myeloma as studied by filter paper electrophoresis. *Am J Med, 18:*462, 1955.
181. Perez-Soler, R., Esteban, R., and Guardia, J.: Urinary monoclonal immunoglobulin in multiple myeloma. *Ann Intern Med, 94:*140, 1981.
182. Perry, M. C., and Kyle, R. A.: The clinical significance of Bence-Jones proteinuria. *Mayo Clin Proc, 50:*234-238, 1975.
183. Pruzanski, W.: Clinical manifestations of multiple myeloma: Relation to class and type of M component. *Can Med Assoc J, 114:*896-897, 1976.
184. Pruzanski, W., and Rother, I.: IgD plasma cell neoplasia: Clinical manifestations and characteristic features. *Can Med Assoc J, 102:*1061-1065, 1970.
185. Smithline, N., Kassirer, J. P., and Cohen, J. J.: Light-chain nephropathy: Renal

tubular dysfunction associated with light-chain protein uria. *N Engl J Med, 294:*71-74, 1976.

186. Solomon, A.: Bence-Jones proteins and light chains of immunoglubulins. *N Engl J Med, 294:*91-98, 1976.
187. Vilpo, J. A., and Irjala, K.: IgD-Lambda myeloma with separate heavy- and light-chain M-components. *Clin Chem, 26:*1760-1761, 1980.
188. Zarrabi, M. H., Stark, R. S., Kane, P., Dannaher, C. L., and Chandor, S.: IgM myeloma, a distinct entity in the spectrum of B-cell neoplasia. *Am J Clin Pathol, 75:*1-10, 1981.
189. Bence-Jones, H.: On a new substance occurring in the urine of a patient with mollities ossium — philos. *Trans Roy Soc Lond* (Biol), *1:*55-62, 1948.
190. Kyle, R. A., Maldonado, J. E., and Bayrd, E. D.: Idiopathic Bence-Jones proteinuria — a distinct entity? *Am J Med, 55:*222-226, 1973.
191. Perrie, H. D., and Kyle, R. A.: The clinical significance of Bence-Jones proteinuria. *Mayo Clin Proc, 50:*234-338, 1975.
192. Bartoloni, C., Flamini, G., Logroscino, C., Guidi, L., Scuderi, F., Gambassi, G., and Terranova, T.: IgD (kappa) "nonsecretory" multiple myeloma: Report of a case. *Blood, 56:*898-901, 1980.
193. Ferraris, A. M., Haupt, E., and Ratti, M.: Multiple myeloma without detectable Ig synthesis. *Acta Haematol* (Basel), *62:*257-261, 1979.
194. Hurez, D., Preud 'Homme, J. L., and Scligmann, M.: Intracellular "monoclonal" immunoglobulin in non-secretory human myeloma. *J Immunol, 101:*263-264, 1970.
195. Jennett, J. C., Wilkman, A. S., and Benson, J. D.: IgD myeloma with intracytoplasmic crystalline inclusions. *Am J Clin Pathol, 75:*231-235, 1981.
196. Luper, W. E., Phillips, L. E., Hamill, R. D., and Rogers, T. E.: Non-secretory myeloma: Report of a case. *Tex Med, 76:*50-53, 1980.
197. Mancilla, R., and Davis, G.: Non-secretory multiple myeloma. Immunohistological and ultrastructural observations in two patients. *Am J Med, 63:*1015-1022, 1977.
198. Mossler, J. A., Wortman, J., Reeves, W., and McCarty, K. S., Jr.: Intracytoplasmic IgM in a non-secretory myeloma. *Arch Pathol Lab Med, 105:*165-166, 1981.
199. River, G. L., Tewksbury, D. A., and Fudenberg, H. H.: Nonsecretory multiple myeloma. *Blood, 40:*204, 1972.
200. Silling, K., Silling, J., Jacobsen, N. O., Thomsen, O. F.: Nonsecretory myeloma associated with nodular glomerulosclerosis. *Acta Med Scand, 207:*137-143, 1980.
201. Stavem, P., Froland, S. S., Haugen, H. F., and Lislerud, A.: Nonsecretory myelomatosis without intracellular immunoglobulin. *Scand J Haematol, 17:*89, 1976.
202. Stites, D. P., and Whitehouse, M. J.: Evolution of multiple myeloma with nonsecreted paraproteins. *Clin Res, 23:*283, 1975.
203. Turesson, I., and Grubb, A.: Non-secretory or low-secretory myeloma with intracellular kappa chains. *Acta Med Scand, 204:*445-451, 1978.
204. Whicher, J. T., Davies, J. D., and Grayburn, J. A.: Intact and fragmented intracellular immunoglobulin in a case of non-secretory myeloma. *J Clin Pathol, 28:*54, 1975.
205. Wille, L. E., Forre, O., Mathiesen, P. M. S., Hovig, T., and Sorteberg, K.: "Non-secretory" plasma cell dyscrasia with normal serum immunoglobulins. *Acta Med Scand, 204:*437-443, 1978.
206. Arend, W. P., and Adamson, J. W.: Nonsecretory myeloma. Immunofluorescent demonstration of paraprotein with bone marrow plasma cells. *Cancer, 33:*721-728, 1974.
207. Hijmans, W., Schuit, H. R. E., and Hulsing-Hesselink, E.: An immunofluorescence study on intracellular immunoglobulins in human bone marrow cells. *Ann N Y Acad Sci, 177:*290, 1971.

208. Hijmans, W., Schuit, H. R. E., and Klein, F.: An immunofluorescense procedure for the detection of intracellular immunoglobulins. *Clin Exp Immunol, 4:*457, 1969.
209. Hijmans, W., Schuit, H. R. E., Van Nieuwkoop, J. A., and Van Camp, B.: Immunofluorescence as an aid in the detection and classification of paraproteinaemia. *Ric Clin Lab, 10:*17-21, 1980.
210. Lhurent, G., Gourdin, M., and Reyes, F.: Immunoperoxidase detection of immunoglobulins in cells of immunoproliferative diseases. A comparison between conjugate and nonconjugate (PAP) procedures. *Am J Clin Pathol, 74:*265-274, 1980.
211. Smetana, K., Busch, R. K., Hermansky, F., and Busch, H.: Nucleolar immunofluorescence in bone marrow specimens of human hematological malignancies. *Blut, 42:*79-86, 1981.
212. Taylor, C. R., and Mason, D. Y.: The immuno-histological detection of intracellular immunoglobulin in formalin-paraffin sections from multiple myeloma and related conditions using the immunoperoxidase technique. *Clin Exp Immunol, 18:*417, 1974.
213. Cline, M. J., and Berlin, N. I.: Studies of the anaemia of multiple myeloma. *Am J Med, 33:*510-525, 1962.
214. Paaske-Hansen, O., Thorling, E. B., and Drivsholm, A.: Serum erythropoietin in myelomatosis. *Scand J Haematol, 19:*106-110, 1977.
215. Wallner, S. F., Kurnick, J. E., Kautzin, K., and Ward, H. P.: The effect of serum from uremic patients on erythropoietin. *Am J Hematol, 3:*45-55, 1977.
216. Castaldi, P. A., and Penny, R.: A macroglobulin with inhibitory activity against coagulation factor VIII. *Blood, 35:*370-376, 1970.
217. Coleman, M., Vigliano, E. M., Weksler, M. E., and Nachman, R. L.: Inhibition of fibrin monomer polymerization by lambda myeloma globulins. *Blood, 39:*210-223, 1972.
218. Harbaugh, M. E., Hill, E. M., and Conn, R. B.: Antithrombin and antithromboplastin activity accompanying IgG myeloma. Report of a case with severe bleeding. *Am J Clin Pathol, 63:*57-67, 1975.
219. Lackner, H.: Hemostatic abnormalities associated with disproteinemias. *Sem Hemat, 10:*125-133, 1973.
220. Perkins, H. A., Mackenzie, M. R., Fudenberg, H. H.: Hemostatic defects in dysproteinemias. *Blood, 38:*695-707, 1970.
221. Rubins, J., Qazi, R., and Woll, J. E.: Massive bleeding after biopsy of plasmacytoma. *J Bone & Joint Surg, 62-A:*138-140, 1980.
222. Sanchez-Avalos, J., Soong, B. C. F., and Miller, S. P.: Coagulation disorders in cancer: II. Multiple myeloma. *Cancer, 23:*1388-1398, 1969.
223. Wright, R. S.: Acute congestive heart failure apparently secondary to solitary plasma cytoma and massive hemorrhage after biopsy. Case report. *J Bone & Joint Surg, 55-A:*1749-1752, 1973.
224. Bayrd, E. D.: The bone marrow on sternal aspiration in multiple myeloma. *Blood, 3:*987-1018, 1948.
225. Graham, R. C., Jr., and Bernier, G. M.: The bone marrow in multiple myeloma: Correlation of plasma cell ultrastructure and clinical state. *Medicine, 54:*225-243, 1975.
226. Rosenthal, N., and Vogel, P.: Value of sternal puncture in diagnosis of multiple myeloma. *J Mt. Sinai Hosp, 4:*1001, 1938.
227. Drewinko, B., Alexanian, R., Boyer, H., Barlogie, B. and Rubinow, S. I.: The growth fraction of human myeloma cells. *Blood, 57:*333-338, 1981.
228. Durie, B. G. M., and Salmon, S. E.: Cellular kinetics, staging, and immunoglobulin synthesis in multiple myeloma. *Ann Rev Med, 26:*283-288, 1975.
229. Durie, B. G. M., and Salmon, S. E.: A clinical staging system for multiple myeloma.

Correlation of measured myeloma cell mass with presenting clinical features. Response to treatment and survival. *Cancer, 36:*842-854, 1975.

230. Merlini, G., Waldenstrom, J. G., and Jayakar, S. D.: A new improved clinical staging system for multiple myeloma based on analysis of 123 treated patients. *Blood, 55:*1011-1019, 1980.
231. Osby, E., Carlmark, B., and Reizenstein, P.: Staging of myeloma. A preliminary study of staging factors and treatment in different stages. *Recent Results Cancer Res, 65:*21-27, 1978.
232. Pruzanski, W., Gidon, M. S., and Roy, A.: Suppression of polyclonal immunoglobulins in multiple myeloma: Relationship to the staging and other manifestations at diagnosis. *Clin Immunol Immunopathol, 17:*280-286, 1980.
233. Salmon, S. E., and Durie, B. G. M.: Cellular kinetics in multiple myeloma. A new approach to staging and treatment. *Arch Intern Med, 135:*131-138, 1975.
234. Vercelli, D., DiGuglielmo, R., Guidi, G., Scolari, L., Buricchi, L., and Cozzolino, F.: Bone marrow percentage of plasma cells in the staging of monoclonal gammopathies. *Nouv Rev Fr Hematol, 22:*139-145, 1980.
235. Salmon, S. E., Mackey, G., and Fudenberg, H. H.: "Sandwich" solid phase radioimmunoassay for the quantitative determination of human immunoglobulin. *J Immunol, 103:*129-137, 1969.
236. Salmon, S. E., and Smith, B. A.: Immunoglobulin synthesis and total body tumor cell number in IgG Multiple myeloma. *J Clin Invest, 49:*1114-1119, 1970.
237. Aliapoulios, M. A., Goldhaver, P., and Munson, P. L.: Thyrocalcitonin inhibition of bone resorption induced by parathyroid hormone in tissue culture. *Science, 151:*330, 1966.
238. Friedman, J., and Raisz, L. G.: Thyrocalcitonin: inhibitor of bone resorption in tissue culture. *Science, 150:*1465, 1965.
239. Rousseau, J. J., Franck, G., Grisar, T., Reznik, M., Heynen, G., and Salmon, J.: Osteosclerotic myeloma with polyneuropathy and ectopic secretion of calcitonin. *Europ J Cancer, 14:*133-140, 1978.
240. Rousseau, J. J., Heynen, G., Franck, G.: Role of calcitonin in osteosclerosis of myeloma? *Arch Intern Med, 140:*1554, 1980.
241. Brown, T. S., and Paterson, C. R.: Osteosclerosis in myeloma. *J Bone & Joint Surg, 55-B:*621-623, 1973.
242. Clarisse, P. D. T., and Staple, T. W.: Diffuse bone sclerosis in multiple myeloma. *Radiology, 99:*327-328, 1971.
243. Engels, E. P., Smith, R. C., and Krantz, S.: Bone sclerosis in multiple myeloma. *Radiology, 75:*242-247, 1960.
244. Evison, G., and Evans, K. T.: Bone sclerosis in multiple myeloma. *Br J Radiol, 40:*81-89, 1967.
245. Himmelfarb, E., Sebes, J., and Rabinowitz, J.: Unusual roentgenographic presentations of multiple myeloma. *J Bone & Joint Surg, 56-A:*1723-1728, 1974.
246. Jeha, M. T., Hamblin, T. J., and Smith, J. L.: Coincident chronic lymphocytic leukemia and osteosclerotic multiple myeloma. *Blood, 57:*617-619, 1981.
247. Krainin, P., D'Angio, G. J., and Smelin, A.: Multiple myeloma with new bone formation. *Arch Intern Med, 84:*976-982, 1949.
248. Langley, G. R., Sabean, H. B., and Sorger, K.: Sclerotic lesions of bone in myeloma. *Can M A J, 94:*940, 1966.
249. Lipper, S., Kahn, L. B., and Hesselson, N.: Localized myeloma with osteogenesis and russell body formation. *S Afr Med J, 49:*2041-2045, 1975.
250. Lowbeer, L.: Occurrence of osteosclerosis in multiple myeloma. *Lab Med Bull Pathol, 10:*396-397, 1969.

251. Mathews, J. W., Jr., and Olivier, C. A.: Osteoblastic multiple myeloma. Case report. *South Med J, 67:*318, 1974.
252. Odelberg-Johnson, O.: Osteosclerotic changes in myelomatosis; report of a case. *Acta Radiol, 52:*139-144, 1959.
253. Rodriguez, A. R., Lutcher, C. L., and Coleman, F. W.: Osteosclerotic myeloma. *JAMA, 236:*1872-1874, 1976.
254. Shin, M. S., Mowry, R. W., and Bodie, F. L.: Osteosclerosis (punctate form) in multiple myeloma. *South Med J, 72:*226-228, 1979.
255. Aguayo, A., Thompson, D. W., and Humphrey, J. G.: Multiple myeloma with polyneuropathy and osteosclerotic lesions. *J Neurol Neurosurg Psychiatry, 27:*562, 1964.
256. Getaz, P., Handler, L., Jacobs, P. and Tunley, I.: Osteosclerotic myeloma with peripheral neuropathy. *S Afr Med J, 48:*1246-1250, 1974.
257. Mangalik, A., and Veliath, A. J.: Osteosclerotic myeloma and peripheral neuropathy. A case report. *Cancer, 28:*1040-1045, 1971.
258. Morley, J., and Schwieger, A.: The relation between chronic polyneuropathy and osteosclerotic myeloma. *J Neurol Neurosurg Psychiatry, 30:*432-442, 1967.
259. Reitan, J. B., Pape, E., Foss, A. S. D., Julsrud, O. J., Slettnes, O. N., Solheim, O. P.: Osteosclerotic myeloma with polyneuropathy. *Acta Med Scand, 208:*137-144, 1980.
260. Talerman, A., and Bateson, E. M.: Multiple myeloma associated with bone sclerosis and peripheral polyneuropathy. *Br J Radiol, 43:*698, 1970.
261. Waldenstrom, J. G., Adner, A., Gydell, K., and Zettervall, O.: Osteosclerotic "plasmocytoma" with polyneuropathy, hypertrichosis and diabetes. *Acta Med Scand, 203:*297-303, 1978.
262. Ell, P. J., Knittel, B., Mahr, G., and Meixner, M.: Whole-body bone scans in patients with plasmacytoma. Typical pattern of "hot-spots" in the rib cage. *Nuklearmedizin, 16:*195-197, 1977.
263. Lindstrom, E., and Lindstrom, F. D.: Skeletal scintigraphy with technetium diphosphonate in multiple myeloma — a comparison with skeletal x-ray. *Acta Med Scand, 208:*289-291, 1980.
264. Monteyne, R., Inderadjaja, N., Schelstraete, K., and Laukens, P.: Scintigraphically "cold" bone lesion due to myeloma. Correlation of scintigraphical and histological findings. *J Belge Radiol, 60:*501-504, 1977.
265. Waxman, A. D., Siemsen, J. K., Levine, A. M., Holdorf, D., Suzuki, R., Singer, F. R., and Bateman, J.: Radiographic and radionuclide imaging in multiple myeloma: The role of gallium scintigraphy: Concise communication. *J Nucl Med, 22:*232-236, 1981.
266. Woolfenden, J. M., Pitt, M. J., Durie, B. G. M., and Moon, T. E.: Comparison of bone scintigraphy and radiography in multiple myeloma. *Radiology, 134:*723-728, 1980.
267. Blom, J., Hansen, O. P., and Mansa, B.: The ultrastructure of bone marrow plasma cells obtained from patients of the disease. *Acta Pathol Microbiol Scand, 88:*25-39, 1980.
268. Maldonado, J. E., Brown, A. L., Jr., Bayrd, E. D., and Pease, G. L.: Cytoplasmic and intranuclear electron-dense bodies in the myeloma cell. *Arch Path, 81:*484, 1966.
269. Stavem, P., Ly, B., and Rirvik, T. O.: Abnormal pattern of the rough endoplasmic reticulum of plasma cells in multiple myeloma with multiple concentric lamellar bodies and "single sac loops." *Acta Med Scand, 208:*115-118, 1980.
270. Alexanian, R.: Treatment of multiple myeloma. *Acta Haematol* (Basel), *65:*237-240, 1980.

271. Bersagel, D.: Treatment of plasma cell myeloma. *Ann Rev Med, 30:*431-443, 1979.
272. Durie, B. G. M., and Salmon, S. E.: Evaluation and treatment of multiple myeloma and related disorders. *Front Rad Ther Onc, 10:*170-177, 1975.
273. Kyle, R. A., and Elveback, L. R.: Management and prognosis of multiple myeloma. *Mayo Clin Proc, 51:*751-760, 1976.
274. Paredes, J. M., and Mitchell, B. S.: Multiple myeloma: Current concepts in diagnosis and management. *Med Clin North Am, 64:*729-742, 1980.
275. Waldenstrom, J. G.: *Diagnosis and Treatment of Multiple Myeloma.* New York, Grune and Stratton, 1980.
276. Lazarus, H. M., Kaniecki-Green, E. A., Warm, S. E., Aikawa, M., and Herzig, R. H.: Therapeutic effectiveness of frozen platelet concentrates for transfusion. *Blood, 57:*243-249, 1981.
277. Lazor, M., and Rosenberg, L.: Mechanism of adrenal-steroid reversal of hypercalcemia in multiple myeloma. *N Engl J Med, 270:*499-455, 1964.
278. Mazzaferri, E., O'Dorisio, T. M., and Lobuglio, A. F.: Treatment of hypercalcemia associated with malignancy. *Sem Oncol, 5:*141-153, 1978.
279. Raisz, L. G.: New Diphosphonates to block bone resorption. *N Engl J Med, 302:*347-348, 1980.
280. Siris, E. S., Sherman, W. H., Baquiran, D. C., Schlatterer, J. P., Osserman, E. F., and Canfield, R. E.: Effects of dichloromethylene diphosphonate on skeletal mobilization of calcium in multiple myeloma. *N Engl J Med, 302:*310-315, 1980.
281. Vanbreukelen, F. J., Bijvoet, O. L., and Vanoosterom, A. T.: Inhibition of osteolytic bone lesions by (3-amino-1-hydroxypropylidene)-1, 1-bisphosphonate (A.P.D.). *Lancet, 1:*803-805, 1979.
282. Kyle, R. A., and Jowsey, J.: Effect of sodium fluoride, calcium carbonate, and vitamin D on the skeleton in multiple myeloma. *Cancer, 45:*1669-1674, 1980.
283. Cohen, P., and Gardner, F. H.: Induction of subacute skeletal fluorosis in a case of multiple myeloma. *N Engl J Med, 271:*1129-1133, 1964.
284. Cohen, P.: Fluoride and calcium therapy for myeloma bone lesions. *JAMA, 198:*583-586, 1966.
285. Case, D. C., Lee, B., and Clarkson, B. D.: Improved survival times in multiple myeloma treated with Melphalan, Prednisone, Cyclophosphamide, Vincristine, and BCNU: M-2 Protecol. *Am J Med, 63:*897-903, 1977.
286. Cavagnaro, F., Lein, J. M., Pavlovsky, S., Becherini, J. O., Pileggi, J. E., Micheo, E. Q., Jait, C., Musso, A., Suarez, A., and Pizzolato, M.: Comparison of two combination chemotherapy regimens for multiple myeloma: Methyl-CCNU, Cyclophosphamide, and Prednisone versus Melphalan and Prednisone. *Cancer Treat Rep, 64:*73-79, 1980.
287. Gobbi, M., Cavo, M., Savelli, G., Raccarani, M., and Tura, S.: Prognostic factors and survival in multiple myeloma. Analysis of 91 cases treated by Melphalan and Prednisone. *Haematologica* (Pavia), *65:*437-445, 1980.
288. Gutterman, J. U., Blumenschein, G. R., Alexanian, R., Yap, N. Y., Buzdar, A. U., Cabanillas, F., Hortobagyi, G. N., Hersh, E. M., Rasmussen, S. L., Harmon, M., Kramer, M., and Pestka, S.: Leukocyte interferon-induced tumor regression in human metastatic breast cancer, multiple myeloma, and malignant lymphoma. *Ann Intern Med, 93:*399-406, 1980.
289. Karp, J. E., Humphrey, R. L., and Burke, P. J.: Timed sequential chemotherapy of Cytoxan-refractory multiple myeloma with Cytoxan and Adriamycin based on induced tumor proliferation. *Blood, 57:*468-475, 1981.
290. Riccardi, A., Merlini, G., and Montecucco, C. M.: Treatment of multiple myeloma with Vincristine. *Acta Haematol* (Basel), *64:*176-178, 1980.

291. Riccardi, A., Merlini, G., Montecucco, C., and Perugini, S.: Vincristine in the treatment of multiple myeloma. *Haematologica* (Pavia), *65:*595-611, 1980.
292. Riccardi, A., Montecucco, C., Cresci, R., Traversi, E., and Perugini, S.: Effect of Vincristine on the bone marrow cells of patients with multiple myeloma: A cytomorphologic study. *Tumori, 66:*319-329, 1980.
293. Van Camp, B., De Bock, B., and Peetermans, M.: Nonsecretory myeloma: Immunological studies during treatment with Melphalan, Methotrexate and Prednisolone. *Br J Haematol, 35:*670, 1977.
294. Salmon, S. E., Hamburger, A. M., Soehnlen, B., Durie, B. G. M., Alberts, D. S., and Moon, T. E.: Quantitation of differential sensitivity of human tumor stem cells to anticancer drugs. *N Engl J Med, 298:*1321-1327, 1978.
295. Baldry, P. E., and Royds, J. E.: Respiratory infections in myelomatosis. *Thorax, 16:*291-296, 1961.
296. Callerame, M. L., and Nadel, M.: Pneumocystitis carinii pneumonia in two adults with multiple myeloma. *Am J Clin Pathol, 45:*258-263, 1966.
297. Eastham, W. N., and Gurr, F. W.: Disseminated aspergillosis as a complication of multiple myelomatosis. *Med J Aust, 2:*329-332, 1970.
298. Glenchur, H., Zinneman, H. H., and Hall, W. H.: A review of 51 cases of multiple myeloma: Emphasis on pneumonia and other infections as complications. *Arch Intern Med, 103:*173-183, 1959.
299. Gordon, H., Bandmann, M., Sandbank, U.: Multiple myeloma associated with progressive multifocal leukoencephalopathy and pneumocystis carinii pneumonia. *Isr J Med Sci, 7:*581-588, 1971.
300. Lazarus, H. M., Lederman, M., Lubin, A., Herzig, R. H., Schiffman, G., Jones, P., Wine, A., and Rodman, H. M.: Pneumococcal vaccination: The response of patients with multiple myeloma. *Am J Med, 69:*419-423, 1980.
301. MacGregor, R. R., Negendank, W., and Schreiber, A.: Impaired granulocyte adherence in multiple myeloma. Relationship to complement system, granulocyte delivery and infection. *Blood, 51:*591-599, 1978.
302. Maritz, F. J., and Joubert, J.: Haemophilus influenzae lobar pneumonia with underlying multiple myeloma: A case report. *S Afr Med J, 57:*1098-1100, 1980.
303. Meyers, B., Hirschman, S. Z., and Axelrod, J.: Current patterns of infection in multiple myeloma. *Am J Med, 52:*87-92, 1972.
304. Norden, C. W.: Infections in patients with multiple myeloma. *Arch Intern Med, 140:*1150-1151, 1980.
305. Twomey, J. J.: Infections complicating multiple myeloma and chronic lymphocytic leukemia. *Arch Intern Med, 132:*562-565, 1973.
306. Zinneman, H. H., and Hall, W. H.: Recurrent pneumonia in multiple myeloma and some observations on immunologic response. *Ann Intern Med, 41:*1152-1163, 1954.
307. Freeman, Z.: Myelomatosis with extensive pulmonary involvement. *Thorax, 16:*378-381, 1961.
308. Gabriel, S.: Multiple myeloma presenting as a pulmonary infiltration: Report of a case. *Dis Chest, 47:*123-126, 1965.
309. Herskovic, T., Anderson, H. A., and Bayrd, E. D.: Intrathoracic plasmacytomas: Presentation of 21 cases and review of literature. *Dis Chest, 47:*1-6, 1965.
310. Kilburn, K. H., and Schmidt, A. M.: Intrathoracic plasmacytoma: Report of a case and review of the literature. *Arch Intern Med, 106:*862-869, 1960.
311. Kintzer, J. S., Jr., Rosenow, E. C., III, and Kyle, R. A.: Thoracic and pulmonary abnormalities in multiple myeloma. A review of 958 cases. *Arch Intern Med, 138:*727-730, 1978.

312. Kleinholz, E. J., Jr., and Tennebaum, M. J.: Pleural plasmacytoma presenting as pleural effusion. *Va Med Mon, 100:*1035-1040, 1973.
313. Monta, L. E., and Ramanan, S. V.: Recurrent pulmonary embolism: A sign of multiple myeloma. *JAMA, 233:*1192-1193, 1975.
314. Romanoff, H., and Milwidsky, H.: Primary plasmacytoma of the lung. *Br J Dis Chest, 56:*139-143, 1962.
315. Ballocchi, S., Bergonzi, G., Dall'Aglio, P., Fontant, F., Gandi, U., Pantano, E., Poisetti, P., and Scarpioni, L.: Tubular proteinuria in myeloma. *Ric Clin Lab, 10:*149-156, 1980.
316. Bardana, E. J., Bennett, W. M., and Porter, G. A.: Multiple myeloma presented as acute renal failure. *Northwest Med, 67:*965-968, 1968.
317. Bear, R. A., Cole, E. H., Lang, A., and Johnson, M.: The treatment of acute renal failure due to myeloma kidney. *Can Med Assoc J, 123:*750-753, 1980.
318. Bell, E. T.: Renal lesions associated with multiple myeloma. *Am J Path, 9:*393, 1933.
319. Border, W. A., and Cohen, A. H.: Renal biopsy diagnosis of clinically silent multiple myeloma. *Ann Intern Med, 93:*43-46, 1980.
320. Borders, W. A., and Cohen, A. H.: Renal biopsy diagnosis of clinically silent multiple myeloma. *Ann Intern Med, 93:*43-46, 1980.
321. Brown, W. W., Herbert, L. A., Piering, W. F., Pisciotta, A. V., Lemann, J., Jr., and Garancis, J. C.: Reversal of chronic end-stage renal failure due to myeloma kidney. *Ann Intern Med, 90:*793-794, 1979.
322. Bryan, C. W., and Healy, J. K.: Acute renal failure in multiple myeloma. *Am J Med, 44:*128-133, 1968.
323. Cohen, A. H., and Border, W. A.: Myeloma kidney: An immunomorphogenetic study of renal biopsies. *Lab Invest, 42:*248-256, 1980.
324. Cohen, A. H., Border, W. A., and Glassock, R. J.: Nephrotic syndrome with glomerular mesangial IgM deposits. *Lab Invest, 38:*610-619, 1978.
325. DeFronzo, R. A., Humphrey, R. L., Wright, J. R., and Cooke, C. R.: Acute renal failure in multiple myeloma. *Medicine* (Baltimore), *54:*209-223, 1975.
326. Healy, J. K.: Acute oliguric renal failure associated with multiple myeloma. *Br Med J, 1:*1126-1130, 1963.
327. Heyburn, P. J., Child, J. A., and Peacock, M.: Relative importance of renal failure and increased bone resorption in the hypercalcaemia of myelomatosis. *J Clin Pathol, 34:*54-57, 1981.
328. Kjeldberg, C. R., and Holman, R. E.: Acute renal failure in multiple myeloma. *J Urol, 105:*21-23, 1971.
329. Kobernick, S. D., and Whiteside, J. H.: Renal glomeruli in multiple myeloma. *Lab Invest, 6:*478, 1957.
330. Martinez, M. M., Yium, J., and Suki, W. N.: Renal complications in multiple-myeloma: Pathophysiology and some aspects of clinical management. *J Chronic Disease, 24:*221-237, 1971.
331. McQueen, E. G.: The nature of urinary casts. *J Clin Pathol, 15:*367-373, 1962.
332. Morris, R. C., and Fudenberg, H. H.: Impaired renal acidification in patients with hypergammaglobulinemia. *Medicine* (Baltimore), *46:*57-69, 1967.
333. Paaske-Hansen, O., and Drivsholm, A.: Inter-relationships between blood volume, venous haematocrit and renal failure in myelomatosis. *Scand J Haematol, 20:*461-466, 1978.
334. Seymour, A. E., Thompson, A. J., Smith, P. S., Woodroffe, A. J., Clarkson, A. R.: Kappa light chain glumerulosclerosis in multiple myeloma. *Am J Pathol, 101:*557-580, 1980.

335. Silva, F. G., Meyrier, A., Morel-Maroger, L., and Pirani, C. L.: Proliferative glomerulonephropathy in multiple myeloma. *J Pathol, 130:*229-236, 1980.
336. Talreja, D., Slater, L. M., Dara, P., Branson, H., and Armentrout, S. A.: Multiple myeloma complicated by myelomatous obstructive uropathy. *Cancer, 46:*1893-1895, 1980.
337. Walgh, D. A., and Ibels, L. S.: Multiple myeloma presenting as recurrent obstructive uropathy. *Aust N Z J Med, 10:*555-558, 1980.
338. Feest, T. G., Burge, P. S., and Cohen, S. L.: Successful treatment of myeloma kidney by diuresis of plasmapheresis. *Br Med J, 1:*503-504, 1976.
339. Humphrey, R. L., Wright, J. R., Zachary, J. B., Sterioff, S., and DeFronzo, R. A.: Renal transplantation in multiple myeloma: A case report. *Ann Intern Med, 83:*651-653, 1975.
340. Johnson, W. J., Kyle, R. A., and Dahlberg, P. J.: Dialysis in the treatment of multiple myeloma. *Mayo Clin Proc, 55:*65-72, 1980.
341. Mod, A., Fust, G., Harsanyi, V., Natonek, K., Poros, A., Szabo, J., and Hollan, S. R.: Plasmapheresis in patients with leukaemia, multiple myeloma and immune complex diseases. *Acta Haematol Pol, 11:*165-171, 1980.
342. Ray, P. K., Besa, E., Idiculla, A., Rhoads, J. E., Jr., Bassett, J. G., and Cooper, D. R.: Extracorporeal immunoadsorption of myeloma IgG and autoimmune antibodies: A clinically feasible modality of treatment. *Clin Exp Immunol, 42:*308-314, 1980.
343. Berkman, E. M., and Orlin, J. B.: Use of plasmapheresis and partial plasma exchange in the treatment of patients with cryoglobulinemia. *Transfusion, 20:*171-178, 1980.
344. Bergsagel, D. E.: Total body irradiation for myelomatosis. *Br Med J, 2:*325, 1971.
345. Fitzpatrick, P. J., and Rider, W. D.: Half body radiotherapy. *Int J Rad Oncol Biol Phys, 1:*197-207, 1976.
346. Jaffe, J. P., Bosch, A., and Raich, P. C.: Sequential hemi-body radiotherapy in advanced multiple myeloma. *Cancer, 43:*124-128, 1979.
347. Maruyama, Y., and Thomson, J., Jr.: Radiotherapeutic response of plasma cell tumors associated with monoclonal gammopathy. *Cancer, 26:*110-113, 1970.
348. Mill, W. B.: Radiation therapy in multiple myeloma. *Radiology, 115:*175-178, 1975.
349. Prato, F. S., Kurdyak, R., Saibil, E. A., Carruthers, J. S., Rider, W. D., and Aspin, N.: The incidence of radiation pneumonitis as a result of single fraction upper half body irradiation. *Cancer, 39:*71-78, 1976.
350. Qasim, M. M.: Techniques and results of half body irradiation (HBI) in metastatic carcinomas and myelomas. *Clin Oncol, 5:*65-68, 1979.
351. Saenger, E. L., Silberstein, E. B., Aron, B., Horwitz, H., Kereiakes, J. G., Bahr, G. K., Perry, H., and Friedman, B. I.: Whole body and partial body radiotherapy of advanced cancer. *Am J Roentgenol Med, 117:*670-685, 1973.
352. Alexanian, R., Balcerzah, S., Bonnett, J. D., Gehan, E. A., Haut, A., Hewlett, J. S., and Monto, R. W.: Prognostic factors in multiple myeloma. *Cancer, 36:*1192-1201, 1975.
353. Cohen, D. M., Svien, H. J., and Dahlin, D. C.: Long term survival of patients with myeloma of the vertebral column. *JAMA, 187:*914, 1967.
354. Durie, B. G., Cole, P. W., Chen, H. S., Himmelstein, K. J., and Salmon, S. E.: Synthesis and metabolism of Bence-Jones protein and calculation of tumour burden in patients with Bence-Jones myeloma. *Br J Haematol, 47:*7-19, 1981.
355. Durie, B. G., Salmon, S. E., and Moon, T. E.: Pretreatment tumor mass, cell kinetics, and prognosis in multiple myeloma. *Blood, 55:*364-372, 1980.
356. Feinleib, M., and MacMahon, B.: Duration of survival in multiple myeloma. *J Natl Cancer Inst, 24:*1259-1269, 1960.

357. Gobbi, M., Cavo, M., Savelli, G., Baccarani, M., and Tura, S.: Prognostic factor and survival in multiple myeloma. Analysis of 91 cases treated by Melphalan and Prednisone. *Haematologica* (Pavia), *65:*437-445, 1980.
358. Ikoku, N. B.: Report of Medical Research Council's Working Party. Analysis of presenting features of prognostic significance. *Br J Haemat, 24:*123-139, 1973.
359. Jansen, J., Huijgens, P. C., and Van Der Velde, E. A.: The prognosis of multiple myeloma. *Neth J Med, 23:*246-251, 1980.
360. Osgood, E. E.: The survival time of patients with plasmacytic myeloma. *Cancer Chemother Rep, 9:*1-10, 1960.
361. Shustik, C., Bersagel, D. E., and Pruzanski, W.: Kappa and lambda light chain disease. Survival rates, and clinical manifestations. *Blood, 48:*41-51, 1976.
362. Gonzales, F., Trujillo, S., and Alexanian, R.: Acute leukemia in multiple myeloma. *Ann Intern Med, 86:*440-443, 1977.
363. Rosner, F., and Grunwald, H.: Multiple myeloma terminating in acute leukemia. *Am J Med, 57:*927-939, 1974.
364. Rosner, F., and Grunwald, H, W.: Multiple myeloma and Waldenstrom's macroglobulinemia terminating in acute leukemia. Review with emphasis on karyotypic and ultrastructural abnormalities. *N Y State J Med, 80:*558-570, 1980.

Index